Tuberculosis of Bones, Joints and Spine

Evidence Based Management Guide

Tuberculosis of
Bones, Joints and
Spine

Evidence Based Management Guide

Chief Editor

Anil K Jain MS, MAMS, FAMS, FRCS (Eng.)

Director Professor and Head
Department of Orthopaedics
University College of Medical Sciences and GTB Hospital
Past President, Indian Orthopaedic Association
Ex-Editor of Indian Journal of Orthopaedics
Deputy Editor, Journal of Bone and Joint Surgery (Am)
Visiting Professor, The Tamil Nadu Dr MGR Medical University

Associate Editor
Rajesh Arora

Forewords
Prof. Keith DK Luk
Prof. Surendra Mohan Tuli

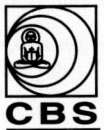

CBS

CBS Publishers & Distributors Pvt Ltd

New Delhi • Bengaluru • Chennai • Kochi • Kolkata • Mumbai
Hyderabad • Nagpur • Patna • Pune

Tuberculosis of **Bones, Joints** and **Spine**

Evidence Based Management Guide

ISBN: 978-93-86310-85-9

Copyright © Author and Publisher

First Edition: 2017

Published by Satish Kumar Jain and produced by Varun Jain for

CBS Publishers & Distributors Pvt Ltd

4819/XI Prahlad Street, 24 Ansari Road, Daryaganj, New Delhi 110 002, India.
Ph: 23289259, 23266861, 23266867 Website: www.cbspd.com
Fax: 011-23243014   e-mail: delhi@cbspd.com; cbspubs@airtelmail.in.
Corporate Office: 204 FIE, Industrial Area, Patparganj, Delhi 110 092
Ph: 4934 4934   Fax: 4934 4935   e-mail: publishing@cbspd.com; publicity@cbspd.com

Branches

- **Bengaluru:** Seema House 2975, 17th Cross, K.R. Road,
  Banasankari 2nd Stage, Bengaluru 560 070, Karnataka
  Ph: +91-80-26771678/79   Fax: +91-80-26771680   e-mail: bangalore@cbspd.com
- **Chennai:** 7, Subbaraya Street, Shenoy Nagar, Chennai 600 030, Tamil Nadu
  Ph: +91-44-26680620, 26681266   Fax: +91-44-42032115   e-mail: chennai@cbspd.com
- **Kochi:** Ashana House, No. 39/1904, AM Thomas Road, Valanjambalam,
  Ernakulam 682 016, Kochi, Kerala
  Ph: +91-484-4059061-65   Fax: +91-484-4059065   e-mail: kochi@cbspd.com
- **Kolkata:** 6/B, Ground Floor, Rameswar Shaw Road, Kolkata-700 014, West Bengal
  Ph: +91-33-22891126, 22891127, 22891128   e-mail: kolkata@cbspd.com
- **Mumbai:** 83-C, Dr E Moses Road, Worli, Mumbai-400018, Maharashtra
  Ph: +91-22-24902340/41   Fax: +91-22-24902342   e-mail: mumbai@cbspd.com

Representatives

- **Hyderabad**   0-9885175004 • **Nagpur**   0-9021734563 • **Patna**   0-9334159340
- **Pune**   0-9623451994

Printed at Magic International Pvt. Ltd., Greater Noida, UP, India

_to_

Shashi Prabha

My wife

To see a smile on her face and sparkle in her eyes

Pragya (Daughter)

Bhushan (Son-in-law)

Aayush (Son)

To remind them that they are the best thing that ever happened to me.

Contributors

Lead Authors

Anil K Jain MS, MAMS, FAMS, FRCS (Eng.)
Director Professor and Head
Department of Orthopaedics
University College of Medical Sciences
and Guru Teg Bahadur Hospital, Delhi

Ravi Sreenivasan MS, DNB
Ex-Senior Resident
Department of Orthopaedics
University College of Medical Sciences
and Guru Teg Bahadur Hospital, Delhi

Navjeevan Singh MD (Pathology)
Director Professor
Department of Pathology
University College of Medical Sciences
and Guru Teg Bahadur Hospital, Delhi

Rumpa Saha MD (Microbiology)
Professor
Department of Microbiology,
University College of Medical Sciences
and Guru Teg Bahadur Hospital, Delhi

Other Contributors

Ish Kumar Dhammi MS
Senior Consultant
Department of Orthopaedics
University College of Medical Sciences
and Guru Teg Bahadur Hospital, Delhi
Editor – Indian Journal of Orthopaedics

Rajesh Arora MS, DNB, MNAMS
Senior Resident
Department of Orthopaedics
University College of Medical Sciences
and Guru Teg Bahadur Hospital, Delhi

SK Saraf MS
Prof. of Orthopaedics
IMS, BHU, Varanasi

Ankur Jain MS
Senior Resident
Department of Orthopaedics
University College of Medical Sciences
and Guru Teg Bahadur Hospital, Delhi

Acknowledgements

Prof. Rakesh Bhargava
Ex. Prof. & Head of Orthopaedics
SMS Medical College, Jaipur

Prof. Aditya N Agarwal
Professor
Department of Orthopaedics
University College of Medical Sciences
and Guru Teg Bahadur Hospital, Delhi

Prof. SK Mukherjee
Ex. Director Medical Education, Govt. of Chhattisgarh
Chhattisgarh

Prof. Sumit Sural
Prof. of Orthopaedics
Maulana Azad Medical College, New Delhi

Mathew Verghese
Consultant Orthopaedic Surgeon
St. Stephen Hospital, Tees Hazari, New Delhi

Amer Nath Jena
Head of PET-MR
Indraprastha Apollo Hospital, New Delhi

Foreword

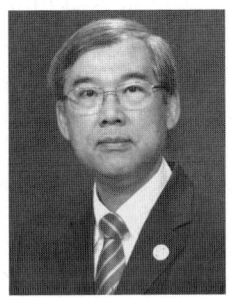

Tuberculosis is a disease known since ancient times and lesions of the spine are well documented in Egyptian mummies. Significant strides have been made to control and treat tuberculosis in the last 6 decades. The disease burden is significantly reduced in high income countries due to improved nutrition, sanitation and elimination of overcrowed inhabitations. However, it still continues to be endemic in low income countries. The emergence of immune deficiency syndrome, and development of drug resistance have added new dimensions to the disease.

Bone and joint tuberculosis poses unique challenges to clinicians as it produces damage to the bones, joints and spine. As a result, inspite of good biological control of the disease, significant biomechanical abnormality does occur and patients are often left with sequelae affecting longevity and quality of life. The early diagnosis of the disease before bony destruction can prevent the development of such sequelae. The end point of treatment that determines the duration of ATT in bone and joint TB is still not clearly defined. The emergence of drug resistance is an additional challenge to the clinicians. Although we have made good improvements in diagnostics, many gaps in the knowledge for early diagnosis, adequate treatment, and prevention and treatment of complications of bone and joint tuberculosis still remains.

It is a privilege to write a foreword for this book by Prof Anil K Jain whom I have known for over two decades. I have heard his thoughts on the subject in international conferences and read his numerous research contributions to the literature. It is most timely for him to put his life-long experience into a textbook.

The book is structured to provide the basic knowledge from the bacteriology, pathology to clinical aspects of osteoarticular and spinal tuberculosis. From Chapter 6 onwards, it includes evidence based management guides to the clinical situations of each joint and the spine. This section is presented in a question–answer form using examples and includes all questions that come to the mind of clinicians while treating these cases at the different stages of the disease. I would recommend this book to all clinicians who are treating osteoarticular tuberculosis. It should have an important place in libraries and on the bookshelves of trainees as well as practicing clinicians.

Prof Keith DK Luk
Immediate Past President of SICOT
President of ISSLS
Tam Sai Kit Professor in Spine Surgery
Chair Professor, Dept of Orthopedics and Traumatology
The University of Hong Kong

Foreword

Tuberculosis has existed in homo-sapiens since the accent of man on Earth. Skeletal tuberculosis constitutes nearly 3% of all clinical tuberculous infections. The treatment of osteoarticular tuberculosis has passed through various phases depending essentially upon the availability of effective drugs for clinical use. The "orthodox treatment" in pre 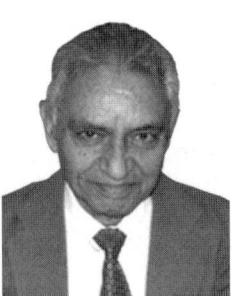 antitubercular era comprised of open air, sunshine, nutritional support, and splintage by plaster of Paris casts to encourage ankylosis/fusion of the involved joint/spine. The end result after 5 years of diagnosis was death (50%), precarious healed status (25%), and clinically healed status (25%). The availability of effective antitubercular drugs encouraged the surgeons to advocate "Universal-Surgical" extirpation for every lesion of skeletal tuberculosis. Observations from countries with high disease burden led to evolution of a more rational "Middle-path-regime", treating most of the patient with antitubercular multidrug therapy and opting for operative procedures for complications and/or for restoring the function of joints. Imaging modalities (MRI) enabled the treating physicians to diagnose the disease at predestructive stage, further improving the results of drug therapy.

Despite commendable progress in the management of skeletal tuberculosis, there are still challenges and problems in many areas like diagnosis at early stage, harvesting of mycobacteria, prevention and treatment of MDR-/XDR-TB, recurrence of tuberculosis, duration of treatment and drug combinations. This book titled "Tuberculosis of Bones, Joints and Spine: Evidence Based Management Guide" by Prof. Anil K Jain has attempted to address these issues and offer evidence based guidelines for effective interventions. I am confident this book will provide robust guides to treat these complex cases and achieve heated status with good functional outcome. I congratulate the authors for this endeavor and I am confident that the book will provide useful tips to the clinicians to evaluate and treat the cases of osteoarticular tuberculosis in various stages of disease.

Surendra Mohan Tuli
Former Chairperson and Professor of
Orthopedics, Institute of Medical Sciences
BHU, Varanasi and University College of Medical Sciences
University of Delhi

Preface

Osteoarticular tuberculosis is one of the most devastating infection in terms of morbidity of active disease and sequelae. Inspite of tremendous strides in imaging, diagnostics, and treatment, it continues to challenge the acumen of any clinician. The disease burden has continued to swell in the world particularly in the low resource countries. At one end, we are able to make better diagnosis and institute effective chemotherapy, on the other hand the drug resistance is adding new complexity to the clinical problem.

The osteoarticular tuberculosis is an extrapulmonary disease which is secondary to hematogenous dissemination following primary pulmonary tuberculosis. The osteoarticular tuberculosis may occur following primary infection or reactivation of healed lesion/dormant bacilli whenever the body immunity is lowered as a result of increased age/under nutrition/co-morbid diseases or acquired immune deficiency syndrome. Osteoarticular tubercular lesion is slowly developing and takes few months to develop classical lesion. The bone lesion takes 3–4 months in pathogenesis before it is appreciated on plain X-rays (bone looses 30–40% calcium content). The diagnosis in this window period when symptoms are vague and instituting ATT can help in achieving healed status with near normal bones, joints and spine. The MRI has made the diagnosis in an early stage (preclassical/predestructive stage) possible.

The bone lesion causes bone destruction and even if it is adequately treated by potent chemotherapeutic drugs it still leaves biomechanical damage and unrecovered neural deficit and/or spinal deformity. The early diagnosis to prevent mechanical damage to load-bearing structures and effective treatment is the key to avoid multiple clinical problems which occur, if disease is allowed to run its full course (natural history of disease). The emergence of multi-drug resistance, association of acquired immune deficiency syndrome (AIDS) and osteo-articular TB have compounded the complexity of the disease.

The literature is full of articles published on various aspect of osteoarticular tuberculosis. Most of studies have emanated from the west while it is a disease of low income countries. During last 15–20 years, lots of articles were also published by Indian authors and by authors from the less resource countries. However, still many questions while treating osteoarticular TB remain unanswered. The issues which a clinician faces while diagnosing and treating osteoarticular TB were listed while interacting in various meetings to develop bone and joint TB guidelines as a part of INDEX TB guidelines. The evidence-based answers are provided so that we could know the current evidence to the clinical practice and know the gap in existing knowledge for future research.

This book is arranged in two sections. Section one gives scientific content in chapter form while section two includes the clinical questions faced by clinicians. The last chapter includes a series of cases diagnosed and treated by us at University College of Medical Sciences and Guru Teg Bahadur Hospital, Delhi over last 25 years. The extensive literature search was performed and it included reading of about 8000 abstracts and 1600 full texted articles. It also includes about 44 articles written by the author. The permission has been obtained for inclusion of few photographs from author's published articles from Indian Journal of Orthopaedics. Most of the work reported in this book by author was conducted in University College of Medical Sciences and Guru Teg Bahadur Hospital.

I would like to express my gratitude to my teacher, mentor Prof Surendra Mohan Tuli who had been my role model since I joined orthopaedics and it is he who inculcated reasoning, biological thought process and third dimension.

I would like to express my thanks to all my postgraduate students who have participated in building clinical data while doing thesis on one or other subject. The patients who reported for treatment and reposed faith while treating them deserve special thanks.

Thanks are due to authors and co-contributors who gave their valuable time while preparing and editing the manuscripts hence deserve special thanks. Dr Ravi Sreenivasan and Dr Rajesh Arora deserve special mention for their continued efforts in collecting and analysing the literature, preparing it as manuscript and editing. I would express thanks to Mrs Ritu Chawla (AGM–Production) and other staff of CBS Publication in producing quality prints as well for following the time line. Mr Amit Pal has contributed in helping me the technical aspect of computer related work at all the time hence deserve my thanks.

The mammoth task could not be completed without the help, encouragement and appreciation by my wife Dr Shashi Prabha Jain, my daughter Dr Pragya, son-in-law Dr Bhushan Shah and son Aayush Jain. Their contribution cannot be expressed in words "Thank you".

I hope this book will prove to be the foundation to build future research on the subject and evolve better treatment outcomes.

Anil K Jain

Contents

Chapter 1

Introduction

India inhabitates one-sixth of world's population and one-third of world's TB cases. India has approximately two to three million people infected with tuberculosis making it a large disease burden country for tuberculosis. India reports approximately 2.2 million new TB cases annually and prevalence is about 2.5 million cases. About 40% of the Indian population is infected with TB bacteria and vast majority of whom have latent rather than active TB. About 2,20,000 patients die every year due to tuberculosis. 5% (4.5–5.4%) of TB cases are HIV positive. This disease has huge socioeconomic impact as it affects the productive age group. These figures are still an underestimate as not all cases are treated/reported under national TB program. Almost 45% patients are treated outside the national program. Multidrug resistance (MDR) and total drug resistance (TDR) is an emerging challenge in the management of tuberculosis. The reported incidence of MDR-TB is 2–3% in new TB cases and 12–17% in retreatment cases.

Bone and joint tuberculosis is extrapulmonary tuberculosis and has special issues attach with it. About 2–3% of all TB cases affect bone and joint, hence approximately 60,000–90,000 new cases are reported from India every year.

The bone and joint TB is unique in many ways.
a. Being a paucibacillary disease, the bacteriological isolation is difficult and low.
b. Being a deep-seated lesion, it is difficult, if not impossible, to procure tissue repeatedly and isolate *Mycobacterium* to conclusively document treatment response/failure to treatment.

c. The primary function of bone is locomotion, weight trans-mission and protection of neural structures. The damage due to tuberculosis produces deformation of load bearing bones and joints as well as spinal deformities. Even after adequate treatment by antitubercular drugs, the spine and limb continue to produce disabilities due to sequalae of deformities and deranged biomechanics.

d. The end point of treatment is still an unresolved issue. It is practically impossible to ascertain that the lesion has become bacteriologically sterile under the influence of ATT and bone has achieved healed status, that is why a controversy exists about the optimum duration of ATT.

e. The emergence of drug resistance has compounded the problem. The suspicion of a case with drug resistance, investigation, final diagnosis and treatment of a drug resistance has added a new dimension to tuberculosis management in India.

Due to biomechanical consideration, it is imperative to diagnose and subsequently treat bone and joint TB in a pre-destructive (inflammatory stage) before an anatomical damage has occurred. If the patients are treated well before the bone destruction has occurred, the patient can be given a limb/spine with near normal alignment and function.

India is a unique country with huge gap in the standard of health care available in different parts of the country. Not all cases are treated correctly and appropriately at first instance. Some of them may not have access to orthopaedic care facilities. These cases report in (a) various stages of pathogenesis of disease, (b) partially and inappropriately treated, (c) with/without various complications.

The literature emnating from the west (developed countries) provide evidence only on the clinical issues which their clinician scientists face. Since developing countries see the natural history of disease, the clinicians have to treat simple to most complicated TB cases. The research has to continue to provide solutions to all clinical stages of disease.

Whenever a patient with suspected or established TB of bone and joint report, the various questions come to the mind of clinicians in order to diagnose and treat them. Spine and various joints affection may present with region-specific clinical issues. The various issues are:

a. How do we suspect osteoarticular tuberculosis (bone or joint wise)?
b. When suspected, how to investigate the case?
c. When can we start ATT with or without bacteriological confirmation of diagnosis?
d. What are the indications of biopsy (percutaneous/open)? What is the ATT regimen (drugs, dosages)?
e. How to monitor the treatment of a case of TB of bone and joint?
f. What are the complications of each region and how should those be prevented. If already report with complications, how should they be evaluated and treated?
g. How to minimize deterioration of biomechanical damage/ deformities of each joint and spine while the patient is on treatment?
h. How to grade the various complications? What are the indications of surgery, type of surgery in TB spine with neurological complications/spinal deformities/late onset paraplegia.
i. How to prognosticate for neurological recovery in spinal TB with neurological deficit?
j. When to stop treatment? (How to define end point of treatment?)
k. How to investigate and treat poor clinical response/no response to treatment?
l. How to suspect, investigate and treat a case of drug-resistance?

Many such questions come to the mind of treating clinicians/ surgeons. This book is a compilation of such bone/joint specific clinical issues and suggested evidence-based answers with supported references. It includes first five chapters providing the basic knowledge on osteoarticular tuberculosis. Chapter 2 discusses microbiology of *Mycobacterium* and microbiological diagnosis of osteoarticular tuberculosis. Chapter 3 covers pathology of osteoarticular tuberculosis which includes the pathology of bone and joint tuberculosis and pathological basis of diagnosis. Chapters 4 and 5 are on osteoarticular tuberculosis and spinal tuberculosis, respectively. These two chapters include the description of disease, clinical features, diagnosis, investigations and management. The complications of osteoarticular TB are also described as a text with prevention, treatment and prognosis. Chapter 6 is an evidence-based regionspecific (spine, hip, knee, ankle and foot, shoulder elbow and wrist and hand) treatment guides. Each part of Chapter 6 includes clinical issues as questions. The answers are provided with supported articles published in literature. Chapter 7 includes a series of cases which were treated over the years and are reported with follow-up. I am sure the clinicians will find it useful while treating a case of bone and joint tuberculosis and report outcome of their experiences as publication.

REFERENCE

1. TB India 2016-Part 1; Ministry of health and family welfare. Ww.tbindia.nic.in.

Chapter 2

Microbiology and Diagnosis of Osteoarticular Tuberculosis

Osteoarticular tuberculosis remains a significant worldwide problem, being a source of subsequent deformities and functional disabilities. Therefore, it should be recognized and treated early, particularly in children, given that appropriate management can lead to a full recovery.[1] This secondary tuberculosis is the result of tuberculous process development in bone, joints or both. Osteoarticular lesions usually occur following a paucibacillary hematological dissemination by the fixation of a colony inside the active bone marrow. The retrograde lymphatic dissemination (i.e. from the mediastinal lymph nodes to the dorsal spine or from the mesenteric lymph nodes to the lumbar spine) or the contiguity disseminations (such as rib tuberculosis following pleurisy or humeral head tuberculosis secondary to a shoulder bursitis) should be mentioned among other less significant mechanisms involved in the pathogenesis of osteoarticular tuberculosis.[2,3] This process may involve any bone or cartilage, i.e. both vertebrae and weight-bearing bones and cartilages. Whether it be a recent exposure or reactivation of dormant bacilli, both can lead to considerable osteoarticular disease.

MICROBIOLOGY

The etiological agents, *Mycobacterium tuberculosis* (MTB) and *non-tubercular mycobacteria* (NTM) are slender rods. They do not readily stain, but once stained, resist de-colorization with dilute, mineral acids and are, therefore, called acid-fast bacilli

(AFB). They are aerobic, non-motile, non-capsulated and non-sporing. Growth is generally slow and takes up to one month.

The genus *Mycobacterium* contains three groups: Obligate parasites, opportunistic pathogens and saprophytes.

A. Obligate Parasites

Mycobacterium tuberculosis complex which includes several species, all probably derived from a soil bacterium:

1. *Mycobacterium tuberculosis*—commonest in humans.
2. *Mycobacterium bovis*—transmitted from consumption of unpasteurized milk.
3. *Mycobacterium africanum*—causing tuberculosis in humans in tropical areas.
4. *Mycobacterium microti*—pathogen for rodents only.
5. *Mycobacterium canetti*—rare causes of tuberculosis in Africa.
6. *Mycobacterium caprae*—cattle pathogen.
7. *Mycobacterium pinnipedii*—pathogens of seals.

Out of all *Mycobacterium tuberculosis, M. bovis* and *M. africanum* are common pathogens in humans.

Mycobacterium leprae: The second human pathogenic *Mycobacterium* is the lepra bacillus causing leprosy. Discovered by Hansen in 1868, though not been possible to culture it *in vitro* so far.

B. Opportunistic Pathogens

Non-tuberculous Mycobacterium (NTM): These are a mixed group of isolates from diverse sources—from skin ulcers, and from soil and water and other environments, birds, cold-blooded and warm-blooded animals. They are opportunistic pathogens and can cause many types of disease. They are broadly categorized based on pigment production and rate of growth:

1. **Group I.** *Photochromogens*: No pigmentation in dark become pigmented on exposure to light—*M. kansasii, M. marinum.*

2. **Group II.** *Scotochromogen*: Pigmented in the dark—*M. scrofulaceum, M. gordonae.*

3. **Group III.** *Non-photochromogens*: No pigments even on exposure to light—*M. avium, M. intracellulare, M. ulcerans* and *M. xenopi.*

4. **Group IV.** *Rapid growers*: Growth within seven days—*M. fortuitum, M. chelonae* and *M. smegmatis.*

C. Saprophytes

These mycobacteria are isolated from number of sources. These include *M. phlepi* from grass and *M. smegmatis* from smegma.

Organism Characteristics

1. Aerobic, non-motile, non-spore forming bacillus.
2. High cell wall content of high molecular weight lipids—mycolic acid.
3. Slow growth rate:
   a. Generation time of 20 hours *vs* 20 minutes in *E. coli.*
   b. 3–8 weeks for growth on solid media
   c. Implications for length of treatment for complete sterilization compared with most bacterial pathogens.

PATHOGENESIS

Sites of TB disease: TB disease can occur in pulmonary and extrapulmonary sites.

Pulmonary: Tuberculosis (TB) most commonly affects the lungs; this is referred to as pulmonary TB.

Although the majority of TB cases are pulmonary, TB can occur in almost any anatomical site or as disseminated disease.

Extrapulmonary: Extrapulmonary TB (EPTB) occurs in places other than the lungs, including the larynx, the lymph nodes, the pleura, the brain, the kidneys, and the bones and joints. In HIV-infected persons, EPTB disease is often accompanied by pulmonary TB.

Mode of Transmission

a. *Transmission*: Lungs are the portal of entry except *M. bovis* in which case unpasteurized dairy products are the source. Infection occurs when a person inhales droplet nuclei containing tubercle bacilli that reach the alveoli of the lungs. These tubercle bacilli are ingested by alveolar macrophages; the majority of these bacilli are destroyed or inhibited. A small number may multiply intracellularly and are released when the macrophages die. If alive, these bacilli may spread by way of lymphatic channels or through the bloodstream to more distant tissues and organs (including areas of the body in which TB disease is most likely to develop, e.g. regional lymph nodes, apex of the lung, kidneys, brain, and bone). This process of dissemination primes the immune system for a systemic response.

b. *Inhalation of droplet nuclei (bacillus 5 microns)*: From infectious person with active pulmonary tuberculosis, NOT just positive purified protein derivative (PPD)/tuberculin test/Montaux test.
  i. *Cough*: Most efficient as 3000 infectious droplet nuclei per cough.
  ii. *Talking*: Similar quantity over 5 minutes.
  iii. *Sneezing*: More efficient than coughing.
  iv. *Singing*: Intermediate between talking and coughing.
  v. *Inoculum size relevant*: Cutting through lung tissue aerosolize millions of bacilli; PPD conversion and progression to active tuberculosis astonishingly high.
  vi. *Virulence of strain*: Kentucky outbreak after minimal contact with index patient.
  vii. Bacillus remains alive and infectious in air for long period; ventilation is the key in preventing transmission; isolation of patient and mandated number of air exchanges in hospital rooms minimizes transmission.

Primary infection (before immune response)
a. Bacillus reaches alveoli.
b. Replicates extracellularly in alveolar space and intracellularly in alveolar macrophage.

c. Lack of immediate host immune response: Alveolar macrophage ingests TB bacillus; bacillus sits in phagosome; phagosome normally incorporates proton-ATPase into membrane leading to decreased pH and acidification within phagosome; acidified phagosome then normally fuses with cell lysosome, exposing organism to lysosome's toxic enzymes but MTB prevents insertion of proton-ATPase into phagosome so phagosome never gets acidified and never merges with lysosome.

d. MTB multiplies for weeks, both in initial focus in alveolar macrophages and in cells transported lympho-hematogenously throughout body.

e. Metastatic foci well established in regional nodes (hilar, mediastinal) and then to tissues which retain bacilli and favor multiplication: Apical posterior areas of lungs, lymph nodes in neck, kidneys, epiphyses of long bones, vertebral bodies, juxtaependymal meningeal areas adjacent to subarachnoid space.

These will be areas of reactivation disease in future as organisms seeded remain alive but dormant once immune response occurs.

Reactivation can occur in any one of these areas of the body with or without reactivation in others, i.e. TB meningitis or "scrofula" with no pulmonary TB.

Development of immune response: Must have intact cellular immune system, including CD4 cells:

a. 6–12 weeks after initial infection alveolar macrophage infected with *M. tuberculosis* releases interleukins 12 and 18.

b. These attract and stimulate T lymphocytes (mainly CD4): All people have native population of CD4 cells which can recognize mycobacterial antigens which have been processed and presented by macrophages.

c. CD4 cell meets mycobacterial antigen presented by macrophage and becomes activated-transformed CD4 cell, which proliferates and produces clone of similarly reactive T lymphocytes.

d. When population of activated lymphocytes is large enough, get cutaneous delayed reaction to tuberculin tissue hypersensitivity: Positive PPD (Implications in AIDS patients with low CD4 cells: Cannot perform this process so no positive PPD response to tuberculin.)

e. Meanwhile, CD4 cells release interferon gamma (INFγ): INFγ stimulates additional macrophage. Phagocytosis and INFγ stimulate macrophage to secrete regulatory factors including tumor necrosis factor alpha (TNFα).

f. TNF α increases macrophages' ability to kill *M. tuberculosis* and is required for granuloma formation. Lack of TNF α results in inability to control initial TB infection and leads to reactivation of latent organisms.

g. The inflammatory lesion is a dynamic environment that is regulated both by the bacteria and by the host. TDM (trehalose dimycolate) is a key bacterial modulator of the immune response while B lymphocytes, T lymphocytes and phagocytes are key host regulators of the inflammatory site.

The protective and pathologic response of host to *M. tuberculosis* is complex and multifaceted, involving many components of the immune system. Because of this complexity, it becomes extremely difficult to identify the mechanism(s) involved in protection and design surrogate markers to be measured as *in vitro* correlate of protective immunity. The type of acquired cellular response that will mediate immunity has till date not been defined and which should, therefore, be induced by vaccination; this severely limits our ability to develop novel vaccines.

Pathology: Tissue response depends on activation of macrophages with secretion of lytic enzymes which cause tissue necrosis and granuloma formation.

Risk of developing TB disease over a lifetime: Without treatment, approximately 5% of persons who have been infected with *M. tuberculosis* will develop disease in the first year or two after infection, and another 5% will develop disease sometime later in life. Thus, without treatment, approximately 10% of persons with normal immune systems who are infected with *M. tuberculosis* will develop TB disease at some point in their lives.

HIV-TB coinfection: HIV infection is the greatest risk factor for the development of TB in persons with latent TB infection (LTBI), due to a weakened immune system. Studies from many parts of the world have shown higher incidence of TB among HIV-infected individuals, ranging from 5 to 10 per year, which is in sharp contrast to the lifetime risk of 10% among people without HIV. Persons with HIV infection are at increased risk of rapid progression of a recently acquired infection, as well as of reactivation of latent infection. Studies from different parts of the country have estimated that 60 to 70% of HIV positive patients will develop TB in their lifetime. Differences in HIV-positive TB, as opposed to HIV-negative TB, include a higher proportion of cases with EPTB or disseminated disease. In HIV-infected persons, EPTB disease is often accompanied by pulmonary TB in which case they usually are infectious. Children younger than 5 years of age are also at increased risk for progression of LTBI to extrapulmonary disease. Though most patients respond very well to antituberculous treatment initially, they develop other opportunistic infections and deteriorate rapidly within a few months. Further, recurrence of TB is more frequent than in immunocompetent population, due to both endogenous reactivation and exogenous reinfection.

TB Control Programs

The National TB control program which was started in 1962 was changed to The Revised National TB Control Program (RNTCP), based on the DOTS strategy. It began as a pilot project in 1993 and was launched as national program in 1997 but the rapid RNTCP expansion began in late 1998 with its firm objectives of universal access to early quality diagnosis and quality TB care for all TB patients. NKSHAY, the web based TB reporting for TB program, has been another notable achievement initiated in 2012 and has enabled capture and transfer of individual patient data from the remotest health institutions of the country. DOTS was scaled up to DOTS Plus to address MDR-TB and other challenges like TB-HIV.

LABORATORY DIAGNOSIS

1. *Sample collection*:
   i. *Sputum*: When to collect sputum samples: For diagnosis of TB, three at least 3–5 mL sputum examination (spot–morning–spot) are performed for three consecutive morning sputum sample.

   To obtain desirable sputum specimen, the patients should be instructed to:
   - Rinse the mouth with water, mouthwash/oral drug might contaminate the specimen or inhibit growth of any AFB present.
   - Collect only the exudative material brought up from the lungs after a deep productive cough.

   Sputum induction: The inhalation of warm, aerosolized hypertonic (5–10%) saline irritates the lungs enough to induce both coughing and the production of sputum.

   ii. *Laryngeal swabs:* May be useful in children and patients who raise no sputum or swallow it.

   iii. *Gastric lavage:* The patients must be hospitalized. The collection of gastric aspirate should be made in the morning after the patient awakens in order to obtain sputum swallowed during sleep. Collect three such specimens on three consecutive days in 1 oz sterile wide mouth container. Immediately after collection of the aspirate, neutralize it with sodium carbonate solution or 10% trisodium phosphate.

   iv. *Bronchial washing, bronchoalveolar lavage, biopsy or brushing and transtracheal aspiration* not only produce a primary specimen, but the procedure causes the patients to produce sputum naturally for several days. Five mL of lavage/washing may be collected into the sterile container.

   v. *Cerebrospinal fluid:* Should be collected (2 mL) under all sterile condition.

   vi. *Body fluid (pleural fluid, pericardial fluid, ascitic and peritoneal fluid):* Collect as much as possible into a sterile large saline bottle or a large screw-capped bottle or large syringe with tip cap.

vii. Collect **blood** specimens into SPS blood-collection tubes. To prevent clotting of fluid, add 2 drops of 10% sodium citrate for every 10 ml of specimens collected.

viii. *Synovial fluid*: It is usually non-hemorrhagic and turbid, with moderate elevation of the white blood cell count, ranging between 10,000 and 20,000 cells/mL with a predominance of polymorphonuclear leukocytes.

ix. *Urine*: The specimen of choice is that total early morning clean voided after proper genital toileting, collected into a large wide-mouthed screw-capped bottle. It should be kept in refrigerator prior to procedure. *Three such specimens should be taken on three different times on three consecutive days.*

x. *Pus*: Adequate volumes of pus should be collected in sterile glass container, *pus swabs should be avoided.* Biopsy specimens from abscess walls may be sent for culture and other biological tests.

xi. *Lymph nodes*: Aspirate from lymph nodes or biopsy material from lymph nodes may be sent in a sterile container without a fixative or a preservatives. Collection should be done under aseptic conditions. *The sample should not be diluted or immersed in saline or other fluid or wrapped in gauze. Freezing decreases yield.*

xii. *Abscess contents and aspirated fluid*: As much volume as possible should be collected into a sterile container under all aseptic conditions. *No swabs are acceptable.*

xiii. *Bone and bone marrow*: A piece of bone in a sterile container without any fixative or preservatives may be sent to the lab. Bone marrow to be collected as such into SPS (sodium polyanethole sulfonate) containing blood collection tube (1.5 mL).

xiv. *Tissue specimens*: Collected as biopsy specimens and sent as such in a sterile container.

2. *Transportation*: Transport samples immediately to laboratories as soon as possible.

3. *Digestion-decontamination procedures (according to CDC 2015)*: Thick mucoid sputum is digested and samples often need to be decontaminated in the laboratory to increase yield. The following may be used: N-acetyl-L-cysteine with 2% sodium hydroxide; 4% NaOH; 10% Zephiran-along with trisodium phosphate; 10% sodium citrate; 5% oxalic acid; sulfuric acid; cetylpyridinium chloride–sodium chloride.

4. *Diagnostic methods*:

 1. **Microscopy:** It is highly specific with 50–80% sensitivity. Sputum smear microscopy requires 10^4–10^5 organism/mL to be readily demonstrated in direct smears. The sensitivity varies according to load of the bacilli in extrapulmonary samples.

    a. *Ziehl-Neelsen technique of staining*: Direct or concentrated smears of sputum are stained and examined for AFB under 100× magnification of light microscope. Sputum microscopy is the most reliable single method in the diagnosis and control of tuberculosis. A Kinyoun's modification of ZN staining can also be used (cold staining) (Fig. 2.1).

    b. *Auramine-rhodamine*: When several smears are to be examined daily it is more convenient to stain with fluorescent dyes (auramine-rhodamine) and examine under ultraviolet illumination using a fluorescent microscope (Fig. 2.2).

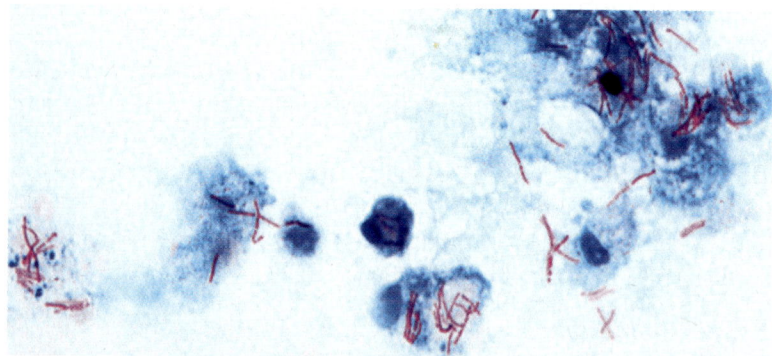

Fig. 2.1: Ziehl-Neelsen stain showing acid-fast (pink) tubercle bacilli (under 100× magnification of light microscope) with the characteristic beaded appearance

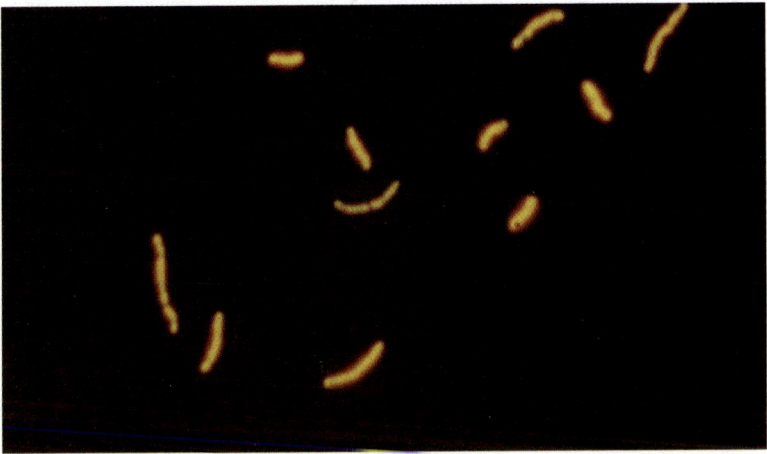

Fig. 2.2: Characteristic yellow fluorescent tubercle bacilli under ultraviolet illumination with auramine–rhodamine stain (100× magnification of fluorescent microscope)

2. **Culture:** Culture is the gold standard diagnostic technique for tubercle bacilli, detecting as few as 10 to 100 bacilli/ mL of specimen. It is now available in most places of the world via WHO reference labs. Culture positivity in the extra-pulmonary samples is often less common than smear positivity. Presence of dead bacilli or viable but non-culturable forms could be the reason for the lower culture positivity rate. Many of patients may have been on treatment at the time specimens were sent for culture, explaining this phenomenon. Many different media have been devised for cultivating tubercle bacilli. The three main groups identified are—egg-based media, agar-based media and liquid media. The ideal media for isolation of tubercle bacilli should:

   • Be economical and simple to prepare from readily available ingredients.
   • Inhibit the growth of contaminants.
   • Support luxuriant growth of small numbers of bacilli.
   • Permit preliminary differentiation of isolates on the basis of colony morphology.

Types of Media

a. *Solid media*:

   i. Egg-based media: For example, Lowenstein-Jensen media.
   - *Advantage*: Can be stored in the refrigerator for several months and it supports good growth of most mycobacteria.
   - *Disadvantages*: When contamination does occur it usually involves the total surface of medium (Fig. 2.3).

   ii. Agar-based medium: For example, Middlebrook 7H-10 or 7H-11 (Fig. 2.4).
   - *Advantage*: Contamination less likely, enables earlier observation of colony morphology.
   - *Disadvantages*: Medium contained in plates has a tendency to dry out during prolonged storage or incubation unless it is kept in plastic bags that retard the loss of moisture; preparation requires great care, expensive.

The concentrated material is inoculated into at least two bottles of LJ medium, examined for growth after incubation at 37°C for 4 days (for rapid growing Mycobacterium, fungi and contaminant bacteria) and at least twice weekly thereafter. It can detect 10–100 organisms/mL; *3–8 week's incubation to detect organisms*, a negative report is given if no growth occurs after 8–12 weeks.

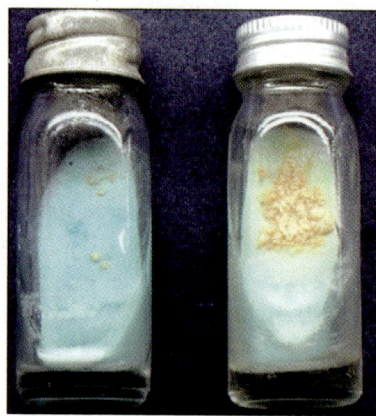

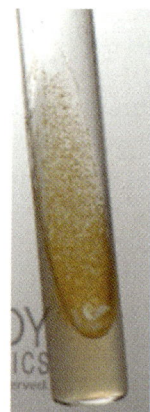

Fig. 2.3: Lowenstein-Jensen medium with showing characteristic rough, buff and tuff colonies of *M tuberculosis*

Fig. 2.4: *Mycobacterium scrofulaceum* Group II (ATCC 19981) colonies growing on Middlebrook

b. *Liquid media*: Middlebrook 7H12, , Kirchner media, Dubos media, Smith media, etc. It takes at least 1–3 weeks of incubation to detect organism.

c. *Automated system*: The use of liquid media with radiometric growth detection such as BACTEC-460 has simplified culture methods and anti-tubercular drug sensitivity and enabled *results to be given in 2–3 weeks*. They were based on radio-isotopes. They have been replaced with other automated continuously monitored systems:

   i. **BACTEC system:** This assay system developed by Becton Dickinson is *based on generation of radioactive carbon dioxide from substrate palmitic acid.*[3] This method has been extensively used all over the world and *growth can be detected in 5–10 days in this system*. Inclusion of NAP (beta-nitro-alpha-acetylamino-beta-hydroxypropiophenone) helps in distinguishing *M. tuberculosis* (inhibited) from other mycobacteria. This system has been widely used for drug susceptibility testing and is currently used as a comparative standard.[4]

   ii. **MGIT (mycobacterial growth indicator tube):** Based on fluorescence detection of mycobacterial growth in a tube containing M7H9 broth together with florescence-based oxygen sensor at the bottom of tube, this method has also been developed by Becton Dickinson for detection and drug screening.[4, 5] This system helps in *early detection (7– 12 days) of mycobacterial growth* and has been reported to be useful for drug susceptibility testing[5] but the experience is limited.

   iii. **MB/BacT:** This system (Organon Technika) is adapted from strategy of *colorimetric detection* earlier tried for detection of bacterial growth in blood cultures. This has been reported to be useful for drug susceptibility testing of *M. tuberculosis.*[6]

   iv. **Septi-Chek:** This is a biphasic medium system (Roche) consisting of an enriched selective broth and a slide with nonselective Middle brook agar on one side and with two sections on other side-one with NAP and egg containing agar, second with chocolate agar for detection of contamination. This system has also been found to be quite useful for rapid detection of growth of mycobacteria.[7]

v. **Reporter phages:** Mycobacterial specific bacteriophages and reporter genes, like luciferase, have been successfully used for detection of growth and for assessing the drug susceptibility to anti-TB drugs.[8-10] Indication of viability could be either emission of light from organism due to activation of luciferase gene or production of a plaque on an indicator strain of mycobacteria.[9,10] Results can be obtained in 48 h and such systems are commercially also available (Biotec/Medispan).

vi. *Other methods*: E-test has been reported to be useful for drug susceptibility testing in *M. tuberculosis*.[11] Flow cytometry has also been observed to be a rapid method for drug susceptibility testing but it is technology-intensive.[12]

New Rapid Drug Susceptibility Methods

i. *Nitrate reductase assay*: Mycobacteria have nitroreducatse enzymes that reduce nitrate to nitrite in the reaction pathway. When griess reagent is added on the 21st day of incubation nitrite in the medium causes pink-purplish color. In the presence of drug, the appearance of a color represents resistance to the drug.

ii. *PHA-B-assay*: Also known as **phage amplified biologically** assay. It is based on the ability of viable mycobacteria to support replication of an infecting mycobacteriophage. Phage assay allows determination of RMP/INH resistance in strains of *M. tuberculosis* within 48 hours from culture.

iii. *Luciferase reporter phage assay*: Viable mycobacteria are with reporter phage expressing firefly luciferase gene. Easily detectable signals are seen a few minutes after the infection of *M. tuberculosis* with reporter phages. Light production requires metabolically active *M. tuberculosis* cells, in which reporter phages replicate and luciferase gene is expressed. When drug susceptible *M. tuberculosis* strains are incubated with specific drug they fail to produce light with luciferase reporter phages. In contrast, drug resistant strains are unaffected by the drugs and produce light (Fig. 2.5).

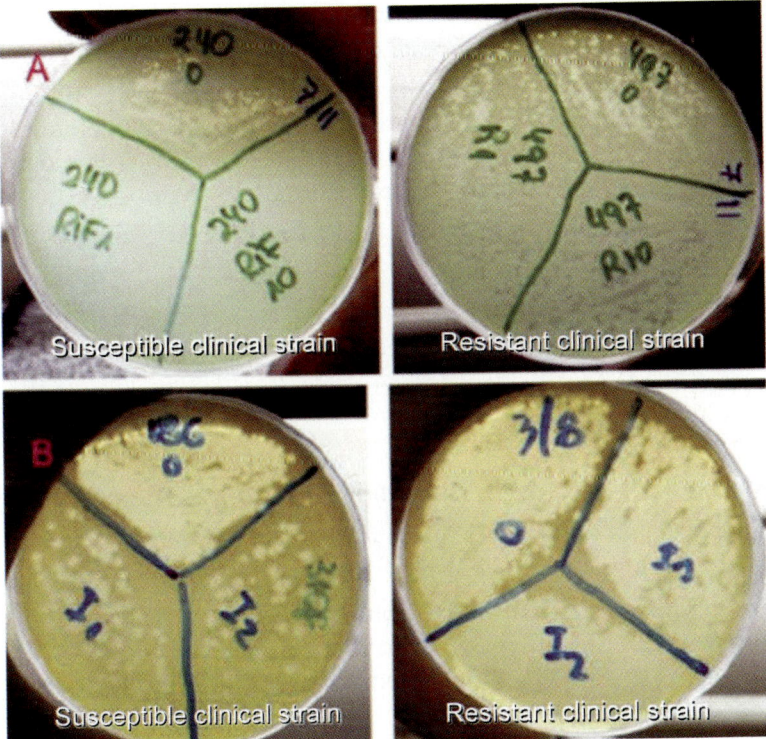

Fig. 2.5: Luciferase reporter phage assay showing light production by resistant strains of *M. tuberculosis*

iv. *Microscopic observation drug susceptibility assay (MODS):* This is a broth based technique for the detection of tuberculosis and multidrug resistant directly or indirectly from sputum. *M. tuberculosis* grows faster in liquid medium than in solid medium. In this cords can be visualized microscopically in liquid medium at an early stage. Incorporation of drugs permits rapid and direct drug susceptibility testing concomitantly with the detection of bacterial growth.

v. *Colorimetric assays:* It involves oxidation reduction with a color change. Liquid medium on 96 well microtiter plates containing the test drug is inoculated with mycobacteria and incubated for 7 days at 37°C. When resazurin reagents are added to wells they give pink color, if bacterial growth is present indicating resistance to the test drug.

vi. *E-test*: It is based on determination of drug susceptibility using strips containing gradients of impregnated antibiotics. There are reports about a high rate of false resistance by this method when compared with other methods.

vii. *Commercial liquid media based culture tests include*:
- BACTEC 460
- MGIT
- BacT/Alert
- Septi-Check
- Reporter phage

Molecular Methods for Detection of Drug Resistance

These are essentially required for the rapid identification of multi-drug resistant (MDR) TB strains.

i. *INNO-LiPA-Rif (Line probe assays)*: It is based on the reverse hybridization principle. Amplified biotinylated DNA material is hybridized with specific oligonucleotide probes and after addition of enzyme substrate complex with chromogen results in a purple/brown precipitates and result is visually interpreted. It is useful to detect resistance against rifampicin and isoniazid.

ii. *LAMP-TB assay (loop mediated isothermal amplification)*: This relies on a novel form of nucleic acid amplification with sufficient efficiency that enough DNA is generated to enable detection by visual inspection of fluorescence. This method has been evaluated on a limited basis and has been shown to have high sensitivity for smear positive specimens but low sensitivity for smear negative specimens (Fig. 2.6).

iii. *PCR single strand conformation polymorphism (PCR-SSCP)*: It is based on the property of single-stranded DNA to fold into a tertiary structure whose shape depends on its sequence. In combination with PCR, SSCP has been applied for the detection of resistance to rifampicin, isoniazid, streptomycin and ciprofloxacin.

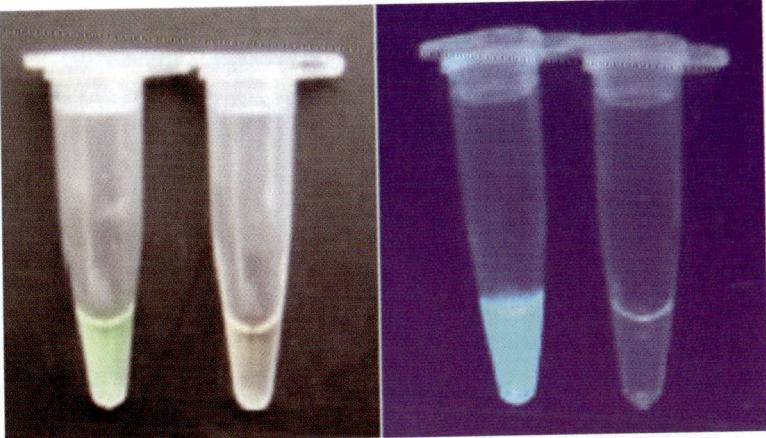

Fig. 2.6: Visual detection of omp25 LAMP reaction using fluorescent metal indicator. (a) Under daylight; (b) under UV light; plus sign denotes positive reaction (with target DNA); minus sign denotes negative reaction (without target DNA)

iv. *Oligonucleotide microarrays*: It allows for the simultaneous detection of multiple genetic sequences which can be used to detect either conserved sequences for detection of microorganism and/or detection of mutation in sequences that confer drug resistance of an isolates.

v. *Xpert MTB/RIF*: It is self-enclosed rapid PCR device that to some extent mitigates many of the limitation of other molecular assays. It is a rapid method to detect resistance against rifampicin with 95% sensitivity for smear positive cases and 55% for smear negative cases (Fig. 2.7).

vi. *Nucleic acid sequence based assay (NASBA)*: It can detect *M. tuberculosis* complex in fresh sample. It is a developed world technology but too costly for resource poor countries. More sensitive and more specific than the AFB smear. *Results available within hours to a few days.* Sensitivity intermediate between acid-fast smear and culture. If AFB smear is negative, nucleic acid amplification is 40–77% sensitive. If AFB smear is positive, nucleic acid amplification is 95% sensitive and nearly 100% specific.

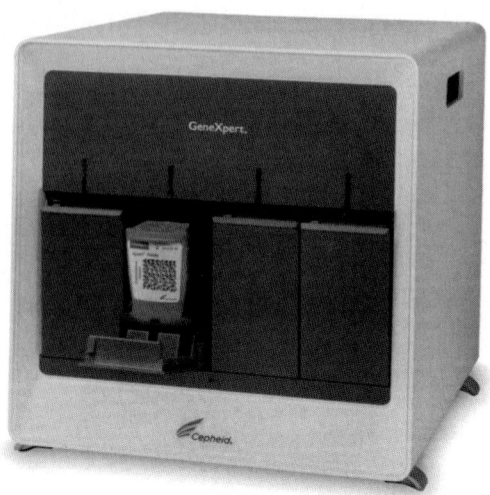

Fig. 2.7: GeneXpert diagnostic machine

Newer Molecular Methods for Detection of Drug Resistance

1. ***Hybridization on DNA chip*:** It can also be used for rapid detection of mutations responsible for drug resistance. It can simultaneously detect different drug resistant mutations in *M. tuberculosis.* It is based on the hybridization of DNA obtained from clinical samples to oligonucleotides immobilized on solid support such as miniaturized glass slides. The overall specificity is 100% and 95% for INH and RMP resistant respectively.[13]

2. ***Molecular beacons*:** It has hairpin-shaped molecules with an internally quenched fluorophore whose fluorescence is restored when they bind to a target nucleic acid.

3. ***PCR pyrosequencing*:** It is a novel method of nucleic acid sequencing by synthesis that is based on the released pyrophosphate (ppi) during DNA synthesis. The cascade of enzymatic reactions generates visible light which is proportional to the number of incorporated nucleotides. It used for detection of RMP resistance and target taken is 180bp region of rpoB gene.

4. ***Heteroduplex analysis (HA)*:** It depends on the conformation of duplex DNA when analyzed in native gels. Heteroduplex

are formed when PCR amplification products from known wild type and unknown mutant sequences are heated and re-annealed. The DNA strands will form a mismatched heteroduplex, if there is a sequence difference between the strands of the wild type and tested DNA.

Drug Resistance in *Mycobacterium tuberculosis*

Terms used to describe drug resistance in TB:

i. *Multi-drug resistant TB (MDR-TB):* Defined as resistant to at least isoniazid (INH) and rifampicin (RMP) both with and without resistant to other drugs.

ii. *Extensively drug resistant TB (XDR-TB):* Resistant to isoniazid and rifampicin, plus resistant to any fluoro-quinolone and at least one of three injectable second-line drugs (i.e. amikacin, kanamycin or capreomycin).

iii. Strains are having resistance to all first- and second-line anti-TB drugs known as **extremely drug resistant TB (XXDR-TB)** and **totally drug resistant TB (_TDR-TB_).**

In 2015, an estimated 9 million people developed TB and 1.5 million died from the disease (WHO Global Report 2015). India and China alone accounted for 24% and 11% of total cases, respectively (TB INDIA 2015 Revised National TB Control Programme Annual status Report). Globally 3.5% of new and 20.5% of previously treated TB cases was estimated to have had MDR-TB in 2015. On average, an estimated 9.0% of patients with MRD-TB had XDR-TB. Almost 50% of MDR-TB cases worldwide are estimated to occur in China and India.

Irrational use of antibiotics by the general physicians, self-medication or non-compliance by patients may be some of the reasons for such high rates of drug resistance. It is important to offer DST (drug sensitivity testing) for patients with EPTB, using criteria similar to what is now recommended for pulmonary TB (Programmatic Management of Drug Resistant TB guidelines—PMDT). Rapid DST methods are now available and it is important that all TB laboratories be equipped to process EPTB specimens which will enable these patients to access MDR-TB treatment, if required.

Risk factors of drug resistance
  i. Low adherence to treatment.
  ii. Inadequate drug regimen.
  iii. Patient dependent pharmacodynamics and pharmaco-kinetic properties of the drug administered.
  iv. Increased bacillary load.
  v. Treatment without drug susceptibility testing or culture.
  vi. Delayed in recognition and diagnosis.

MDR treatment regimen: WHO recommends the following 5 agent treatment regimens for MDR-TB: Pyrazinamide, fluoro-quinolone, ethionamide, cycloserine and one parenteral agent (amikacin/kanamycin).

Types of drug resistance: According to WHO criteria define:
  i. *Primary/acquired drug resistance*: As the isolation of a drug resistant strain from a patient without a history of previous treatment for one month.
  ii. *Secondary drug resistance*: It is the main cause of primary drug resistance due to transmission of resistant strains. Or inadequate drug delivery is main cause of secondary drug resistance.

Development of drug resistance: Two steps: Mutation and Selection

1. *Mutation*: In any prokaryotic genome, mutations are constantly occurring due to base changes caused by exogenous agents, DNA polymerase errors, deletions, insertion, and duplications. The antibiotic resistance genes encoding fundamental replication functions of the organism such as *rpoB* and *gyrA* are typically highly conserved. It confers drug resistance which occurs in individual organism at a very low rate. With high numbers of organism, small population resistant to each drug will exist.

2. *Selection*: Organism with resistant mutations to a particular drug will have an advantage over susceptible organisms when all are exposed to that drug. The resistant organism can outgrow the susceptible organism.

TB Drug Susceptibility Testing (DST) Methods

a. *Direct method*: Done on solid media either where a set of drug containing and drug free media are *inoculated directly with concentrated specimen*. The advantage—*results* are available sooner *within 3 weeks* on agar plates.

b. *Indirect method*: The *pure cultures are inoculated* in drug containing and drug free slopes either on LJ medium or 7H11 medium.

Indirect Methods (Phenotypic)

a. *Proportion method*: Enables a precise estimation of the proportion of mutants resistant to a given drug. May be performed on L-J or agar media (Middlebrook 7H10 and 7H11). Proportion of resistant bacilli determined by expressing resistant portion as a percentage of total population tested.

b. *Absolute concentration method*: Standardized inoculum grown on drug free media and media containing graded concentration of the drug to be tested. Resistance expressed in terms of lowest concentration of drug inhibiting growth, i.e. MIC.

c. *Resistance ratio method*: Compares unknown strain of TB bacilli with a standard laboratory strain (H37Rv). Parallel sets of media, drug are inoculated with a standard inoculum prepared from both the unknown and standard strains of tubercle bacilli. Resistance expressed as the ratio of MIC-s of test and control strains.

Molecular Methods

To overcome the limitations of traditional culture and identification, chemical methods based on lipid profiles,[13] hybridization with specific gene probes,[14-20] polymerase chain reaction—restriction fragment length polymorphism (PCR-RFLP) methods such as gene for hsp 65 kDa protein,[21] *katG*,[22] and rRNA genes[23-25] and sequencing of 16S rRNA[26] have been described.

a. *Analysis of lipid profiles by chromatographic techniques*: Characteristic mycobacteria lipid profiles can be analyzed by HPLC or HP-TLC[13] and quick identification of mycobacterial isolates can be done.

b. *DNA probes*: Based on information about specific gene sequences, well-defined oligonucleotide probes for identification of various clinically relevant mycobacteria have been developed[14-20] and are readily available for rapid confirmation of the identity of mycobacterial isolates including *M. tuberculosis*, *M. avium* and several other mycobacteria.

c. *Ribosomal RNA-based probes*: In recent years, rRNA gene region has been extensively explored for designing systems for ribosomal DNA fingerprinting and for development of probes/as well as gene amplification assays for various of mycobacterial species including *M. tuberculosis, M. leprae* and *M. avium, etc.*[2,14,15] which target *r*RNA, ribosomal DNA, spacer and flanking sequences. rRNA targeting probes are 10–100-fold more sensitive and may be used to confirm the diagnosis directly in the clinical specimens; the lowest detection limit is around 100 organisms.

d. *Gene amplification methods for identification*: Strategies to identify isolates from cultures and also directly from the clinical specimens include amplification of specific gene regions followed by hybridization with species specific probes,[6, 7] sequencing and RFLP analysis such as hsp 65 kDa gene,[21] *kat*G[22] and rRNA genes. While PCR-sequencing approach can be applied by reference laboratories,[26] the hybridization and RFLP approaches are easily practicable in clinical mycobacteriology laboratories.

e. *Gene amplification methods for direct detection of M. tuberculosis sequences from clinical specimens*: These methods may be classified as those based on polymerase chain reaction (PCR) and others based on isothermal amplification reactions,[2, 27] and are highly sensitive and *under optimum conditions may detect 1–10 organisms in paucibacillary extrapulmonary forms of tuberculosis.*[27,28]

f. *PCR*: Variety of PCR methods, e.g. conventional DNA-based PCR, nested PCR and RT-PCR, have been developed and can be used for confirming the diagnosis and also monitoring the progress.

Advantages of molecular assay are:
i. Highly sensitive and specific
ii. Rapid results
iii. Widely used

Disadvantage of molecular assay are:
i. Needs a laboratory infrastructures
ii. Continued need for culture for AST
iii. Costly

Other Test

Tuberculin skin test: The Mantoux test is the recommended standard tuberculin skin test (TST). Tuberculin is commercially available in 1, 2, and 5 tuberculin unit (TU) PPD (purified protein derivative, RT23 equivalent) forms.[10,11] For the test, it is important to raise a wheal of approximately 6 mm after the intradermal injection. The test is read 48–72 hours after an injection. Marking with a ball-pen or palpatory methods are used to read the induration. The influence of a prior BCG vaccine on the test depends on conditions such as the interval between the BCG vaccination and the TST and the age at vaccination. If the prevalence of TB infection is high enough, the positive predictive value of the TST is also high.[12, 13] If the patient returns for a reading beyond 72 hours but before the 7th post-injection day, a positive test can still be read. A repeat test may be needed, if there is no induration and the wheals present beyond the stipulated time for reading in which case should preferably be performed on the other arm. Limitations— sensitivity may be decreased in malnutrition and immuno- deficiency and cross-reaction with NTM or with *Mycobacterium bovis* vaccine strains.[14,15]

Immunological Test

Interferon gamma release assays (IGRAs by quantiferon assay): In addition to the traditional TST, which is known to lack both sensitivity and specificity, blood-based assays have recently become available. These T cell assays rely on the stimulation of host blood cells with *M. tuberculosis*-specific antigens and measure the production of interferon γ (**IFN-γ**). Although more specific than the TST, **but they are currently unable to distinguish between active disease and latent TB infection (LTBI)**. Therefore, interpretation of the results remains dependent on the clinical context. Two new IGRAs may offer improved specificity and sensitivity over the TST for the diagnosis of LTBI. One of these, quantiferon gold (QFT-gold), showed encouraging results in low-risk BCG-vaccinated subjects and patients with active TB.[16,17] QFT-gold overcomes some of the shortcomings of the TST, such as the need for return visits, reader variability, variable specificity, and cross-reactivity with BCG vaccination and NTM infections.[18–20]

A Note for Clinicians

Both routine and AFB cultures (before starting anti-TB treatment), using automation, are essential in the accurate diagnosis of osteoarticular TB. Even in disease endemic countries, only a clinical suspicion and imaging results are not accurate enough to diagnose and treat osteoarticular TB. Nested PCR has great potential to improve the clinicians' ability to diagnose clinically suspected TB rapidly. This will ensure early treatment for patients and prevent further transmission of the disease. Although MGIT and PCR increase the number of definite diagnoses, they are expensive and not routinely available in TB endemic countries, except in the larger cities.

In contrast, conventional culture is cost-effective. Minimally, AFB smear, LJ culture and histopathology of tissue specimens can be done at a much lower cost and can increase the number of definite diagnoses.

Empirical therapy leads to needless treatment, compounds problem of drug resistance in tuberculosis, and does not accurately address the actual etiology. Drug susceptibility testing of all culture isolates should be the basis for treatment of resistant cases. Using reporter genes and bacteriophages (e.g. Biotec/Medispan), diagnosis and drug susceptibilty results can be obtained within 4–8 hours.

Mycobacterial cultures using liquid media with susceptibility should form the backbone of management of osteoarticular TB.

Nested PCR enhances the sensitivity, if performed in addition to culture.

REFERENCES

1. Titov AG, Vyshnevskay A, Mazurenko SI, *et al.* Use of polymerase chain reaction to diagnose tuberculous arthritis from joint tissues and synovial fluid. *Arch Pathol Lab Med* 2004, 128(2):205–209.

2. Teklali Y, El Alami ZF, EL Madhi T, *et al.* Peripheral osteoarticular tuberculosis in children: 106 case-reports. *Joint Bone Spine* 2003, 70(4):282–286.

3. Barbu Z. Tuberculoza secundară osteoarticulară. în: Moisescu V. (ed), Tratat de Ftiziologie, ed. dacia, cluj-napoca, 1977, 220–228.

4. Gorse GJ, Pais MJ, Kusske JA, *et al.* Tuberculous spondylitis. *Medicine* 1983, 62:178.

5. Berney S, Goldstein M, Bishko F. Clinical and diagnostic features of tuberculous arthritis. *Am J Med* 1972 Jul; 53(1):36–42.

6. Tuli SM. Epidemiology and prevalence. Tuberculosis of the skeletal system. 2nd ed. Jaypee, New Delhi; 1997.

7. Karen B, Tuli SM. Severe kyphotic deformity in tuberculosis of the spine. *Int Orthop* 1995;19(5):327–331.

8. Chen SC and Chen KT. *J Emerg Med Trauma Surg Care* 2014, 1:002.

9. Chan PC, Chang LY, Wu YC, *et al.* Age-specific cutoffs for the tuberculin skin test to detect latent tuberculosis in BCG-vaccinated children. *Int J Tuberc Lung Dis* 2008, 12:1401–1406.

10. Wang PD. Assessment of the need for universal BCG vaccination of children in Taipei. *Public Health* 2009, 123:74–77.

11. Menzies D. What does tuberculin reactivity after bacille Calmette-Guérin vaccinations tell us? *Clin Infect Dis* 2000, 3:71–74.

12. McFadden JJ, Kunze Z, Seechum P. DNA probes for detection and identification. In: McFadden J, editor. *Molecular biology of the mycobacteria*. UK: Surrey University Press; 1990 p. 139–72.

13. Araujo Z, de Waard JH, de Larrea CF, *et al.* The effect of Bacille Calmette-Guérin vaccine on tuberculin reactivity in indigenous children from communities with high prevalence of tuberculosis. *Vaccine* 2008, 26:5575–5581.

14. Chen SC, Chen KL, Chen KH, *et al.* Updated diagnosis and treatment of childhood tuberculosis. *World J Pediatr* 2013, 9: 9–16.

15. Dhanasekaran S, Jenum S, Stavrum R, *et al.* Effect of non-tuberculous Mycobacteria on host biomarkers potentially relevant for tuberculosis management. *PLoS Negl Trop Dis* 2014, 8:3243.

16. Ewer K, Deeks J, Alvarez L, *et al.* Comparison of T-cell-based assay with tuberculin skin test for diagnosis of Mycobacterium tuberculosis infection in a school tuberculosis outbreak. *Lancet* 2003, 361:1168–1173.

17. Brock I, Weldingh K, Lillebaek T, *et al.* Comparison of tuberculin skin test and new specific blood test in tuberculosis contacts. *Am J Respir Crit Care Med* 2004, 170:65–69.

18. Mori T, Sakatani M, Yamagishi F, *et al.* Specific detection of tuberculosis infection: an interferon-gamma-based assay using new antigens. *Am J Respir Crit Care Med* 2004, 170:59–64.

19. Mazurek GH, Villarino ME. CDC Guidelines for using the Quantiferon-TB test for diagnosing latent Mycobacterium tuberculosis infection: Centers for Disease Control and Prevention. *MMWR Recomm Rep* 2003, 52: 15–18.

20. Mazurek GH, Jereb J, Lobue P, *et al.* Guidelines for using the Quantiferon-TB Gold test for detecting Mycobacterium tuberculosis infection, United States. *MMWR Recomm Rep* 2005, 54:49–55.

21. Pai M, Riley LW, Colford JM Jr . Interferon-gamma assays in the immunodiagnosis of tuberculosis: a systematic review. *Lancet Infect Dis* 2004, 4:761–776.

22. Costantino F, de Carvalho Bittencourt M, *et al.* Screening for Latent Tuberculosis Infection in Patients with Chronic Inflammatory Arthritis: Discrepancies Between Tuberculin Skin Test and Interferon-γ Release Assay Results. *J Rheumatol* 2013, 40:1986–93.

23. Ahmed N, Caviedes L, Alam M, *et al.* Distinctiveness of *Mycobacterium tuberculosis* genotypes from human immunodeficiency virus type 1-seropositive and -seronegative patients in Lima, Peru. *J Clin Microbiol* 2003; 41:1712–6.

24. Vaneechouttee M, De Beenhouwer H, Claeys G, *et al.* Identification of *Mycobacterium* species by using amplified ribosomal RNA restriction analysis. *J Clin Microbiol* 1993; 31:2061.

25. Roth A, Reischl U, Streubel A, *et al.* Novel diagnostic algorithm for identification of mycobacteria using genus specific amplification of 16S-23S rRNA gene spacer and restriction endonucleases. *J Clin Microbiol* 2000; 38:1094–1104.

26. Rogall T, Flohr T, Bottger EC. Differentiation of *Mycobacterium* species by direct sequencing of amplified DNA. *J Gen Microbiol* 1990; 136: 1915–20.

27. Forbes BA, Hicks KES. Direct detection of *Mycobacterium tuberculosis* in respiratory specimens in a clinical laboratory by polymerase chain reaction. *J Clin Microbiol* 1993; 31:1688–94.

28. Verma A, Rattan A, Tyagi JS. Development of a 23S rRNA based PCR assay for the detection of mycobacteria. *Indian J Biochem Biophys* 1994; 31:288–94.

Chapter 3

The Pathology of Osteoarticular Tuberculosis

Tuberculosis (TB) is a major health problem globally with a very high disease burden in developing countries; 9.6 million new TB cases and 1.5 million TB deaths were reported in 2014. India and China alone accounted for 24% and 11% of total cases, respectively. TB is broadly divided into pulmonary TB and extrapulmonary TB (EPTB); extrapulmonary TB comprising of disease of lymph nodes, pleura, bones and joints, genitourinary system, meninges, abdomen and other sites.

Osteoarticular TB accounts for 4–5% of the total TB burden. Accurate and early diagnosis of osteoarticular TB is difficult because lesions are often deep, inaccessible, and the disease is often paucibacillary. It is true for almost every form of EPTB that there is a tendency to initiation of empirical therapy based on clinicoradiological suspicion. Pulmonary TB, in contrast, is often multibacillary. Sputum samples are easier to obtain, repeated sampling is possible, and the multibacillary nature of the disease makes microscopic detection of acid-fast organisms simpler.

Involvement of the musculoskeletal system by TB occurs generally by hematological dissemination of *Mycobacterium tuberculosis* (MTB) from a primary visceral focus (lungs, kidney or lymph nodes). It can also be a result of direct extension from a focus of tubercular osteomyelitis. In the joints, the disease usually begins with synovial seeding of the bacilli, resulting in synovial hypertrophy and effusions. The granulomatous inflammation proliferates from the periphery to the centre resulting in loss of articular cartilage and bony erosions; which may culminate in joint destruction, subluxation, or dislocation. It may also present as a cold abscess, or sinus tract. Neurological dysfunction is a dreaded complication of TB spondylitis; hence, early diagnosis and timely intervention can significantly improve the outcomes of the patients.

Pathogenesis and Clinical-pathologic Correlations

"We dance round in a ring and suppose, but the secret sits in the middle and knows".

—Robert Frost: The Secret Sits

Over one-third of the world population is infected by MTB; only a small proportion develops the disease. To explain this phenomenon, it is attractive to invoke immunity in the context of host–parasite balance; however, this explanation is probably simplistic, and there is more to it. Much progress has been made in understanding how immunity works; however, putting that knowledge into practice to benefit the patient is frustratingly difficult.

Granulomatous inflammation is the result of an immune response to poorly soluble antigens, often lipid. The mycobaterial cell wall contains lipids that render them poorly soluble; TB is thus primarily a granulomatous disease. Granulomatous inflammation destroys existing tissue, and therefore, must heal with scarring and fibrosis; as the scar tissue contracts permanent deformity follows because fibrosis is irreversible, and refractory to treatment.

Immune responses are mediated through cell-to-cell signaling via cytokines, which are chemical substances produced by cells. Antigen recognition, presentation, and processing; immune cell recruitment, multiplication, and memory; phagocytosis, bacterial killing, degradation, and elimination of breakdown products are important pathways in containing the infection and protecting the body from succumbing to it. The interested reader may find excellent detailed accounts of these events in specialized texts; here I shall restrict myself to some basic concepts relevant to osteoarticular TB.

The predominant immune response to MTB in the immunocompetent host is type IV hypersensitivity—which consists of two arms: **Delayed type hypersensitivity (DTH), and cell-mediated immunity (CMI)**. In an apparent attempt to destroy infective organisms in tissue affected by TB, DTH, the predominant response in most patients with TB, destroys every cell in the vicinity of an infected focus resulting in what is described as caseation necrosis. The destruction is so complete that no trace of pre-existing tissue can be recognized in areas of caseation. This DTH response to MTB may appear inappropriately large in relation to the number of organisms because bacteria are difficult to find in areas of caseation.

In what appears to be an effort at containment, caseating foci are often surrounded by granulomas which are cohesive collections of epithelioid cells, which are thought to be predominantly secretory in nature, i.e. they produce cytokines. Necrosis and giant cells may or may not be present. Under the influence of appropriate stimuli epithelioid cells are also thought to be capable of turning into macrophages, and several of them may merge to form giant cells.

Giant cells in epithelioid cell granulomas are described as Langhans type giant cells on the basis of their microscopic appearance; however, they are not prerequisite to the recognition of the inflammation as granulomatous. In common with many other types of giant cells, particularly the foreign body type, they probably help in clearing effete cells and necrotic tissue through phagocytosis. Eye catching though they are because of their size, they are not known to have diagnostic significance.

In a further attempt at containment by the granuloma, there may be an outer zone of fibrosis. If the balance tilts in favor of the bacteria, tell-tale signs are visible to the microscopist: the granulomas are large and confluent, with large areas of necrosis. The epithelioid cell collections are less cohesive, the outer ring of fibrosis is poorly developed, and stainable acid-fast bacteria are easier to find indicating that they are present in greater numbers. Thus, there is a correlation between tissue reaction patterns and bacterial density which may help the microscopist in searching for organisms.

Epithelioid cell granulomas and fibrosis indicate strong DTH. In this scenario, the host may well be able to contain the disease, but MTB may still eventually outsmart the host. MTB may survive in a dormant state in foci of caseation or the calcification that may result from successful containment, apparently for many years until conditions are again favorable for growth. Indeed, stainable acid-fast organisms can sometimes be demonstrated in fine-needle aspirate smears from calcified lymph nodes. This phenomenon, one of the enduring enigmas of TB, is called **"reactivation TB"**. Alternately, adequately treated patients may be re-exposed and reinfected, often with a different, more virulent strain of MTB in what is called **"reinfection TB"**. In yet another gruesome twist, inadequate or failed treatment may result in recurrence of the disease as in **"recurrent TB"**, often with drug-resistant clones of MTB. By employing multiple subversive strategies against the host MTB presents a formidable challenge that begs better understanding of how it works.

For the patient with skeletal TB widespread destruction of tissue translates to catastrophic collapse of the supporting function of bone, say collapse of a vertebral body, or fracture of a long bone, and the attendant morbidity. To complicate matters, the necrotic tissue may undergo liquefaction under the influence of various cytokines such as interleukin-2 (IL-2), interferon-γ (IFN-γ), and tumor necrosis factor (TNF) derived mainly from macrophages. The liquefied material tracks along paths of the least resistance giving rise to cold abscesses—"cold" because there are no accompanying signs of acute inflammation. This act of treachery allows explosive proliferation of MTB because pus from cold abscesses is a conducive environment for their growth. Ironically, pus from cold abscesses also gives the investigating team a better opportunity to clinch the diagnosis because organisms are present in larger numbers, they are easier to find in direct smears of pus, and to isolate by culture. As a corollary, it may be a good ploy to look for cold abscesses in patients suspected to have spinal TB, and to attempt diagnostic aspiration, if one can be found. Delay might be counterproductive because the cold abscess may break through the skin by creating a sinus, or scrofula that drain the abscess. MTB are mostly impossible to find in smears from the persisting, watery discharge.

TB of the joints may result in an initial sterile effusion in the joint space which may progress to a frankly purulent inflammation with necrosis. For poorly understood reasons, the synovial inflammation is often an acute inflammation representing a type I hypersensitivity response. It is probable that healthy joint spaces being sterile, they are protected sites; the entry of MTB into joints, therefore, results in explosive proliferation and elicits a neutrophilic response as in the immunologically naïve individual. It is not uncommon to see phagocytosis of acid-fast organisms by neutrophils in direct smears of pus aspirated from joints and stained by the Ziehl-Neelsen (ZN) stain.

Like leprosy, TB is also a disease with a spectrum; at one end is paucibacillary disease in the host with good immunity and strong DTH, manifesting the effects of the widespread tissue destruction described above. The other end of the spectrum may be seen in anergic patients, where the disease involves many organs, but with little, or no tissue destruction. In between are several permutations and combinations.

Paradoxically, it is paucibacillary disease which presents to the practitioner of orthopedics, whose job becomes doubly difficult because definitive diagnosis by the gold standard is often elusive, the disease leaving behind only a trail of uncertainty and unreliable circumstantial evidence. **Resort to a variety of diagnostic techniques—from clinical suspicion, through radiological, pathological, and microbiological techniques, as well as serological and molecular methods, and often recourse to therapeutic response—is not surprising.** We congratulate ourselves on our diagnostic excellence when patients are cured by our antituberculous therapies, not realizing that **by working with populations in areas of high endemicity, it is chance that saves the day.** In this ocean of TB, the skilled physician is the one who recognizes non-tuberculous disease at first encounter; just as the skilled physician working in low-endemic areas is the one who recognizes TB at first presentation.

Mycobacteria, like all forms of life barring some humans, being illiterate, will not read this. They will happily continue to follow the laws of nature while we struggle to comprehend what is going on.

Diagnostic Workup

Osteoarticular TB may present as tubercular spondylitis, arthritis of the hip, knee, or other joints, osteomyelitis, and occasionally as tenosynovitis and myositis. The clinical differential diagnosis may include neoplasms, pyogenic arthritis and fungal infections.

TB is a bacterial disease and the gold standard for the diagnosis of active TB is the isolation of MTB by culture. The task of establishing the diagnosis in every patient by this gold standard is frustrating because it is so often unrewarding; over time a situation evolves where no effort is made to procure tissue for microbiological methods. Instead, reliance is placed on clinical-radiological examination and histopathology or cytopathology, even therapeutic response, all of which provide only circumstantial evidence of the diagnosis at best. A workup that does not include culture must be condemned.

The laboratory tests should include a culture (conventional or rapid), direct smear for ZN and Gram's stain, tissue examination by cytopathological and histopathological methods, and the newer serological and molecular methods. Attempt to obtain tissue for conventional smear microscopy, culture and drug sensitivity testing must be made in all patients. Every patient with clinicoradiologically suspected vertebral osteomyelitis should be screened for the presence of active pulmonary or other foci of extrapulmonary tuberculosis. If present, and if microbiologically confirmed, the patient should be treated for osteoarticular TB. However, if its nature has not been confirmed microbiologically, the bone lesion should be biopsied percutaneously. Patients without any other, more easily accessible, foci and/or needing surgical management should undergo surgical biopsy. Patients who do not have any indication for surgical management should also undergo percutaneous biopsy.

All biopsy samples which show necrotizing granulomas or smear positivity or which show positive results with direct DNA probes should be considered to be osteoarticular tuberculosis. Waiting for definitive culture reports is advisable for those with negative results.

Samples can be collected of pus from cold abscess, synovial biopsies, percutaneous vertebral biopsies, surgical biopsies, synovial fluid, or tissue from sinus tracts. In our experience, pus aspirated from cold abscesses, pus, and necrotic tissue, not fluid effusions, from joint spaces, offer the best probability for the demonstration of acid-fast bacilli in direct smears stained with the ZN stain. The best results are obtained when the pus is immediately smeared on to glass slides, allowed to air-dry, and fixed in methanol for 30 minutes before being transported to the laboratory. Samples must be handled with due diligence to universal precautions to prevent hazardous exposure to clinical and laboratory personnel. Other tissue—synovial biopsy, percutaneous biopsy, and tissue from sinus tracts, sequestra, and abscess walls are often unrewarding; however, when they are the only options available, they must be utilized for histopathological examination. As little as 0.2 mL of tissue can be handled by the histopathology laboratory; however, the pathologist is always happier with as much tissue as possible. Before putting the tissue into 10% formalin, it might be useful to crush some of it between two slides and smeared for cytological examination. If the tissue is hard and cannot be crushed and smeared into a thin film, imprints should be made by gently pressing the cut surface of tissue on to several different areas of a slide, and then processed as usual. Cytological examination delivers quicker preliminary results.

For patients undergoing surgery without a clear preoperative diagnosis, intraoperative cytological examination of pus and necrotic material can be helpful. The cytopathologist, using both May-Grünwald-Giemsa (MGG) and ZN stains, may be able to exclude a cancer, and demonstrate AFB within the hour. Intraoperative consultations must not be undertaken on impulse. To succeed, an intraoperative consult requires planning, dedication, teamwork, and excellent communication between the orthopedic and the pathology teams. Pathologists and the orthopedic surgeon working together promotes bonding, as also sense of ownership and belonging to the team, all of which contribute better outcomes. A visit by the pathology team to the operation theatre to get a first-hand feel of what goes on, and a reciprocal visit by the surgeons to understand what goes on behind their backs in the laboratory can go a long way in boosting morale and motivation. A request for an intraoperative consult can be anticipated in most instances. The earlier the pathologist is informed, the better prepared he/she will be to handle the consult. Unlike surgeons, most pathologists are not used to working under pressure.

The pathologist needs to ensure that a good, committed technician is available when the sample arrives, that the staining reagents are ready and working, and that communication with the reporting pathologist is established well in time. The surgical team must know how to identify representative tissue, how to prepare a good quality smear—not a difficult job once it is learned—air dry it and, to save time, immerse it in a jar of methanol while it is being transported to the laboratory. Both teams must understand that the consult may not result in a definitive diagnosis; therefore, back-up plans must be in place. The common platform thus created should be used to prepare need based checklists to ensure that procedures are followed, and no step is omitted. Over time, as the intraoperative consult is fine-tuned for efficiency, it can have very satisfying results.

Laboratory Tests

Ziehl-Neelsen staining for acid-fast bacilli has the advantages of being rapid, easy to perform and requiring minimal infrastructure; however, it requires a minimum load of 5,000–10,000 bacilli/mL, and species differentiation is not possible. For *sputum* smears, the WHO recommends that the smears are reported as negative only after scanning a minimum of 100 oil immersion fields over 10 minutes. Since osteoarticular TB is so often paucibacillary, adequate extension of these limits is necessary to search for bacilli. Examination of smears by fluorescence microscopy can also detect AFB.

Fluorescence microscopy utilizes a fluorescent dye to stain the organisms; when excited by ultraviolet light using a special microscope the bacteria appear as bright rods in a dark background. It has been used successfully for the rapid diagnosis of pulmonary TB; however, its use in the diagnosis of EPTB, particularly paucibacillary disease, is not clearly established. Fluorescence microscopy has been claimed to be faster and more sensitive than conventional light microscopy, but the expense, the need for a dark room, and poor specificity limit its usefulness.

Culture: Isolation of the organism on culture is the gold standard for the diagnosis of TB. The culture media available are egg based (Lowenstein-Jensen medium), agar based (Middlebrook 7H10, 7H11), and liquid based (Mycobacterium growth indicator tube). Culture can detect as little as 10–100 bacilli/mL of *sputum*, can distinguish between different mycobacterial species, can be used for drug sensitivity testing and is useful in symptomatic smear negative patients; however, isolation of organisms from samples of tissue or fluids of patients with osteoarticular TB is far more difficult and far less rewarding. Conventional methods of culture are time consuming taking 6–8 weeks and require strict quality control. Rapid culture methods like BACTEC which detect Mycobacteria based on metabolism rather than visible growth give results within 7–14 days. The BACTEC system detects C14 labelled CO_2 and reports it in terms of Growth Index (GI) value.

Tissue biopsy for histopathological examination may show a mononuclear and granulomatous reaction pattern. Sections show granulomas with or without central caseation necrosis. Demonstration of organism requires ZN staining, which, compared to direct smears, is difficult to do well in tissue sections. Inflammatory reaction patterns seen on histopathologic examination of tissue are of secondary importance to the diagnosis because other conditions such as fungal infections, foreign body reactions, and sarcoidosis may be associated with granulomatous inflammation. Histopathologic evidence for diagnosis of TB is adjunctive, always circumstantial, and never a replacement for culture.

Cytological examination of smears: Direct smears may be stained with May-Grünwald-Giemsa (or other Romanowsky dyes) and ZN for cytopathologic examination allowing for the recognition of inflammatory patterns (Figs 3.1–3.4) and detection of acid-fast organisms. If the tissue is representative of the pathology, a tentative diagnosis can be established in a day, or even in an intraoperative consultation; however, as with histopathology, the diagnosis is always circumstantial, never definitive.

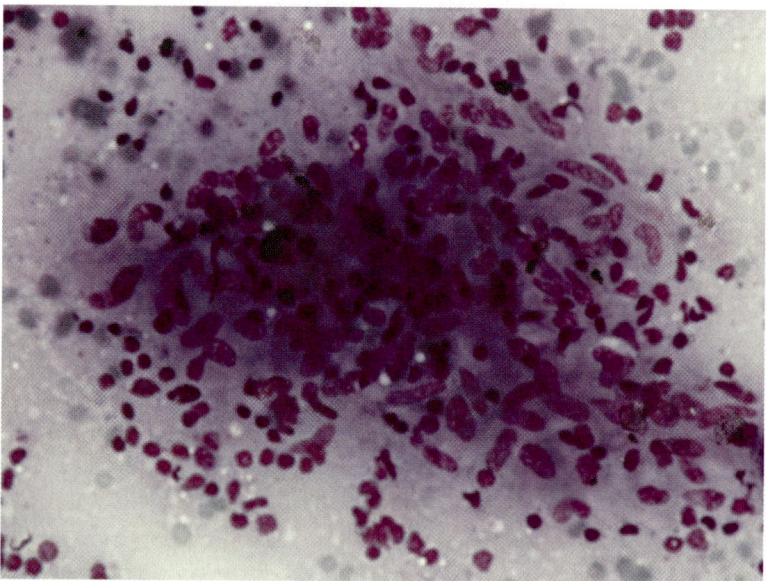

Fig. 3.1: Smear from fine-needle aspiration of an inguinal lymph node in a patient suspected to have spinal tuberculosis. The pale cells with slipper-shaped nuclei are epithelioid cells representing the DTH response. Note the cohesion between these cells: in spite of the shearing force used when aspirated material was smeared, the cells have not dissociated. The darker, round nuclei are lymphocytes representing the CMI. This pattern is associated with paucibacillary disease. MTB will be difficult or impossible to find in smears stained with the Ziehl-Neelsen stain. The evidence of tuberculosis here is circumstantial, and the degree of diagnostic confidence is very low. May-Grünwald-Giemsa ×400

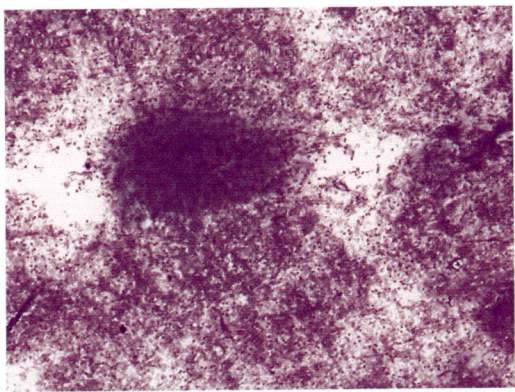

Fig. 3.2: Smear from tissue obtained from the spine in an intraoperative consult. There is an epithelioid cell granuloma in a necrotic background. Some lymphocytes are seen in scattered in the background. Small numbers of acid-fast bacilli were found in smears stained with the Ziehl-Neelsen stain. This tissue reaction also represents paucibacillary disease. The demonstration of acid-fast bacilli in smears constitutes circumstantial evidence of TB; however, the degree of confidence in the diagnosis does not match positive culture. May-Grünwald-Giemsa x100

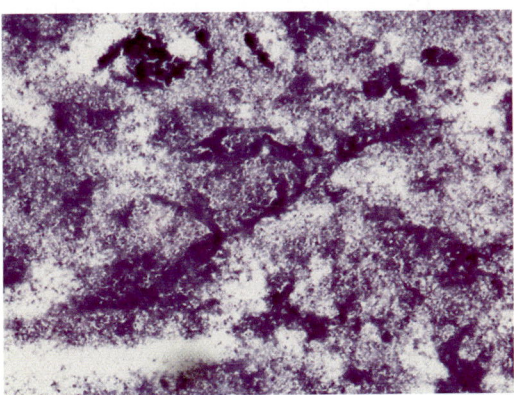

Fig. 3.3: Smear from tissue obtained from the spine in an intraoperative consult. There is only acellular necrotic tissue in this smear. Demonstration of acid-fast-bacilli may provide circumstantial evidence of tuberculosis. Tumor necrosis can be indistinguishable from the necrosis of tuberculosis; therefore, necrosis alone, without AFB, must not be interpreted as evidence in favor of TB. May-Grünwald-Giemsa x100

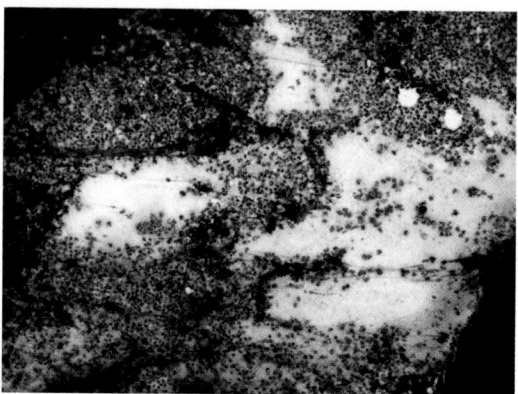

Fig. 3.4: Smear from a knee joint from which thick pus was aspirated. There is a purulent exudate consisting of neutrophils. Acid-fast bacilli were demonstrated in neutrophils in a Ziehl-Neelsen stained smear, providing circumstantial evidence of tuberculosis. This inflammatory response can also be seen in acute purulent synovitis in which Gram's stain may provide a clue to the infective organism. It is important to recognize that culture is the gold standard for diagnosis of any infective disorder. May-Grünwald-Giemsa x100

Serological testing can be used for antigen and antibody detection; however, serological tests are expensive, require trained personnel, have low sensitivity, are affected by BCG vaccination and previous infection, and cannot distinguish between MTB and non-tubercular mycobacteria. **(Serological tests have, therefore, been banned in India since 2012.)**

Molecular methods: Detection and identification of mycobateria directly from clinical samples can be done by polymerase chain reaction (PCR) and nucleic acid amplification test. PCR can provide rapid diagnosis within 48 hours, has high sensitivity, can identify the species and requires very small volume of specimen; however, it cannot differentiate between live and dead mycobacteria. High cost and the infrastructure required limit its usage.

GeneXpert MTB/RIF automates and integrates sample processing and PCR in a single disposable plastic cartridge, giving accurate results within 2 hours. It simultaneously detects MTB and resistance to rifampicin. WHO recommends its use as the initial diagnostic test in adults and children suspected of having MDR-TB or HIV associated TB.

In conclusion, regardless of the organ affected, microbiologic methods are the mainstay in the diagnosis of TB. In the hierarchy of evidence for the diagnosis of TB culture remains the gold standard. Every attempt must, therefore, be made to obtain representative samples for culture, and the recently available molecular tests should be performed when available. Pathologic testing is of secondary importance because the diagnosis is, at best, circumstantial; however, the tools of the pathologist, histopathology and cytopathology, can offer important clues to the diagnosis of TB in the form of demonstration of AFB, and recognition of tissue reaction patterns.

The Hierarchy of Evidence for the Diagnosis of TB

1. Culture.
2. Molecular testing (probable): GeneXpert, nucleic acid amplification testing, PCR, other tests in development.
3. Demonstration of AFB in direct smears or tissue sections.
4. Tissue reaction patterns: Necrotizing granulomas → non-caseating granulomas → necrosis alone without AFB positivity.
5. Radiological examination and imaging studies.
6. Physical examination of the patient.
7. Therapeutic response.

The reader may do well to remember that as one goes down this scale from 1 to 7, the diagnosis of TB becomes less and less certain. Careful consideration and decision making are required to get the best evidence.

SUGGESTED READINGS

1. Lakhanpal VP, Tuli SM, Singh H, Sen PC. The value of histology, culture and guinea pig inoculation examination in osteo-articular tuberculosis. *Acta Orthop Scand* 1974; 45: 36–42.
2. Dannenberg AM, Sugimoto M. Liquefaction of caseous foci in tuberculosis. *Am Rev Respir Dis* 1976; 113: 257–9.
3. Agashe V, Shenai S, Mohrir G, Deshmukh M, Bhaduri A, Deshpande R et al. Osteoarticular tuberculosis – Diagnostic solutions in a disease endemic region. *J Infect Dev Ctries* 2009; 3: 511–516.
4. Colmenero JD, Ruiz-Mesa JD, Sanjuan-Jimenez R, Sobrino B, Morata P. Establishing the diagnosis of tuberculous vertebral osteomyelitis. *Eur Spine J* 2013; 22: 579–586.
5. Kamara E, Mehta S, Brust JCM, Jain AK. Effect of delayed diagnosis on severity of Pott's disease. *Int Orthop* 2012; 36: 245–254.
6. Ministry of Health and Family Welfare G of I. INDEX-TB GUIDELINES: Ministry of Health and Family Welfare. Government of India.
7. World Health Organization. Global Tuberculosis Report 2016.

Chapter 4

Tuberculosis of Bone and Joint (Other Than Spine)

Tuberculosis of bone and joint is important cause of morbidity and functional disability in developing countries. The bone and joint tuberculoses constitute 2–3% of all tuberculosis cases and around 10–35% of extrapulmonary tuberculoses. Spinal TB is most common form of osseous tuberculosis and constitute 50% of all cases of bone and joint affection followed by TB of hip (17%) than foot, knee, elbow, hand, shoulder and others in that order. The introduction of effective (ATT) drugs and improvement in socioeconomic conditions (improved sanitation, hygiene, nutrition) have lead to decrease in the incidence of tuberculosis. But in economically developing countries, it still reports in endemic proportions, and remains a major health problem. The emergence of acquired immune deficiency syndrome (AIDS) pandemic, immigration and chronic debilitating diseases have lead to more and more new cases of tuberculosis.

The causative microbe is the tubercle bacillus (*Mycobacterium tuberculosis*). The following factors predisposes bone for development of a tubercular focus:

a. *Trauma*: Every patient of tubercular affection of the bone gives a history of minor trauma. The minor injury may be a predisposition to form a locus of decreased resistance to develop tubercular lesion.

b. *Disease*: Any viral infection such as measles/chickenpox/ AIDS/malignancy/congenital immune deficiency/chemo- therapy/radiotherapy/immunosuppressant drugs weaken the the immune mechanism and consequently increases the probability of developing tubercular lesion.

c. *Puberty and pregnancy*: It is a common observation that the tubercular lesions are reactivated during pregnancy (Chapter 7; Case No. 3).

d. *Poor socioeconomic condition*: Poor ventilation, sanitation and hygiene and unbalanced diet are other factors associated with increased occurrence of tuberculosis.

PATHOLOGY

Although it has been discussed in separate chapter, the bone and joint tuberculosis occurs following hematogenous dissemination after primary tubercular lesion in lung. Usually, primary complex develops in lungs within 2 years of age. The intial infection occurs in lung in human type and in intestine in bovine type of mycobacterial infection. Once the primary complex occurs and heals still it leaves an immunological memory for future infection. Whenever secondary infection occurs the immune allergy response occurs in the form of acute inflammatory one, i.e. polymorphonuclear leukocytosis and necrosis.

Bony and Synovial Involvement

Bone and synovium are involved secondary to hematogenous dissemination of tubercular bacilli following a primary lung disease. Once tubercle bacilli are lodged itself in active bone marrow and reaches synovium via subsynovial vessels, the destruction starts in the periphery of the joint at attachment of synovium in articular cartilage. The articular surfaces are preserved for long since the tubercular granulation tissue does not have proteolytic enzymes. Initially, the disease may start in synovium or bone but eventually both are infected in a short time. Most of the time lesions heal, due to good immunity of individual. In the presence of insufficient defense to control allergic exudative response to TB bacillii, the implantation occurs and disease starts.

Usually TB bone lesion starts in metaphyseal area because of rich and slow blood supply. The acute inflammatory exudative reaction and a caseation occurs. The decalcification and localized rarefaction is appreciated on plain X-rays which occurs due to reactive hyperemia secondary to inflammation.

Generally, the granulation tissue is limited by fibroblastic healing response. However, when destruction extends up and down the shaft and to the periphery, it reaches subperiosteal space. The exudates may travel and follow the path of least resistance through the soft tissue and forms chronic discharging sinus on skin draining caseous material, particles of bone and partially liquefied straw-colored (yellow) substance. The abscess may remain collected under skin and subcutaneous tissue in the form of cold abscess before formation of discharging sinus. Although with effective antitubercular treatment, the prolonged persistent drainage of sinus does not occur. In preantitubercular era, the persistent drainage of pus for many years used to lead to amyloidosis and death. The cold abscess may migrate along fascial planes (path of least resistance) and may erupt at a distance. The cold abscess from a dorsolumbar vertebral lesion may travels along psoas muscle and may reach up to thigh (*see* Fig. 5.1).

The tuberculosis may also disseminate by retrograde lymphatic dissemination and direct contiguity dissemination. The dorsal spine may be affected by mediastinal tubercular lymphadenopathy and lumbar spine by mesenteric tubercular lymphadenopathy. The affection of rib by tuberculosis may occur following direct contiguity dissemination from pleurisy and humeral head tuberculosis following shoulder bursitis.

The physeal plate is generally not destroyed in the initial stage. Later on, the damage to calified cartilage affects the growth and assymetric damage leads to deformity. In adult, the infection enters the joint through damage to subchondral area where synovium joins the cartilage. In children, the subperiosteal infection in metaphyseal area enters the joint directly (hip, knee, shoulder) or after penetrating the capsule.

Synovial Disease

The synovium is involved first, in a low-grade infection. The synovium becomes congested and swollen due to granulation tissue. The initial disease starts near the attachment of synovial membrane to articular cartilage. This area is full of translucent tubercle, deposits of fibrin and neovascularization and is termed 'pannus' (ring of granulation tissue). The caseation necrosis of the synovium and capsule is rare. At this stage, joint has moderate effusion with clear fluid, hence is called reactive fluid or reactive arthritis. Once disease process is progressed, the inflammatory synovitis produces nonspecific increase of joint fluid containing rice bodies (small accumulation of fibers and articular cartilage). In view of absence of caseation necrosis of synovium and the capsule, a negative synovial biopsy does not necessarily rule out tuberculosis. TB synovitis generally heals with fibrosis and marked synovial thickening. However, if the granulation tissue has exudative response, it erodes the cartilage and infection extends up and down the shaft and in the periphery to reach subperiosteal space.

CLINICAL PICTURE

Bone and/or joint tuberculosis is a low-grade infection and has insidious onset. The degree of local and general reaction depends on the intensity of infection and the defense response. The joint tuberculosis is a monoarticular or mono-osseous involvement and may have other visceral lesions (e.g. pulmonary, intestinal, renal). The family history of TB may be present. History of minor injury preceding the current disease may be available. The constitutional symptoms including low-grade evening rise fever, anorexia, weight loss, night sweats, malaise, tachycardia, anemia may be present.

If the joint is allowed to pass through natural history of disease without intervention, then it passes through a sequence of early synovitis, early and advanced arthritis. In early stage of disease, patient presents with insidious onset pain, increased local temperature, muscle wasting on clinical examination. The limb develops 10–15° flexion deformity. There may be boggy swelling (caused by synovial inflammation), tenderness, muscle spasm, night cries in children (due to relaxation of muscle spasm with deep sleep which allows painful motion and generate severe pain), stiffness, actual limitation of active and passive motion due to fibrous ankylosis. There could be various deformities of joint. The lymphadenopathies (matted local draining lymph nodes) are frequently observed.

The clinical diseases may be (a) granular, which is mild, non-destructive, and fibrosing type and (b) caseous and exudative type, which is destructive and abscess forming. Both types may occur simultaneously but one may predominate the other.

The osseous (granular) lesion, generally involves the metaphysis or the epiphysis, often following a minor injury. The clinical presentation is with mild vague pains, limp and fatigue and minimal constitutional symptoms. The slight rise in temperature, tenderness, bony thickening, effusion in adjacent joint (non-specific) is elicited on clinical examination. There may be wasting adjacent to the joint with restriction of joint movements. A fluctuant abscess formation may be present.

The osseous (exudative or caseous) lesion has insidious onset. The patient presents with marked constitutional symptoms like fever, anorexia, weight loss, malaise, and night sweats. Pain is much more marked and worst at night. The local temperature is raised with indurated tense, thin and shiny skin. The movements of adjacent joint elicit muscle spasm. The abscess may rupture and form sinus, which may remain discharging for months. When the abscess penetrates joint, it causes infectious arthritis.

The synovial (granular) lesions are predominantly observed in children. The children gradually develop mild pain in the joint with minimal effusion. Generally, the constitutional symptoms are absent or very mild. The wasting of muscles around joint appears after few months. The synovial thickening and effusion is less with terminal restriction of range of motion. Synovitis may last for years or rarely bone may also be involved. Very rarely it may become exudative type with increase in local symptoms and constitutional symptoms. There could be sub-luxation of joint once arthritis develops.

These patients with synovial (exudative) lesions have poor general condition and generally these lesions have an intense course. The synovitis presents with signs of intense acute inflammation and marked constitutional symptoms. On examination, the joint is diffusely swollen and has raised temperature and marked tenderness. The joint movements are painful with marked spasm. The draining lymph nodes are swollen. If not treated, joint passes through natural history of disease and develops the stages of early arthritis to advanced arthritis with or without complications. The joint may develop fibrous ankylosis, when abscess ruptures externally, and necrotic cartilage is lost. The draining fistula invites secondary infection, which over the years leads to amyloidosis. Although with the advent of potent ATT drugs, this end point is not observed.

ROENTGENOGRAPHIC FINDINGS

The bone and joint TB is a slowly developing disease. It takes 3–4 months of disease process to show radiological features. The first radiological sign of an active disease is a localized rarefaction/osteoporosis. The speed of decalcification depends on reactive hyperemia, which is most intense in exudative infections. As the disease advances, the articular margin starts losing sharpness and become fuzzy. Even if the lesion is located in one carpal/tarsal bone, the remaining carpals/tarsals also rapidly decalcify, suggesting on X-ray examination that the infection affects all.

The X-ray findings in stage of synovitis are:
a. Epiphyseal and metaphyseal areas show decalcification.
b. Swollen synovial shadow may be visible. The synovial affection or inflammation secondary to adjacent bony focus shows indistinguishable findings.
c. The recalcification on treatment is suggestive of reduction of disease activity.

X-ray findings in arthritic stage:
a. Joint space narrowing secondary to destruction of articular cartilage.
b. A small zone of osteolytic area suggestive of granular foci surrounded by diffuse osteoporosis.
c. In caseating lesions, the osteolytic foci is very clear.
d. Secondary to healing, the perifocal bone is thickened as a calcified ring.
e. In an exudative central lesion, the decalcified trabeculae start calcifying.

In central caseation, calcium gets deposited to give the dense image of a sequestrum (coke-like sequestrum) which is surrounded by an osteolytic ring representing the fibrous wall. The bone is osteoporotic/normal/or dense, depending on the defense reaction. The radiological signs at this stage may resemble as osteomyelitis. Joint effusion shows a soft tissue shadow. The abscesses may be seen as vague irregular densities in surrounding soft tissues. The destructive process may produce collapse of bone/subluxation/dislocation/migration and deformity of the joint. The damage to growth plate produces angular deformities due to irregular growths. The synovitis stimulates the osteogenesis of the epiphysis, which may lead to premature appearance/enlargement of the ossific nuclei. The lesion adjacent to the epiphyseal growth plate may stimulate longitudinal growth. When it damages the growth plate and encroaches on the area of endochondral ossification, growth is irregularly retarded and deformity results. The periosteal ossification is seen when the focus is superficial and bone looks thicker on palpation as happens in the small long bones of the hand and the foot. The newly formed bone (periosteal reaction) may encircle and enlarge the diaphysis in small long bones of hand/foot. The centre of tuberculous cavity may show a sequestrum of cancellous bone or following calcification of caseous tissue (irregular soft, feathery, coke-like sequestrum).

Computerized Tomography

- Useful to show smaller destroyed area of bone erosion.
- Detects disease in those areas of skeleton not appreciated on plain xrays such as craniovertebral spine, cervicodorsal spine, rib, sternum, sacroiliac joint, posterior elements of vertebrae.
- Intraspinal encroachment and dystrophic calcification is well appreciated by CT scan.
- Guided biopsy/aspiration provides tissue for histological/cytological/microbiological diagnosis.

MRI

- More sensitive and specific than X-rays and CT scan to detect tubercular lesion. The disease can be diagnosed in predestructive stage of disease.

- MRI can show abscess/granulation tissue/caseous tissue in multiple planes.
- Encroachment of the vertebral canal, localized tuberculoma, and generalized granuloma are better appreciated.
- The spinal cord changes, such as myelitis, myelomalacia, syrinx, can be appreciated.

Ultrasonography (USG)

It is a useful non-invasive modality to detect soft tissue mass which may be solid or liquid and is useful to detect deep-seated abscesses and perform guided aspiration.

INVESTIGATION

- X-ray chest-PA view should be done in all cases with osteo-articular TB.
- X-ray of the region affected is useful to make diagnosis and a baseline X-rays for follow-up evaluation of response to the ATT.
- HIV testing should be performed in all cases.
- Suitable imaging CT/MRI/USG should be performed to evaluate the lesion and perform guided biopsy.
- The diagnosis should be ascertained as best as possible by imaging before starting ATT. Wherever possible all patients should have a biopsy of the lesion to procure tissue for diagnosis, rule out other diagnosis and perform drug sensitivity testing.
- The specimen obtained should be sent for: (a) Microscopy and culture for pyogenic bacteria and *Mycobacterium TB*, (b) histology and cytology and molecular diagnosis.

COURSE AND PROGNOSIS

The potent antitubercular drugs have changed the prognosis and outlook in tuberculosis of bones and joints. The tubercular lesion which is mild granular can heal before the bone necrosis has occurred without residual joint scarring and ankylosis. The tubercular lesions usually heal by fibrosis. An epiphyseal caseous lesion may spread into the joint and widely infect the synovium. These cavities may undergo fibrous encirclement to effect a clinical cure. The living bacilli in the central area may reactivate the infection at any time. The recalcification of bone and, bony ankylosis in a joint is the best form of healing. The joint tuberculosis, if untreated in its natural course, passes through following stages (Tuli):

i. *Stage of synovitis*: In this stage, soft tissue swelling and synovial effusion in the joint is appreciated on clinical examination. The range of joint motion is restricted by 25% or less. The soft tissue shadow (swollen soft tissue) and regional osteoporosis may be the only finding on X-rays.

ii. *Stage of early arthritis*: The patient presents with pain, limp, swelling and deformity. The limitation of movements is between 25 and 50%. On X-rays, the joint space is diminished with marginal erosion of articular surfaces with no gross destruction of articular bone.

iii. *Stage of advanced arthritis*: The patient presents with similar clinical features as in early arthritis but in severe form and of longer duration. There is gross restriction (up to 75% in all directions) of joint motion. The marked diminution of joint space and gross destruction of articular margins is seen on X-rays.

iv. *Stage of advanced arthritis with subluxation or dislocation*: In addition to stage III, the restriction of joint motion is gross (more than 75%). The joint deformities are severe due to subluxation or dislocation. The wandering/migrating acetabulum or pathological dislocation of hip, triple deformity of knee, anterior subluxation of wrist, subluxation of ankle are some of the complications observed in various joints.

v. *Stage of sequelae of arthritis*: The ankylosis of the joint is the usual sequelae. Fibrous ankylosis allows painful jog of movement at joint, however, sound bony ankylosis is painless.

TREATMENT

General Care

High protein and vitamin diet should be given to improve the body resistance. Fresh air, warm dry climate and a good nursing care is advisable.

Bone and Joint Lesion

The bone and joint lesions are treated by antitubercular treatment, rest, intermittent mobilization of the joint and surgery for well-defined indications to gain the range of movement. The drainage of abscess, excision of sinus tract, joint debridement, aspiration of cold abscesses, synovectomies, excisional arthroplasties of the hip, compression arthodesis of joints (knee/ankle), anterolateral decompression of the spine, etc. are performed when indicated.

Chemotherapy and Antibiotics

The osteoarticular tuberculosis is primarily a medical disease and surgery is reserved for complications. Discovery of ATT (a) streptomycin in 1943, its clinical introduction (1947), (b) para-aminosalicylic acid in 1949, (c) isoniazid in 1952 improved the outcome of tuberculosis and these drugs formed the mainstay of conventional long-course chemotherapy. Pyrazinamide was invented in 1956 but was introduced to short course regimen in 1980 while Ethambutol (1962) and rifampicin (1967) were relatively late entrants as antitubercular drugs. The surgery used to be performed on the belief that antitubercular drugs do not penetrate well into osseous tubercular lesions. Many studies using radioactive isotopes of streptomycin and isoniazid among others have demonstrated that antitubercular drugs effectively penetrate into osseous lesions/cavities/abscesses and dry caseous lesions. Isoniazid, rifampicin and pyrazinamide have been found even in foci inside the sclerotic wall.

Short Course or Long Course Treatment?

Rifampicin, ethambutol, pyrazinamide and isoniazid based multidrug short-course chemotherapy has shown positive results which compare favorably with the conventional 18–24-month therapy. The addition of rifampicin to treatment regimens for pulmonary tuberculosis reduced the duration of therapy needed for active disease from 12 to 6 months and the duration of therapy needed for latent infection from nine months to between 2 and 3 months. Presently, the World Health

Organization recommends a daily dosage regimen and an intermittent short course (duration: 8–9 months) as the treatment of choice.

Rationale of Intermittent ATT Regimen

In vitro, exposure of tubercle bacilli to antituberculous drugs is followed by a lag period of several days before bacterial multiplication begin again. Hence, maintenance of a continuous inhibitory concentration of the drug is not necessary to kill or inhibit growth of *Mycobacterium tuberculosis*. Antitubercular therapy for 6–9 months, with surgical excision of the lesion and bone grafting, produced clinical and radiological results comparable to those at 18 months. Even in the presence of paraplegia, a combination of surgery when indicated and a short course of drug treatment for nine months was effective. The short-course intermittent regimen for pulmonary tuberculosis has a scientific rationale. After sputum conversion, four months of ATT is considered adequate treatment. However, bone and joint tuberculosis is a paucibacillary disease. Healing of tubercular lesions is generally clinicoradiological and X-ray pictures lag behind the biological process. There are no well established markers suggestive of end point of treatment hence, the optimum duration of ATT for osteoarticular tuberculosis in general and deep-seated lesions of spinal tuberculosis in particular continues to be debated.

Standardized or Individualized Treatment

Tuberculosis is a public health problem due to endemicity and transmission risk to the community. Ensuring regular intake of all the drugs by the patient is a responsibility of the health staff and of the National Tuberculosis Programmes. WHO developed standardized treatment to tackle the problem of defaulting and inadequate treatment. It was visualized that by giving a standard regimen of drugs one can ensure compliance, coverage and completion of treatment and facilitated analysis of treatment outcomes on a mass scale. The Directly Observed Treatment (DOTS) was introduced to ensure treatment in pulmonary tuberculosis where sputum conversion is a reliable marker for drug efficacy and monitoring of treatment. There are no such markers available for extrapulmonary TB. As a result, a wide variation in the treatment regimens practised by the treating surgeons for skeletal tuberculosis. Agarwal et al studied the prescribing pattern of antitubercular therapy from treating surgeons by a questionnaire and found 30 different prescriptions from 50 surgeons.

Treatment: The current INDEX TB guidelines (for extra-pulmonary TB) recommendations are: There is uncertainty surrounding the optimum duration of treatment for TB of the bones and joints. Some older trials suggested that 6 months treatment may be sufficient, but more advanced diagnostic imaging has led to uncertainty whether these patients are cured for spinal TB at the end of that time. All cases of bone and joint TB should be treated with extended courses of ATT with a 2-month intensive phase consisting of four drugs (isoniazid, rifampicin, pyrazinamide and ethambutol), followed by a continuation phase of rifampicin, isoniazid and ethambutol lasting 10–16 months, depending on the site of disease and the patient's clinical course. Since the monoresistance against ethambutol have been reported in significant percentage hence, ethambutol is now given for full duration of continuation phase.

The current recommendations include: 2RHZE/10RHE. The total treatment duration: 12 months (extendable to 18 months on a case-by-case basis).

The drug therapy in children is also similar to adults. The dosage schedule in children can be divided into 4 weight categories (a) less than 10 kg, (b) 10–17 kg, (c) 18–25 kg and (d) more than 25 kg. The rifampicin and isoniazid are advised as 75 mg each and pyrazinamide 250 mg and etambutol 250 mg/day for a child weighing less than 10 kg. The dosages are doubled, tripled and quadrapuled for the above mentioned weight categories. The children gain weight once on ATT and quickly move from one category to other. Hence, it is advised that the weight of children should be measured on every visit and drug dosage should be adjusted according to weight.

Table 4.1 listing the first-line drugs with side effects

Table 4.1: Antitubercular drugs: First-line drugs

ISONIAZID

Daily dosage (max. dose)	max 300 mg
Children, in mg/kg	10
Adults, in mg/kg	5
Adverse reactions	• Rash, hepatic enzyme elevation/ hepatitis, peripheral neuropathy • Mild CNS effects • Drug interactions resulting in increased phenytoin/disulfiram levels
Monitoring	Baseline measurements of hepatic enzymes for adults. Repeat LFT if • baseline results are abnormal • patient is at high risk for adverse reactions • patient has symptoms of adverse reactions
Comments	• Hepatitis risk increases with age and alcohol consumption • Pyridoxine (vitamin B$_6$) may prevent peripheral neuropathy and CNS effects. • Also used for latent TB infection

RIFAMPICIN

Daily dosage (max. dose)	max 600 mg
Children, in mg/kg	10–12
Adults, in mg/kg	10
Adverse reactions	• GI upset, drug interaction hepatitis • Bleeding problems, flu-like symptoms, rash • Renal failure • Fever
Monitoring	Baseline measurements of CBC, platelets, and hepatic enzymes. Repeat measurements if • baseline results are abnormal • patient has symptoms of adverse reactions
Comments	Causes reddish orange discoloration of body fluids. May permanently discolor soft contact lenses. Drug interactions with methadone and oral contraceptives Contraindicated/cautioned use with protease inhibitors/non-nucleoside reverse transcriptase inhibitors (NNRTIs)

(Contd...)

(Contd…)

PYRAZINAMIDE

Daily dosage (max. dose)	max 2000 mg
Children, in mg/kg	30–35
Adults, in mg/kg	25
Adverse reactions	Hepatitis, rash, GI upset, joint aches, hyperuricemia, gout (rare)
Monitoring	Baseline measurements of uric acid and hepatic enzymes Repeat measurements if • baseline results are abnormal • patient has symptoms of adverse reactions
Comments	Deranges blood sugar and control in diabetics Asymptomatic hyperuricemia needs no treatment

ETHAMBUTOL

Daily dosage (max. dose)	1500 mg
Children, in mg/kg	20–25
Adults, in mg/kg	15
Adverse reactions	Optic neuritis, red-green color blindness Rash
Monitoring	Baseline and monthly tests of visual acuity and color vision
Comments	Not recommended for children too young to be monitored for changes in vision unless TB is drug resistant Optic neuritis may be unilateral, check each eye separately

STREPTOMYCIN

Daily dosage (max. dose)	1 gram/day
Children, in mg/kg	15
Adults, in mg/kg	15
Adverse reactions	Ototoxicity (vestibular/auditory loss) Renal toxicity Pain, rash, induration around injection site
Monitoring	Baseline and repeat tests of hearing, vestibular function and renal function
Comments	Contraindicated in pregnancy Reduced dosage needed for patient of renal failure/patients more than 45 years age. Warm compresses reduce pain around injection site

ATT AND THEIR ADVERSE EFFECTS

Antitubercular drugs have various adverse effects, which have been only briefly discussed below. For a detailed description, one is advised to read appropriate pharmacology textbooks and guidelines. They have been divided into two groups chiefly: Minor (does not need stoppage of treatment, Table 4.2) and major (needs stoppage of modification of drugs, Table 4.3).

Table 4.2: ATT—minor adverse effects, drugs responsible and management

Minor adverse effect	Drug responsible	Management
Nausea, abdominal pain	Usually rifampicin	Reassurance to the patient
Burning sensation in foot	Isoniazid	Add pyridoxine 50–75 mg. Continue INH
Drowsiness	Usually related to isoniazid	Reassurance to the patient
Gastrointestinal upset	Any drug	Reassurance to the patient, Give drugs with less water and over longer period of time; give some amount of food with drugs. If all these fail, add antiemetics
Joint pain	Pyrazinamide	Continue using pyrazinamide, give NSAIDs and hypouricemic diet. Intermittent drug regimens have lesser chances
Reddish discoloration of urine	Rifampicin	Reassurance to the patient
Females on oral contraceptives	Rifampicin	As rifampicin reduces the effectiveness of oral contraceptives, alternative methods of contraception should be used
Itching without rash/mild rash	Any drug	Give antihistaminics. Keep close watch with each dose. Reassurance of patient

Table 4.3: ATT—major adverse effects against the drug responsible with management

Major adverse effect	Drug responsible	Management
Hearing loss	Streptomycin	Replace streptomycin with ethambutol, needs audiometry and ENT opinion
Dizziness	If true vertigo with nystagmus, streptomycin induced	Replace streptomycin with ethambutol if persistent even after one week dose reduction of streptomycin
Jaundice	Drug-induced hepatitis	Stop all ATT till jaundice subsides and liver enzymes revert to normal levels. Interim streptomycin and ethambutol can be given
Moderate-severe skin rash	Can be with all antitubercular drugs	Stop all drugs, may need steroids if systemic effects or mucosal involvement is seen. Gradual reintroduction of drugs to be done
Visual impairment	Ethambutol	Ophthalmologist's opinion; Stop ethambutol
Vomiting/confusion	Can be drug-induced hepatitis	Urgent liver function tests, if not available, stop all drugs and observe
Generalized reactions like purpura, shock, etc.	Rifampicin, pyrazinamide and/or streptomycin	Stop all medicines, need special regimen under physician's guidance

ANTITUBERCULAR DRUGS IN SPECIAL SITUATIONS

Pregnancy

Isoniazid, rifampicin, ethambutol and pyrazinamide—these four first-line drugs are non-teratogenic and are safe for use in pregnancy. A team work by treating obstetrician, orthopedic surgeon and physician is must for successful treatment of tuberculosis. Use of daily pyridoxine (10 mg) is advisable in pregnancy. Aminoglycosides (i.e. streptomycin), ethionamide and fluoroquinolones are teratogenic. For patients on second-line drugs, a decision is taken on the basis of gestational age after detailed discussion with the patient and her spouse, by the treating team.

Lactation

There is no need to stop breastfeeding. Both mother and child should be allowed to stay together. If child is asymptomatic, he/she should be given prophylactic isoniazid (5 mg/kg body weight) daily for 6–9 months.

Patients of Chronic Renal Failure

Isoniazid, rifampicin and pyrazinamide have chiefly hepatic route of excretion. They can be given in patients of renal failure, but a close watch should be kept of serum uric acid (high chances with pyrazinamide in kidney diseases). Daily pyridoxine (10 mg) should be given to prevent INH associated peripheral neuropathy.

Ethambutol, streptomycin and thioacetazone are to be given carefully in such patients after keeping a close watch of creatinine clearance, under the supervision of a physician. The safest regimen is 2HRZ/4–8HR for pulmonary TB. The duration will be longer for osteoarticular TB.

Patient with Liver Disorders

• *Established chronic liver disease*: Pyrazinamide is contra-indicated. Isoniazid plus rifampicin plus one/two non-hepatotoxic drugs like streptomycin and ethambutol can be used. The commonly recommended regimens are 2HRES/ 6HE, 2HRE/6HE or 2HSE/10HE. These regimens are for pulmonary tuberculosis, for osteoarticular tuberculosis the duration will likely be longer. A team work with physician is mandatory for successful treatment.

• *Acute viral hepatitis*: It is not uncommon clinical scenario. One should allow hepatitis to settle, but if antitubercular treatment cannot be withheld; an interim non-hepatotoxic regimen of streptomycin and ethambutol can be given for up to three months (along with fluoroquinolones for extensive disease). Later, HR can be added for continuation phase.

Sinuses

Sinuses arise from a deep-seated lesion containing sequestra and caseous masses. The sinuses start healing and generally heal within 6–12 weeks once patient is put on ATT. Rarely, the sinuses are evacuated surgically by curetting and excising the sinus fibrous wall. Firm healing is usual in about 6 weeks. An alternative procedure is to administer antibiotics and chemo-therapeutic agents and to withhold surgical intervention until the possibility of spontaneous healing can be determined.

Roentgenographic evidence of gross destructive lesions and the presence of sequestra justify immediate surgery.

Abscesses and Effusions

The abscesses and joint effusion generally regress under the influence of systemic ATT and heal by primary intention. The local instillation of streptomycin is rarely indicated as the local concentration of drug are well above MIC for Mycobacterium. Rarely open drainage of abscess is required when aspiration has failed to clear it off. The drainage of abscesses is also performed when abscess size suddenly increases. Paravertebral abscess of cervical spine is drained when retropharyngeal abscess causes difficulty in respiration and deglutition.

Sacroiliac abscesses may be drained and bone grafts immediately inserted to effect an arthrodesis. Paravertebral abscesses can be opened and necrotic bone curetted out of the vertebral body when the lesions are debrided. Occasionally, the juxta-articular lesion may be resected, joint debrided and motion preserved.

Paradoxical reaction: It is labelled when a patient with confirmed or probable skeletal TB on ATT, who initially improves and then subsequently has worsening constitutional symptoms or signs of TB in the absence of another diagnosis or drug resistance. Features include increased size of lesion, appearance of new lesions, recurrent fever and night sweats, or development of another form of TB.

In drug-resistant cases, the patient usually fails to improve from the start of ATT, or deteriorate further. There will be no improvement until an effective second-line ATT regimen is started.

In paradoxical reaction, there is usually an initial improvement, followed by deterioration. The patient will usually begin to improve again without changes to the ATT regimen; ATT should not be stopped or altered. NSAIDs and other supportive treatment are usually sufficient. The situation becomes complicated when we are dealing with cases of relapse, recrudescence, and therapeutically refractory cases. Standardized treatment cannot be applied to such cases as the drug susceptibility of the bacilli varies from person-to-person and from region-to-region as do the adverse reaction and drug toxicity profiles. Compounding the problem is the fact that since osteoarticular tuberculosis especially spinal tuberculosis is a paucibacillary disease, adequate tissue material may not be available for drug susceptibility testing.

So the dilemma remains: Do we tailor the treatment according to drug susceptibility testing in all refractory cases or do we formulate empirical second-line regimens that take into account regional drug resistance profiles?

DRUG RESISTANCE

Second-Line Therapy: Evolution of Drugs and Treatment Regimens

Drug resistance to antitubercular drugs was reported as early as 1948. Multidrug-resistant tuberculosis occurs when the organism develops resistance to rifampicin and isoniazid. Resistance to any other drug is described as "other drug resistance". At five years, the survival rate for patients with multidrug-resistant tuberculosis is 50%, similar to the pre-antibiotic era. The patient may show a poor response to treatment due to noncompliance or a faulty drug regimen in drug combination, drug dosage, duration or spurious drugs. Drug resistance is one of the causes of treatment failure. During the inception of the DOTS protocol by WHO, the cases of pulmonary TB with relapse or refractory disease were started on Category 2 DOTS which consisted of 60 doses of injectable streptomycin in addition to the standard 4 first-line drugs. (2HRZES + 1HRZE + 5HRE). However, this retreatment strategy with 5 first-line drugs for such cases is being relooked, given the rising incidence of MDR-TB cases. The current recommendation by WHO for pulmonary TB is to have 3 regimens: One for fresh cases, one for cases that default treatment and one for MDR cases. The previous 4 category scheme has been abolished for this new classification where it is mandated that all cases not responding to standard drugs at the end of 5 months should undergo drug susceptibility testing to rule out resistance.

The MDR-TB can be diagnosed only if it is suspected. The pulmonary TB lesion in view of high oxygen concentration has abundant *M. tuberculosis* organism. When a case of pulmonary TB continues to remain sputum positive under CAT I or RNTCP DOTS treatment at 5 months or under CAT II at 4 months the drug resistance is suspected.

The problem with osteoarticular and spinal TB is that it is a paucibacillary disease and chances of demonstrating *Mycobacterium* on smear and culture vary between 25 and 75% in a virgin case. The chances of the culture showing growth and demonstrating culture positivity are very low. Spinal TB is a deep-seated lesion where the tissue cannot be procured repeatedly; hence, it is difficult to suspect and diagnose drug resistance. So, our suspicion has to be clinicoradiological, which is not reliable. If a patient does not show clinical improvement or there is deterioration of spinal deformity or a new lesion appears or ulcer/sinus fails to heal or if wounds undergo dehiscence after surgery at 5 months, they should be considered as therapeutically refractory or suspected MDR-TB cases (presumptive drug resistance). MDR-TB can only be labeled once drug resistance is demonstrated after culture. The lesion should be debrided and subjected for histology, smear and BACTEC cultures and molecular methods such as GeneXpert and Line Probe Assay.

The prescriptions for drug resistant TB vary as greatly as the presentation of the disease itself. Various combinations of the drugs such as ethionamide, para-aminosalicylic acid, cycloserine and thioacetazone along with rifampicin and isoniazid were in vogue.

In the last few years, the fluoroquinolone group of drugs has added a new dimension to the chemotherapy of TB. Quinolones have significant *in vitro* activity against M. *tuberculosis,* and they have been used as part of regimens to treat patients with MDR-TB. There is limited data on the use of fluoroquinolones in the treatment of patients with drug-susceptible TB. However, they are not a substitute for the first-line drugs and there is rapid development of resistance in monotherapy with quinolones. In fact, ciprofloxacin is no longer recommended as a second-line drug owing to its improper use.

Ofloxacin, levofloxacin and moxifloxacin are the recommended fluoroquinolones for use in second-line therapy. They act by blocking the enzyme DNA gyrase which has 2 coding genes Gyr A and Gyr B. Mutation in any one of the genes leads to resistance to ofloxacin. However, levofloxacin and moxifloxacin resistance requires mutation in both the genes which is so far relatively rare; thus, making them reserve drugs for ofloxacin resistance.

Ever since the discovery of streptomycin by Waksman in 1943, aminoglycosides have been one of the mainstays for treating refractory tuberculosis. Newer aminoglycosides, such as amikacin, capreomycin and kanamycin, are highly potent drugs with significant bactericidal activity. But they are highly toxic and the incidence of ototoxicity and nephrotoxicity makes them double-edged swords in the battle against tuberculosis.

The second-line drugs have been grouped into 5 groups by WHO:
Group 1: First-line oral agents
• Pyrazinamide (Z)
• Ethambutol (E)
• Rifabutin (Rfb)

Group 2: Injectable agents
• Kanamycin (Km)
• Amikacin (Am)
• Capreomycin (Cm)
• Streptomycin (S)

Group 3: Fluoroquinolones

- Levofloxacin (Lfx)
- Moxifloxacin (Mfx)
- Ofloxacin (Ofx)

Group 4: Oral bacteriostatic second-line agents

- Para-aminosalicylic acid (PAS)
- Cycloserine (Cs)
- Terizidone (Trd)
- Ethionamide (Eto)
- Protionamide (Pto)

Group 5: Agents with unclear role in treatment of drug resistant-TB

- Clofazimine (Cfz)
- Linezolid (Lzd)
- Amoxicillin/clavulanate (Amx/Clv)
- Thioacetazone (Thz)
- Imipenem/cilastatin (Ipm/Cln)
- High-dose isoniazid (high-dose H)
- Clarithromycin (Clr)

In planning an individualized treatment regimen, the following guidelines have been recommended:

- Use at least 4 drugs certain to be effective.
- Use any of the first-line oral agents (Group 1) that are likely to be effective.
- Use an effective aminoglycoside or polypeptide by injection (Group 2).
- Use a fluoroquinolone (Group 3).
- Use the remaining Group 4 drugs to complete a regimen of at least four effective drugs.
- For regimens with fewer than four effective drugs, consider adding two Group 5 drugs.

The total number of drugs will depend on the degree of uncertainty, and regimens often contain five to seven drugs.

IMMUNOMODULATION, IMMUNOTHERAPY AND BIOLOGICAL AGENTS

The bacille Calmette–Guérin (BCG) vaccine has existed for over 80 years since its first use during the First World War in 1921 and is one of the most widely used of all current vaccines, reaching >80% of neonates and infants in countries where it is part of the national childhood immunization programme. BCG vaccine has a documented protective effect against meningitis and disseminated TB in children. It does not prevent primary infection and, more importantly, does not prevent reactivation of latent pulmonary infection, the principal source of bacillary spread in the community. The impact of BCG vaccination on transmission of *M. tuberculosis* is, therefore, limited.

Immunotherapy aims to "realign" or improve the immune response either by promoting protective (Th1) immunity or by blocking harmful immune (Th2) responses. TB patients have a large Th1 response in their lungs. Furthermore, boosting the Th1 responses may induce systemic release of Th1-associated cytokines resulting in necrosis of TB lesions (Koch's phenomenon). Therefore, it is not necessarily better to induce more protective immunity. It may be better to optimize the Th1 response by downregulating the Th2 response.

There are two types of immunotherapy agents. Some enhance protective immunity and/or downregulate Th2 activity; others facilitate access to, or activity of chemo-therapeutic agents in, the bacilli by disrupting bacteriostatic pathways or fibrosis.

Immunotherapeutic agents can be classified according to whether they have been studied in mice (Hsp65 DNA vaccine, anti-TGF-b, anti-IL-4), humans (human immunoglobulin), or both (killed *M. vaccae*, HE2000, rh-IFNg, rh-IL-2, *Mycobacterium w*). *Mycobacterium vaccae* was discovered in cowdung (*vacca*: cow in Latin). Earlier reports including a Cochrane review by de Bruyn *et al.* suggested that it has no benefits as an immunotherapy agent, newer studies suggest that it may still have a role in improving the outcome of tuberculosis.

Drugs that facilitate drug access and bacillary responsiveness include CC-3052 (a thalidomide analogue), etanercept (soluble TNF-α receptor) and high dose prednisolone. All agents are under investigation in Phase I and Phase II trials conducted worldwide in association with the WHO Stop TB Partnership.

Tuli recommended immunomodulation as an adjunct to conventional chemotherapy. It consists of:
1. 2 doses of BCG vaccine 0.1 mL intradermal at 0 and 1 month
2. Followed by 2 doses of bivalent DT or TT vaccine at 2 and 3 months
3. Along with levamisole 150 mg/day for 3 consecutive days per week for 6 weeks.

Conclusions
The tubercular bacilli have been eating the same set of drugs for the last 40 years ever since the discovery of rifampicin in 1967, the last first-line agent to be developed. Although there are a large number of drugs under investigation under the aegis of the Working Group on New TB Drugs (www.newtbdrugs.org), they are still in Phase 1 or Phase 2 trials and no first-line agent has been introduced over the last 40 years.

The incidence of tuberculosis has declined with improved sanitation, nutrition and hygiene. However, two-thirds of the world's population still live in an environment where *Mycobacterium tuberculosis* flourishes. Increasing global travel with frequent migration, co-infection with HIV and declining immunity of an aging population worldwide has made tuberculosis common even in the Western population and a global threat to mankind. Medical science and bacteria are evolving and until such time as all pockets of malnutrition, unhygienic living and immunocompromised conditions are eliminated, we shall have to face the disease consequences of the *Mycobacterium* unabated. Each time scientists feel they have conquered the *Mycobacterium*, it propagates the disease with more vengeance by developing drug resistance.

SUGGESTED READINGS FOR ATT

1. Toman's Tuberculosis: Case detection, treatment and monitoring. Second edition (2004). World Health Organization.

2. Index Tb guidelines: Guidelines on extrapulmonary tuberculosis for India (2016). WHO and Ministry of health & family welfare, Govt of India.

3. RNTCP guidelines (2014). WHO and Ministry of health & family welfare, Govt of India.

4. National Guidelines on Diagnosis and Treatment of Pediatric Tuberculosis. 2012; Available from: http://www.tbcindia.nic.in/ Paediatric guidelines_New.pdf.

(The Bibliography is given at the end of next Chapter)

Chapter 5

Spinal Tuberculosis

Tuberculosis of spine is the most common and dangerous form of skeletal tuberculosis and it constitutes 50% of osteoarticular tuberculosis. It was a common disease in the middle of 19th century, however, with improved sanitation, hygiene, nutrition and after invention of antitubercular drugs, the disease is practically non-existent in developed countries, but continues to be rampant in developing countries. In the recent time, due to acquired immune deficiency syndrome, tuberculosis is again showing rising trends in developed countries also. Historically tuberculous spondylitis was observed in ancient mummies from Egypt and Peru. Hippocrates (400 BC) correlated spinal deformity, paralysis and tuberculosis of spine. Ancient Indian literature mentions it as 'Yakshma' and has been described in Sushruta Samhita and Charak Samhita (600 BC and 1000 BC). Sir Percivall Pott (1779) termed tuberculous spondylitis as "Pott's diease" and described it as a kind of palsy associated with deformity of the back.

Bacillus Calmette–Guerin (BCG) vaccine for tuberculosis was developed (1921) by Calmette and Guerin. Waksman and Schatz introduced streptomycin in 1943 and subsequently other drugs effective against *Mycobacterium* were invented. The introduction of ATT had improved the outcome in spinal TB. In middle of twentieth century, there were two different opinions to treat spinal tuberculosis. (a) Ambulent chemotherapy: where the patients were treated with non-surgical treatment with two or three antitubercular drugs, bed rest and/or ambulation with braces. (b) Universal surgical extripation group where the radical excision of the lesion was advocated to all cases of tuberculosis of the spine. Both the Groups reported almost similar results. The Tuli's "middle path regimen" (1975) was introduced, advocating surgery only when there is specific indication during the course of drug treatment. This regimen was based on the observation of improved neural outcome of disease under cover of ATT when these patients were waiting for surgery in view of poor general condition due to concomittent lung disease and/or non-availability of infrastructure to perform spinal surgery. The usual outcome was healing of the lesion with or without spinal deformity or neural complications.

The newer imaging modalities, like bone scan/USG/CT scan/MRI/PET CT, have led to early diagnosis. Thus spinal tuberculosis outcome has dramatically improved with healing of the lesions with almost near normal spine when diagnosed early. In late stages, when deformity is already present, correction of spinal deformity is advocated to prevent sequelae of spinal deformity and paraplegia. The use of metal undercover of ATT has further improved outcome with better neural recovery and spinal deformity corrections.

PATHOPHYSIOLOGY OF VERTEBRAL TUBERCULOSIS

Spinal tuberculosis usually spreads by hematogenous route and is a secondary infection from a primary site in the lung or genitourinary system. Lower thoracic and lumbar vertebrae are the most common sites followed by mid-thoracic and cervical vertebrae. Paradiscal lesion or contiguous two vertebral body lesion is most commonly observed, however, several contiguous body involvement as well as skip lesions are also seen. The skipped lesions and tubercular meningitis in spinal tuberculosis are observed when spread is through Batson's perivertebral venous plexus.

The infection spreads and destroys the endplates of the adjacent vertebrae. It may spread beneath the anterior longitudinal ligament to reach neighboring vertebrae. The vertebral body becomes soft and gets easily compressed to produce either wedging or total collapse. Anterior wedging is

Table 5.1: Differential diagnosis for spinal tuberculosis

1. Bacterial infections
   a. *Staphylococcus aureus (tubercular botryomycosis presents similar to staphylococcal variety)*
   b. Brucellosis
   c. Syphilis
   d. Anaerobes

2. Mycobacterial infections
   a. *M. tuberculosis complex*
   b. Atypical mycobacteria such as *M. avium intracellulare*

3. Fungal infections
   a. Candidiasis (*Candida albicans*)
   b. Cryptococcosis
   c. Histoplasmosis (*Histoplasma capsulatum*)
   d. Coccidioidomycosis
   e. Paracoccidioidomycosis
   f. Aspergillosis (*Aspergillus fumigatus*)
   g. *Blastomyces dermatitides*

4. Parasitic
   a. Hydatid disease (*Echinococcus granulosus*)

Others
a. *Neoplastic*: Ewing's sarcoma, metastatic unknown primaries, rhabdomyosarcoma, neuroblastoma, chondroblastoma
b. *Lymphoproliferative diseases*: Lymphomas, leukemia, multiple myeloma
c. *Rheumatological*: Systemic lupus erythematosus, rheumatoid arthritis
d. *Miscellaneous*: Sarcoidosis, hyperparathyroidism (Brown tumors), Paget's disease

commonly seen in the thoracic spine where the line of gravitational force passes anterior to the body. This also explains the minimal wedging in cervical and lumbar vertebrae where line of gravitational force passes posterior to vertebral body.

Cold Abscess (Fig. 5.1)

Vertebral tuberculosis leads to caseous necrosis and forms cold abscess consisting of serum, leukocytes, caseous material, bone fragments and tubercle bacilli. This penetrates the ligaments and follows the path of least resistance along preformed fascial planes, blood vessels and nerves, to distant sites from the original bony lesion.

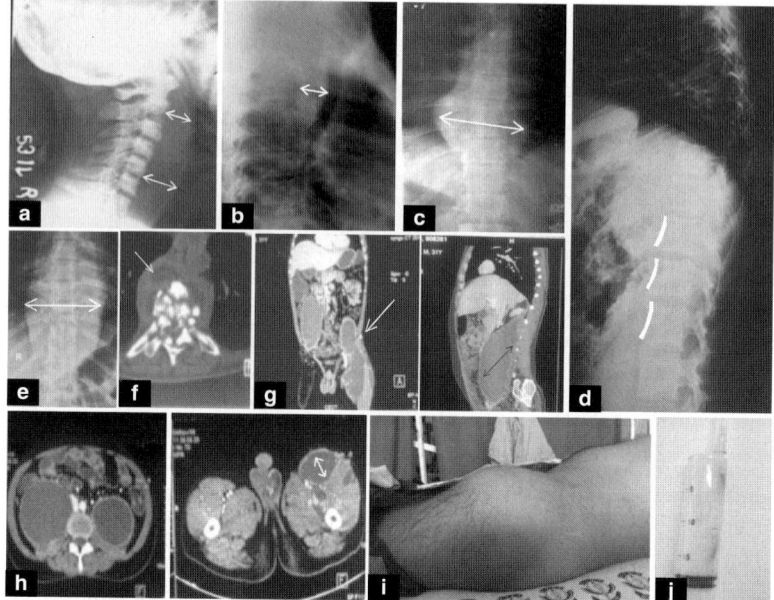

Fig. 5.1: Showing various presentations of cold abscess:

a. Increased prevertebral soft tissue shadow in cervical spine.
b. Increased prevertebral soft tissue shadow anteriorly displacing tracheal shadow in upper dorsal spine.
c. Increased paravertebral shadow seen in AP view of dorsal spine.
d. Anterior scalloping of vertebral body due to abscess (aneursymal phenomenon).
e. Increased paravertebral shadow seen in AP view of dorsolumbar spine.
f. Fragmentary destruction of vertebral body with paravertebral collection
g. CT scan coronal and sagittal sections showing psoas abscess communicating beneath inguinal ligament extending into thigh (arrow).
h. CT scan axial sections showing bilateral psoas abscess and paravertebral abscess.
i. Clinical photo of patient discussed in g and h, showing thigh abscess.
j. Pus aspirated from cold abscess in patient showing in i.

In the cervical spine, the exudate traverses the prevertebral fascia and forms retropharyngeal abscess or may track down in mediastinum to enter into the trachea, esophagus or the pleural cavity. It may spread laterally into the sternomastoid muscle and form an abscess in the neck, which may bulge in the anterior or posterior triangle of the neck.

In the thoracic spine, the exudate may remain confined locally and may appear in the radiographs as a fusiform or bulbous paravertebral shadow. Tension may force the exudate to enter into the spinal canal and compress the spinal cord. A thoracic cold abscess may follow the intercostal nerve to appear anywhere along the course of nerve and can also penetrate the anterior longitudinal ligament to form a mediastinal abscess or pass downwards through medial, middle or lateral arcuate ligament.

In the lumbar vertebrae, the exudate formed commonly enters the psoas sheath to form a psoas abscess. It may also gravitate beneath the inguinal ligament to appear on the medial aspect of the thigh or can spread laterally beneath the iliac fascia to appear near the anterior superior iliac spine. Tracking along the femoral or the gluteal vessels, the abscess can emerge at the Scarpa's triangle, thigh and the gluteal region as well.

Types of Vertebral Lesions

1. The vertebral body is diseased in 98% instances whereas in the remaining 2% the lesion is located in the posterior complex such as laminae, spinous process, transverse process and pedicle.

   The most common lesion is **paradiscal** which affects 2 halves of vertebrae on contiguous side of disk. This is explained by the embryological basis of blood supply to the vertebral bodies. Each vertebral body develops from fusion of distal half of denser part and proximal part of less dense part of distal sclerotome. The paradiscal parts of vertebrae develop from one sclerotome. The vertebral lesion occurs following a hematogenous dissemination and inoculation of tubercular bacilli, thus affects the adjacent halves of two vertebrae. The other varities are **central type**—starting in center of vertebral body, **anterior type**—starting beneath anterior longitudinal ligament, **appendicular type**—affecting posterior element and least common is **synovial variety**—affecting facet joint.

2. **Atypical presentation of spinal tuberculosis** is defined as compressive myelopathy with no visible or palpable spinal deformity and without any classical radiological changes **(spinal tumor syndrome)** suggestive of vertebral destruction. Such lesions are relatively uncommon, mimic low-grade

pyogenic infection, brucella and sickle-cell spondylitis, hydatid disease, lymphoma and malignant deposits and are difficult to diagnose and treat in the early stage of disease. There are more chances of developing neurological complications.

PATHOLOGY OF TUBERCULOUS PARAPLEGIA

The incidence of paraplegia (para- or tetraplegia, hemiplegia or monoplegia) is 10–30% in spinal tuberculosis. The dorsal spine is affected in 50% cases of spinal tuberculosis with neural complications while lumbar and cervical spine in about 25% each.

Tuberculous paraplegia was traditionally classified as "early onset paraplegia" (developing within first 2 years of the onset of disease) and "late onset paraplegia" (developing more than 2 years of the onset of disease) by Seddon (1935). Hodgson replaced this terminology with: Paraplegia with active disease (early onset paraplegia) and paraplegia with healed disease (late onset paraplegia).

The cord terminates at L1, hence paraplegia below L1 level is rare. The spinal canal is spacious below L1 and contains only cauda equina. In dorsal spine affection, neurological complications are more because: (i) Bony spinal canal is narrow, (ii) physiological kyphosis forces the diseased tissue (exudates) to enter inside the spinal canal, and (iii) abscess tends to remain localized under anterior longitudinal ligaments and enters the spinal canal through intervertebral foramina to cause cord compression unlike in lumbar spine where it trickles down in psoas muscle.

Paraplegia with active disease may be caused by mechanical pressure on the spinal cord by an abscess, granulation tissue, tubercular debris and caseous tissue, or by mechanical instability produced by pathological subluxation or dislocation. 76% of canal encroachment is compatible with an intact neural state when no other cause such as mechanical instability or pathological subluxation/dislocation coexists. The direct involvement of the meninges and cord by tubercular infection and inflammation, infective thrombosis or endarteritis of spinal vessels may also lead to neural loss. The spinal cord may show edema of the spinal cord and/or myelomalacia on MRI.

Paraplegia with healed disease may occur in severe deformity of spine 10 to 20 years after healing of the initial lesion. These patients present with old healed severe kyphosis (more than 60°). The spinal cord gets stretched over an internal anterior bony projection (internal salient), producing gliosis. MRI shows severe atrophy of the spinal cord and/or syringohydromyelia, or constricting scarring around the dura. Reactivation of the disease is found in 30 to 40% of cases on exploration. Symptomatic severe stenosis of the lumbar spinal canal and ossification of the ligamentum flavum adjacent to severe kyphosis may produce an incomplete neurological deficit and/or lumbar canal stenosis (Fig. 5.2).

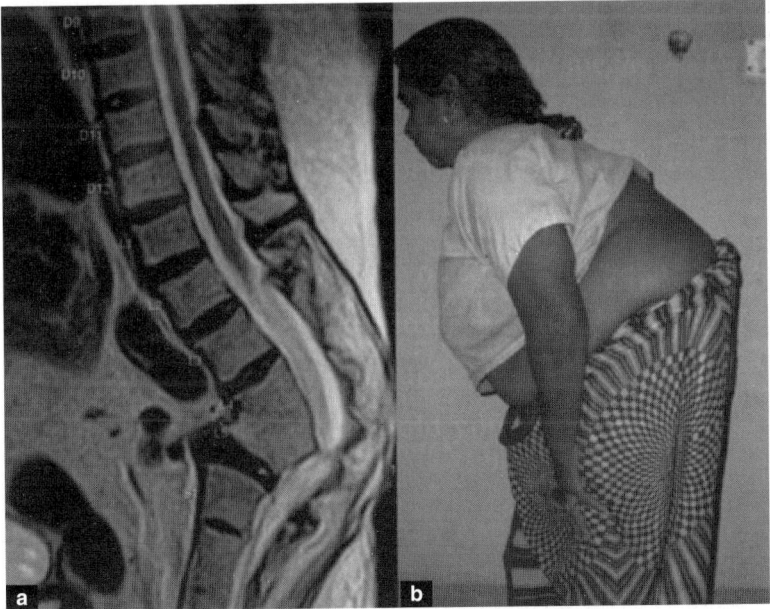

Fig. 5.2: T2-weighted MRI of lumbosacral spine (a) shows a healed kyphosis with lumbar canal stenosis. Clinical photograph (b) of the same patient shows the posture with forward bending due to severe neurogenic claudication. (Adapted from Jain AK, Dhammi IK, Jain S, Mishra P. Kyphosis in spinal tuberculosis—prevention and correction. *Indian J Orthop.* 2010 Apr;44(2):127–36)

March of Neural Deficit in TB Spine

In a typical paradiscal disease of the vertebral column at the level of spinal cord, i.e. up to D12, when compression starts anterior to the cord and affects anterior column of the spinal cord. It shows earliest manifestation as gradual increase in the spasticity which may be appreciated only by the clinician who detects exaggerated reflexes and plantar extensor. As compression further increases, anterior column of spinal cord is compressed more and patient starts losing motor power gradually from partial motor weakness to complete motor loss with signs of UMN lesion. By the time, compression is severe enough to cause complete block to conduction in anterior column (complete motor paralysis), lateral column is also affected partially, thus, producing some reduction of sensation (pain, temperature and crude touch). When compression is further increased, even posterior column of the spinal cord is also affected leading to complete loss of sensation and distur- bances of sphincters, loss of posterior column sensation (fine touch, vibration, 2-point discremination, and proprioception) also. In long-standing compression, the spasticity is replaced by flaccidity and/or flexor spasm. The paradiscal affection will typically show this march of neural deficit. However, if in a panvertebral (all three-column disease) lesion or in a case with pathalogical subluxation/dislocation, this march of neural deficit may not be observed and patient may directly develop severe paraplegia.

Grading of Neural Deficit

The paraplegia is divided into four grades by **Goel, Tuli and Kumar**.

Grade I. Patient is not aware of any motor deficit on clinical examination, the clinician detects the plantar extensor and ankle clonus.

Grade II. The patient complains clumsiness, spasticity or jumpiness while walking. He/she has some weakness, however, he manages to walk.

Grade III. Patient had severe motor weakness and is bedridden. The clinical examination reveals spastic paraplegia in extension. Sensory deficit, if present, is less than 50%.

Grade IV. Patient presents with complete paralysis with paraplegia in flexion, flexor spasms or flaccid paraplegia. There is more than 50% sensory loss with or without sphincteric disturbances. The position sense, vibration sense, fine touch (post-column involvement) are also affected.

Almost 95% cases of tetraplegia/paraplegia in tuberculosis could be classified according to the above pattern of neural deficit. Lesions around conus and cauda equina usually present with sphincter involvement very early in the disease process and also have UMN/LMN/mixed paraparesis/plegia with more sensory loss (bizarre neural deficit).

Neural deficit associated with intraspinal granuloma and with atypical location of lesions may not always fit in the above classification.

ASIA Score (Scale)

The ASIA scale is used to classify neural deficit in spinal trauma. It does not classify all types of neurological deficit associated with Pott's spine, such as: (a) Cases where the patient does not appreciate weakness but the clinician detects signs of upper motor neuron lesion, (b) paraplegia with bladder and bowel involvement, (c) paraplegia in flexion/flaccidity, and (d) paraplegia with flexor spasms.

The differentiating feature between Tuli's grade III and IV is the severity of motor deficit only, hence are inseparable as far as the sensory deficit is concerned. Jain *et al.* evaluated both the classifications (ASIA and Tuli) and opined that both are not complete classification for neural deficit in tuberculosis of the spine.

An ideal classification system should assess the functional status of the paraplegic/tetraplegic patient and should reflect the severity of cord compression. The neural deficit should be staged and each stage should have numeric sensory–motor scoring to differentiate early deterioration or improvement of neurological status. The motor scoring should be performed as for the ASIA score. Sensory deficit at each root level should be recorded as: Grade 0—complete loss of sensation; Grade 1—impairment of lateral as well as posterior column sensations;

Grade 2—impairment of lateral column sensations; Grade 3—normal sensory appreciation. The paraplegia/tetraplegia in TB of the spine should be classified into five stages.

Stage I. The patient does not appreciate weakness but clinician notices clumsiness of gait and signs suggestive of UMN lesion (plantar extensor and ankle clonus). It is the same as Tuli's grade I.

Stage II. The patient has spasticity with motor deficit but is a walker. He is able to lift the upper limb against gravity in tetraparesis. The anticipated motor score in tetraparesis would be between 60 and 100. In paraparesis, it would be between 80 and 100. The sensory impairment of the lateral column is present at all root levels. The sensory score is a summation of sensations at all root levels at and below the level of cord involvement. The sensory score for a particular level of involvement can be calculated by using the formula: Total sensory score = no. of involved root segments × grade of sensation × 2 (for both sides). The sensory score of a patient is expressed as total sensory score/maximum sensory score.

Stage III. Bedridden spastic patient. Anticipated motor score for quadri-/tetraplegia is 0–30, and for paraplegia it is 50–80. Sensory scoring is the same as in stage II.

Stage IV. Bedridden patient with severe sensory loss, and/or pressure sores. Anticipated motor score in tetraplegia is 0 and in paraplegia is 50. There is impairment of both lateral and posterior column sensations.

Stage V. Same as stage IV and/or bladder and bowel involvement, and/or flexor spasms/flaccid tetraplegia/paraplegia. There is usually no motor power below the involved cord segment. There are no sensations distal to the level of involvement. If the bladder/bowel are affected or flexor spasm is present, then in spite of some preservation of motor power or sensation it will be considered as stage V.

CLINICAL PRESENTATION OF TUBERCULOSIS OF SPINE

Spinal tuberculosis most commonly presents in the first three decades, however, no age is immune. A significant delay of weeks to months is common in the diagnosis of TB spine. Both sexes are equally involved. The patients give a history of back pain at the disease site or along the course of a nerve. The pain aggravates on movement of spine and even turning in the bed. This pain is acute and stabbing or dull aching. It persists despite bed rest, and night cries are present, the pain may not be relieved with analgesics. Constitutional symptoms in the form of evening rise of temperature, loss of appetite, weight loss, malaise may be present. Usually some severity of kyphotic deformity may be visible with severe paraspinal spasm. There could be loss of cervical or lumbar lordosis, with wasting of paraspinal muscles. One should also inspect for usual sites of cold abcesses. On palpation, the local temperature is mildly raised. There could be direct tenderness on spinous process of affected vertebra or there could be rotatory tenderness at level of affected vertebrae. The wasting and muscle spasm is confirmed on palpation. There could be knuckle (1–2 VB involvement), angular kyphosis (2–3 VB involved) or rounded kyphosis (4 or more vertebral bodies involved). Upper cervical spinal tuberculosis involvement (C1-C2-C3) can cause hoarseness because of recurrent laryngeal nerve paralysis, dysphagia, and respiratory stridor due to retropharyngeal abscess. These symptoms may result from anterior abscess formation in the neck. Sudden death has been reported with cervical disease after erosion into the great vessels. Neurologic findings may vary from meningeal signs to mild weakness and to paraplegia/tetraplegia.

In a significant percentage of cases, particularly in developing countries, the appearance of weakness brings the patient to the clinician for the first time. On examination, these patients walk with a cautious and clumsy gait. The patient has weakness of all four limbs with cervical spine tuberculosis. In thoracic disease, paralysis of the lower limbs occurs with or without sphincter involvement with signs of upper motor neuron type of paraplegia. In lumbar spine affection, the paraplegia is of lower motor neuron (LMN) type. One of the earliest findings of spinal cord involvement from tuberculosis is sustained clonus in the ankle.

There may be palpable fluctuant swelling in different parts of spine depending on the affection of different segments of vertebral column, e.g. in retropharynx, posterior and anterior triangle of neck in cervical spine disease, along with intercostal nerve in thoracic disease, in the loin, iliac fossa, groin gluteal and ischiorectal region in lumbar disease. Iliac fossa abscess presents with flexion deformity at hip with normal rotation called pseudo hip flexion deformity.

Healed Stage

Once the disease heals, the patient neither looks ill nor feels ill, with no fever and night sweats. There is weight gain. Paravertebral spasm resolves with no tenderness in spine. ESR attains normal value. The neural deficit may improve but spinal deformity that has occurred during active disease, however, persists.

Atypical Lesions (Fig. 5.3)

The atypical lesions are:

1. Intraspinal extramedullary tuberculous granuloma
2. Intramedullary tuberculoma
3. Single vertebral disease
4. Large paravertebral abscess with little or no demonstrable bony focus
5. Isolated epidural abscess with no demonstrable bony focus
6. Isolated involvement of neural arch and appendages
7. Sclerotic lesions and intervertebral bony bridging
8. Multifocal (skipped) lesion
9. Rarely, a herniated intervertebral disk and a failed back syndrome

Atypical location of the disease such as single vertebral affection, posterior complex disease are rare lesions with the advent of MRI some of them may not remain as atypical lesions. These patients have pain on standing with/or without constitutional symptoms. These cases present more often with neurological complications. Clinically, they have tenderness with or without midline or paramedian fluctuant swelling (posterior complex disease), mild kyphosis (single vertebral

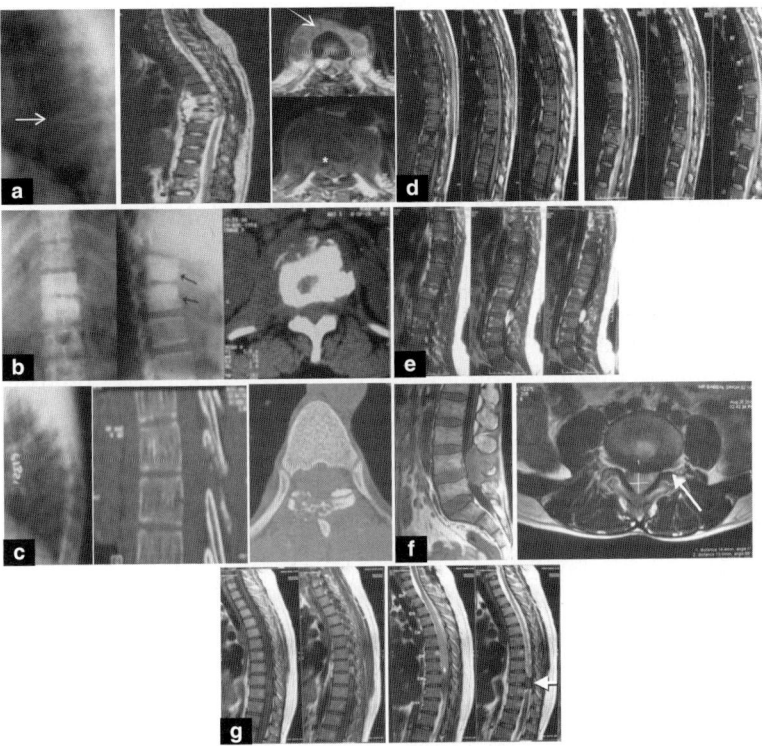

Fig. 5.3: Showing atypical presentations of TB spine:

a. X-rays showing destruction of dorsal vertebra with preservation of disc space (vertebra plana). MRI with T2WI midsagittal scan showing involvement of 3 vetebral bodies in the same patient suggesting lesion is more extensive than seen on X-ray. T2WI and T1WI show paravertebral collection(arrow) and intraspinal collection[*] (T1 hypointense and T2 hyperintense signals) helping in diagnosing as TB spine.

b. TB spine (biopsy proven) presenting with sclerotic vertebra rather than osteopenic vertebra.

c. X-ray and CT of patient with posterior complex disease involving lamina and spinous process.

d. MRI showing skipped lesions in spine which were later confirmed to be of tubercular etiology.

e. MRI showing single vertebral disease, CT-guided biopsy proved it to be Koch's spine with intraspinal lipoma at L1.

f. MR images of patient with TB spine showing posterior element involvement. The collection is pushing the thecal sac anteriorly (arrow).

g. MR images of patient with tuberculosis presenting as intradural granuloma (arrow).

affection). These cases usually present with compressive myelopathy or cauda equina lesion with sphincter involvement in their first attendance. On examination, usually they have no spinal deformity. The direct tenderness is marked when posterior elements are involved. The localization of the level of compression before deciding surgical intervention by any imaging mode is mandatory.

LABORATORY INVESTIGATIONS

In active disease the ESR is raised with relative lymphocytosis and anemia. The Mantoux test is non-diagnostic in endemic area and may be negative in an immunodeficient state. The staining for acid-fast bacilli is positive in 25–75% cases. Culture of acid-fast bacilli requires 4 to 6 weeks incubation period, although BACTEC radiometric culture takes less than 2 weeks. The culture is positive in 40 to 88% cases in osteoarticular TB. Polymerase chain reaction (PCR) is an efficient rapid method and can differentiate typical and atypical mycobacteria, however, it is positive even with presence of DNA from a dead bacteria. A positive PCR test has been observed in tissue samples taken from egyptian mummies. The GeneXpert assay has been recommended by WHO recently for rapid (<2 hrs) detection of the bacilli and rifampicin resistance. A CT/fluoroscopic-guided fine niddle aspiration cytology/biopsy is useful to obtain tissue for diagnosis of spinal lesion.

Whenever a tissue from biopsy is obtained it should always be subjected to AFB staining, culture and sensitivity, a polymerase chain reaction and other molecular diagnostic tests and histopathological examination.

IMAGING OF A CASE OF TUBERCULAR SPINE

Plain Radiography (Fig. 5.4)

Plain radiography can provide information about number of vertebrae involved, the level of bone destruction and angle of kyphosis.

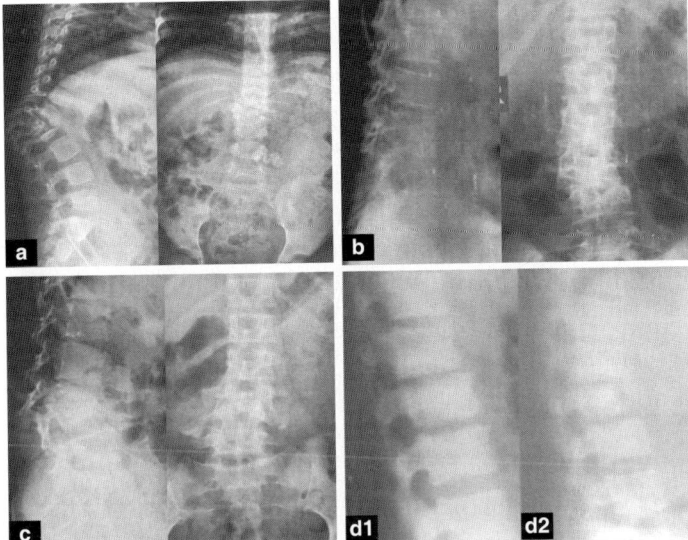

Fig. 5.4: X-ray pictures of various presentations of TB spine:

a. In a case of partially treated case of TB spine, X-rays (lateral and AP views) show affection of 4 vertebrae (D11–L2) with severe kyphotic deformity. D11–L1 vertebrae are destroyed. AP view shows scoliosis suggestive of instability. Left side psoas shadow shows dystrophic calcification (arrow).

b. X-rays (lateral and AP views) in another case show L3–L4 disease with regional osteopenia, obliteration of disk space, scoliosis in AP view suggestive of panvertebral disease (instability).

c. Similar findings in another case of TB spine showing kyphotic deformity at lumbar spine.

d. (d1) Lateral X-ray showing radiodense L2–L4 with destroyed disc margins. The patient has LMN paraplegia. The anterior decompression could not be achieved due to hard vertebral body. The histology was diagnostic of TB spine. (d2) X-ray after obtaining tissue from L3. The bones were hard and spinal decompression could not be achieved. Second stage laminectomy showed extradural granuloma. The patient recovered neurologically.

The classical radiological findings are defined as follows:

1. Regional osteoporosis of affected vertebrae
2. Fuzziness of adjacent disk margins
3. Obliteration of intervertebral disk space
4. Anterior wedging of vertebrae (particularly in thoracic spine)
5. Kyphosis of vertebral column
6. Increase in prevertebral soft tissue shadow in cervical spine
7. Paravertebral soft tissue shadow in dorsal spine

Classical well-established radiological findings, if present and if they correlate with clinical symptoms, one can confidently diag-nose Pott's spine clinicoradiologically.

A lesion of vertebrae can only be seen on plain radiograph when bone loses 30 to 40% of calcium content and is certainly more than 3 months old in its pathogenesis. The limitations of plain radiography in evaluating a TB spine lesion are:

1. The involvement of neural arch is not well appreciated.
2. The lesion less than 1.5 cm may not be observed on X-rays.
3. The integrity of spinal canal and the degree of neural compression cannot be judged.
4. The paravertebral caseous material and psoas abscesses cannot be correctly assessed.
5. The lesions in transitional zones such as at atlantoaxial region, cervicodorsal junction and lumbosacral junction may not be appreciated due to overlap shadow of adjacent bones in plain X-rays.
6. One cannot assess health of cord in cervical and dorsal lesions.

Myelography (Fig. 5.5)

With the introduction of MRI, the myelography is now seldom performed, however, it can still be used to assess adequacy of surgical decompression when patient does not show neural recovery after surgical decompression and presence of stainless steel implant does not allow MRI to be undertaken. The thinning of dye column or complete obstruction to the flow of dye suggests inadequate surgical decompression.

CT Scan (Fig. 5.6)

CT scan is useful to show vertebral destruction early even when the lesions are not seen on plain X-rays and when the lesions are less than 1.5 cm in size. The isolated neural arch lesions are better visualized on CT. The axial view by CT is of value in assessing the progress of disease during treatment such as increasing or decreasing zone of abscess, healing of bony lesion or incorporation bone graft. CT-guided fine-needle aspiration cytology is a useful and minimally invasive method of ascertaining histological diagnosis of vertebral lesions.

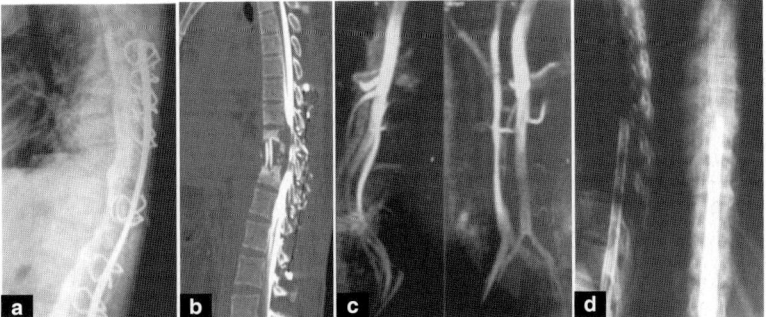

Fig. 5.5: Showing use of myelographic studies for follow up of patients showing unsatisfactory/no improvement post-surgical decompression.

a. Plain myelogram showing free flow of dye beyond the level of disease in a postoperative case.

b. CT myelogram showing partial block in flow of dye with anterior rib graft *in situ*.

c MRI used to give myelographic image in lower lumbar spine.

d. Plain myelogram showing block in CSF flow in a case of intraspinal granuloma. The myelogram was done when MRI was not available.

Various types of vertebral destruction described are:

1. *Osteolytic:* This type of bone destructions are seen in 33% cases of tuberculosis of vertebrae and also seen in pyogenic vertebral osteomyelitis, lymphoma and secondaries. The evidence of tuberculosis elsewhere, painless nature of lesion, large soft tissue swelling and their calcified content are suggestive of a tuberculous lesion.

2. *Fragmentary:* It is the most common pattern found in 47% cases. The destroyed area of vertebral body and appendages shows numerous small residual bone fragments. The fragments are migrated into the associated soft tissue mass and epidural space.

3. *Subperiosteal:* The anterior margins of vertebral body have irregular ragged appearances. The psoas muscle may show hypodense abscess with rim calcification. This type of presentation is rare (10% of total tuberculous lesions).

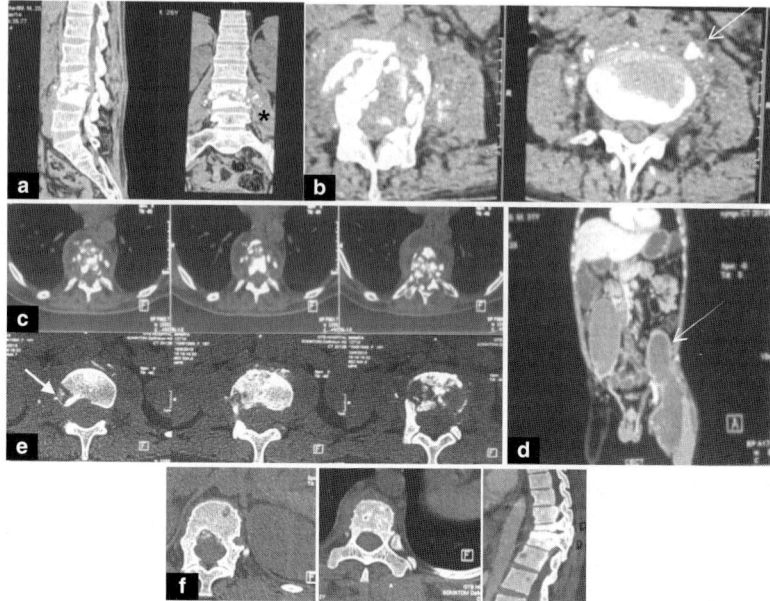

Fig. 5.6: Various findings in computed tomography (CT) scan in TB spine:

a. Sagittal and coronal sections showing anterior vertebral body destruction L3–L4, anterior wedging of vertebra with sclerosis due to reparative response with disk space narrowing. The dystrophic calcification is seen in the psoas abscess (arrow).

b. Fragmentary destruction of vertebral body with paraveterbral collections with calcifications (arrow) outside the vertebral boundary (dystrophic cacification).

c. Fragmentary type of destruction with large pre- and paravertebral collection.

d. Rim enhancement (arrow) of soft tissue collections in psoas major, after administration of intravenous contrast.

e. Osteolytic type of destruction of vertebra (arrow).

f. Sclerotic type of destruction of vertebra (arrow).

4. *Localized and sclerotic:* It is a rare occurrence (less than 10%) in osseous tuberculosis. The destruction is localize with sclerotic margin. Few residual bone fragments are seen within the lytic area. This type is observed in cases with slow destruction or long-standing infection with good immune response.

Evaluation of soft tissue: On CT, the granulation tissue is seen as high attenuation lesion while abscess, and caseous tissue are seen as low density lesion. The paravertebral mass with pus and debris is observed in 88% cases of spinal TB. The differential diagnosis includes brucellosis, sickel cell disease and lymphoma. The information about location extent and size of paravertebral and psoas abscess and their relation to the destroyed vertebral body, aorta, iliac vessels, trachea and esophagus can be visualized, which is useful before operation to indicate the side of abscess in planning surgical approach and guidance to fine-needle aspiration of abscess and to procure tissue for histopathology. Intraspinal extent of abscess (bony as well as in soft tissues) can also be visualized by CT scan.

Magnetic Resonance Imaging (Fig. 5.7A)

MRI is more sensitive than plain radiograph and more specific than scintigraphy. MRI possesses high tissue contrast resolution with multiplanar capabilities that displays all compartments in and around spine in comparision to CT. MRI is a noninvasive modality and without the risk of ionizing radiation hence is well suited for follow-up studies.

Because of its higher contrast resolution, MRI is better to show soft tissue topography. It delineates soft tissue masses in both sagittal and coronal plane. The MRI features are as follows:

a. The extent of disease and spread of tubercular debris under anterior and posterior longitudinal ligament and subligamentous spread of a paraspinal mass can be better appreciated on MRI.

b. The abscess expresses relatively low signal on T1-weighted images and high signal in T2-weighted images due to increased water content and prolong T1 and T2 relaxation time.

The cold abscess in TB spine has smooth margin because of its subligamentous spread, while pyogenic abscess has irregular margin because it destroys the paraspinal ligament and invades the paraortic or precaval space.

On gadolinium DTPA enhancement, MRI shows either an irregular thick or a uniform thin rim enhancement around paraspinal or intraosseous abscess suggesting either caseative necrosis or a cold abscess in tuberculosis, while pyogenic abscess shows diffuse enhancement. The granulation tissue shows uniform enhancement.

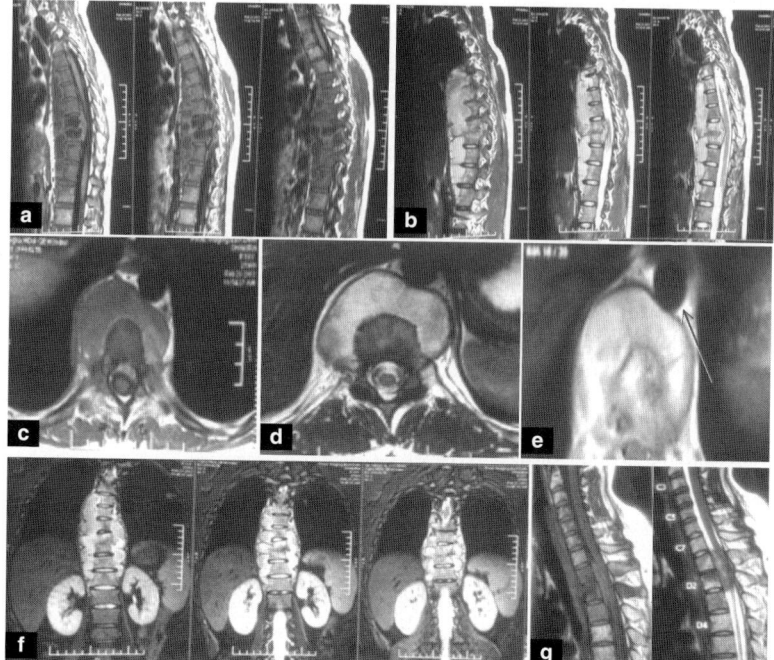

Fig. 5.7A: MR images of patients of TB spine. They show classical findings of tubercular spine, i.e. contiguous vertebral body involvement, relative preservation of disk space, subligamentous extension, large pre- and paravertebral abscess, epidural involvement, vertebral intraosseous abscess, and septate paravertebral shadows.

Figures (a) and (b) are sagittal section of the dorsal spine showing low signal in T1WI and bright signal in T2WI in contiguous vertebral bodies with preservation of intervertebral disk space. The subligamentous watery collection (low signal in T1WI and bright on T2WI) spanning 7 vertebral body height. Figures (c) and (d) are of axial sections T1WI, T2WI showing paravertebral collection and epidural encroachment by the liquid compression. Figure (e) showing MRI axial sections of TB spine. The aorta (arrow) has been pushed away from the vertebral body by the prevertebral collection. On the contrary, in case of neoplasia, the vessels would be surrounded by the growth. Figure (f) shows coronal images of the patient shown in Figs (a) and (b), showing paravertebral collection of seven vertebral body height with preserved disk spaces and loss at only one level. Figure (g) showing sagittal sections of T1WI and T2WI of upper dorsal spine showing involvement of 3 vertebral bodies with epidural encroachment in case of TB spine with neurological deficit.

c. The epidural extension of pus, granulation tissue and hard material such as bone or disk are better appreciated on MRI.

d. The cranial and caudal level of obstruction without the need of intrathecal injection of contrast material above and below is appreciated as a myelographic effect on fast spin echo technique.

e. MRI can delineate isolated extradural lesion (granuloma) from intramedullary lesions such as tuberculoma, spinal cord cavitation and cord edema.

MRI detects tuberculousis of spine in predestructive stage before bone destruction and deformity occurs. MRI has sensitivity of 96%, specificity of 92% and accuracy of 94% in the diagnosis of pyogenic vertebral osteomyelitis. The MRI observation differences in tubercular and pyogenic osteomyelitis are:

1. The relative preservation of IV disk is observed in tuber-culosis as compared with pyogenic infection.

2. The cortical definition of the affected vertebrae being lost in tuberculosis in contradiction to pyogenic.

3. Pyogenic spondylitis is confined to vertebral marrow with no significant extension into intraspinal region with infrequent epidural spread while epidural encroachment is common with tuberculosis. The calcification rarely presents in nontuberculous infection.

Infection of bone and soft tissues on MRI is detected by decrease in signal intensity in T1-weighted images and increase signal intensity in T2-weighted images. Marrow edema, contiguous vertebral body involvement, pre- and paravertebral septate loculated collections, subligamentous collections and endplate erosions with epidural extension are among the most consistent findings in tubercular spondylodiscitis seen on MRI and has been reported to be present as a constellation in 83% cases. Preservation of disks despite extensive bone destruction is virtually pathognomonic for spinal TB. The resolution of bone edema, paravertebral abscess and fatty replacement of bone marrow are observed with healing of TB lesion of the spine (Fig. 5.7B).

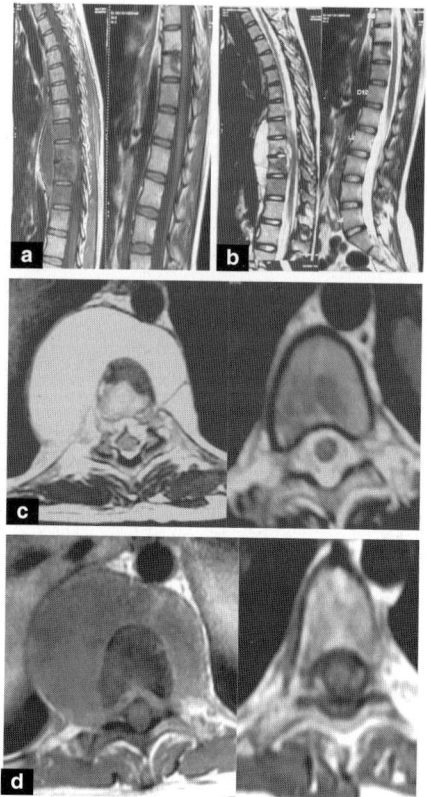

Fig. 5.7B: Healing of tuberculous lesion on MRI. Figure (a) showing mid-sagittal scan T1WI of the patient with low signal prevertebral shadow and low signal in vertebral bodies suggestive of inflammation. At one year follow-up, prevertebral collection disappeared and vertebral bodies showed bright signal suggestive of fatty replacement of marrow. Figure (b) shows mid-sagittal scan of spine in T2WI shows bright signal prevertebral shadow and from vertebral bodies. T2WI at one year follow up shows complete disappearance of prevertebral shadow and reduction of bright signal (bone edema). Figure (c) T2WI axial scan shows bright prevertebral and intraspinal shadow and the vertebral body also shows bright signal. T2WI at one year follow-up on ATT shows complete disappearance of prevertebral and intraspinal shadow and reduction of bone edema. Figure (d) shows axial scan T1WI shows low signal prevertebral shadow which at one year follow-up shows complete disappearance. The vertebral body also showed low signal in pretreatment scan which turned bright on follow-up at one year suggestive of fatty replacement of bone marrow.

MRI Observations in Tuberculous Para- /Quadriplegia

The changes also occur in spinal cord in spinal tuberculosis. Normally, the CSF column is observed as gray column in T1WI and white in T2WI. The following changes are reported in spinal TB (Fig. 5.8):

1. *Cord edema:* The spinal cord shows diffuse hyperintensity in T2-weighted images and diffuse hypo- or isointensity in T1-weighted images.

2. *Myelomalacia:* The spinal cord shows irregularity which is associated with patchy hyperintensity in T2-weighted images (T2WI) and hypointensity in T1-weighted images (T1WI).

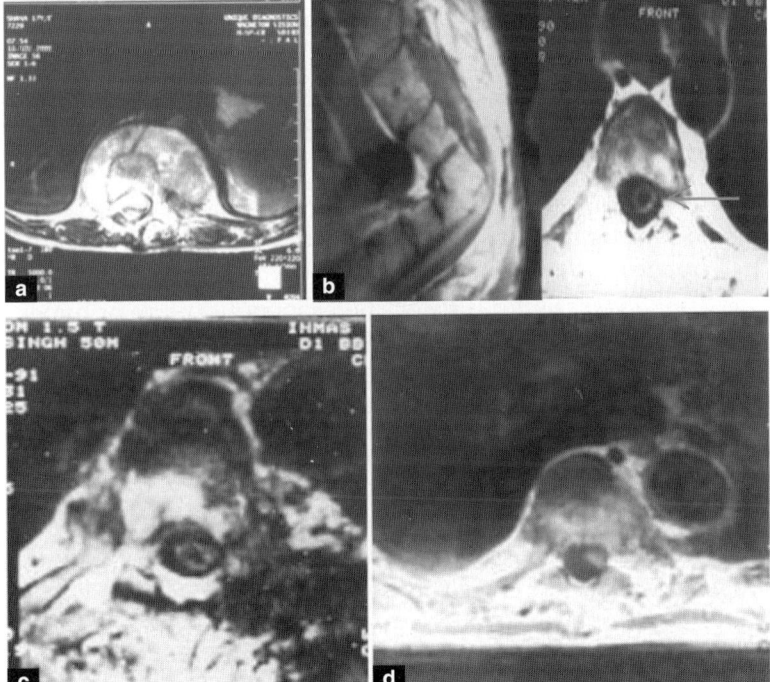

Fig. 5.8: Various cord changes seen in MRI of TB spine:
a. Cord compression due to abscess and bright signal from spinal cord (cord edema)
b. Syringomyelia (syrinx marked using arrow)
c. Myelomalacia and cord atrophy
d. Cord atrophy

3. *Cord atrophy:* It is described as apparent loss of cord size with relative increase of subarachnoid space.

4. *Syringomyelia:* Dilatation of central canal with changes in its signal intensity as that of CSF in T1- and T2-weighted images. It is observed in late onset paraplegia.

5. *Thickening to dura–arachnoid complex:* It is observed as thick hypointense ring in T2-weighted images around spinal cord obliterating the CSF space with relative increase of sub-arachnoid space.

6. *Arachnoiditis:* When normal CSF signal is replaced with irregular hypointense in T2-weighted images.

7. *The extradural compression is of three types:*
   a. *Fluid:* It appears as diffuse hyperintense in T2-weighted images and hypointense in both T1- and T2-weighted images which suggests predominantly fluid in extradural compression. (Fig. 5.7A(c))
   b. *Caseous tissue:* Predominantly caseous tissue appears as mildly hyperintense in both T1- and T2-weighted images.
   c. *Granulation tissue:* It shows heterogenous hypo- or hyper-intensity in T2-weighted images.

Imaging Correlates for Good Neural Outcome

Patients showing:
- Relatively preserved cord size
- Evidence of myelitis/edema of the spinal cord
- Predominantly fluid collection in extradural space which resolves well with ATT alone.

In all such cases, a conservative trial is likely to be rewarding who along with this finding has apparently normal cord parenchyma at the inception of treatment.

Imaging Correlates for Nonfavorable Outcomes

- Patients have significant cord compression showing constriction/strangulation of the spinal cord by granulation tissue.

- Evidence of myelomalacia indicates that irreversible changes have already set in and are not likely to show favorable response even after surgical decompression.
- Patients with extradural collection of mixed or granulomatous (dry) nature showing entrapment of a normal size cord or a constriction of cord with features suggestive of myelitis. The patients with these findings should be undertaken for early surgical decompression.

Mild cord atrophy may be observed in all patients who had shown excellent neural recovery after nonoperative/operative treatment. In paraplegia with healed disease, cord was found atrophied with edema in patients having mild neural deficit. In patients with severe neural deficit, cord atrophy may be associated with myelomalacia/syringomyelia.

Ultrasonography

Ultrasonography (USG) is a valuable non-invasive diagnostic tool for precise anatomic delineation of deeper abscesses in muscles, joints, parenchymatous organs and body cavities. Aspiration under USG guidance is helpful. It is helpful for differentiating the solid mass or cystic nature of the abscess/hematoma. It is particularly useful in follow-up evaluation of psoas abscess when patient is under cover of ATT to document resolution of psoas abscess.

Positron Emission Tomography (PET) Scan (Fig. 5.9)

PET-CT scan helps in picking up the residual inflammation in cases where the signs of healing on contrast MRI are ambiguous. 18F-fluorodeoxyglucose (^{18}F-FDG) labeled scan uptake in diseased area is a sign of persisting disease activity. PET-CT scan has recently been shown to differentiate between pyogenic and tubercular spondylitis.

TREATMENT

The treatment is best described into: **(A) Prechemotherapy era,** and **(B) Post-chemotherapy era:** Which is further subclassified into three philosophies—(a) universal surgical extirpation where surgery was universally advocated along with chemotherapy,

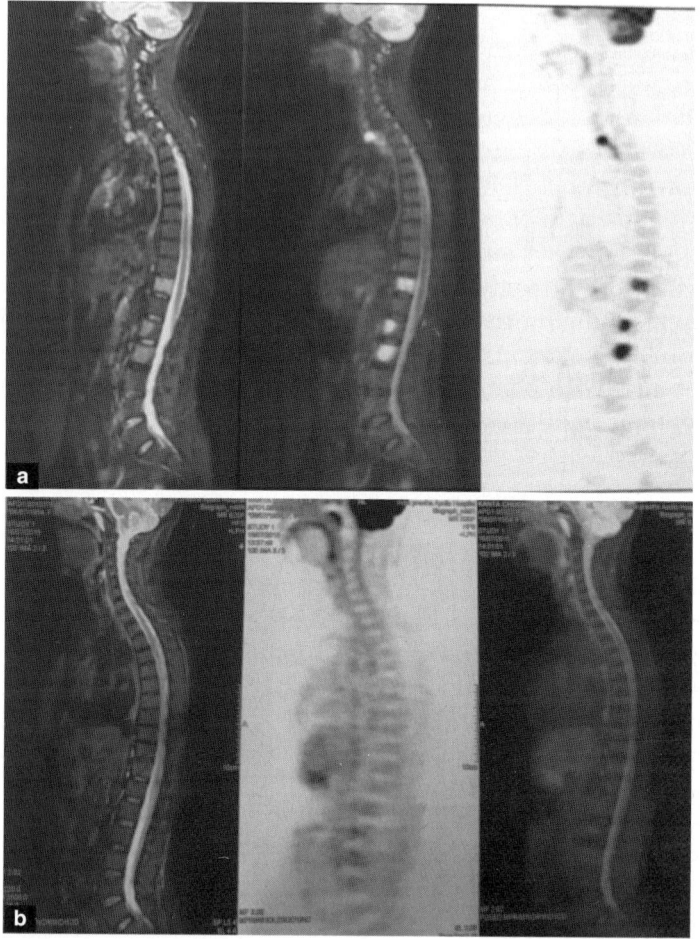

Fig. 5.9: Use of FDG PET for evaluation of disease, to look for skipped lesions and monitor healing of disease.

a. PET images showing multiple level disease with increased FDG activity.
b. After 18 months of drug therapy, there was no activity seen on PET following which ATT was stopped.

(b) middle path regimen where ATT was advocated for all with surgery only for neural complications and (c) recent trends where besides ATT, surgery was advocated for complications such as spinal deformity and neural deficit.

A. Prechemotherapy Era (Orthodox Conservative Treatment)

Ancient Indians (Atharva Veda period 3500 BC–1800 BC) used herbal medicines ("Sipudru"), along with exposure to sunshine to treat tuberculosis. Hippocrates (400 BC)and Galen (131–201 AD) unsuccessfully attempted correction of kyphotic deformities secondary to spinal tuberculosis by forceful maneuvers and manipulation. Rest, immobilization by braces, plaster beds and heliotherapy gained popularity in the late 18th century as the treatment of choice for spinal tuberculosis. In the late 19th and early 20th century, sanatoria or specialized tuberculosis hospitals in the countryside were developed where patients were admitted for 1–5 years and were treated with sunshine, good food and rest. The disease was allowed to run its 3–5 years natural course. This course consisted of three 1–2-year stages (onset, destruction or active stage, repair and ankylosis stage). The primary aim of orthodox conservative treatment was to achieve ankylosis in the least disabling position by rest and immobilization. Only one-third of these patients regained function. The remainder either died or were paralyzed and severely crippled. Kyphotic deformity typically increased and nonsurgical treatment failed to prevent paraplegia and relapse. Surgical drainage of abscesses and sinuses produced more complications and risk of death. Extra lesional surgery in the form of posterior spinal fusion offered only a slight reduction in mechanical pain. The overall prognosis was very poor.

B. Postchemotherapy Era

The antitubercular drugs have changed the outlook for spinal tuberculosis. The streptomycin was introduced into the clinical practice in 1947 while para-aminosalicylic acid in 1949 and isoniazid in 1952. These drugs formed the mainstay of conventional long-course chemotherapy. Pyrazinamide was introduced in 1956 but was popularized when it was added in the early 1980s to then newly developing short-course regimens. Ethambutol (1962) and rifampicin (1967) were relatively late entrants into the armamentarium of antitubercular drugs. Antitubercular drugs only bolstered the trend that was slowly gaining acceptance in the early 1950s, i.e. radical surgical excision for all cases of spinal tuberculosis. The sinuses, ulcers and abscesses despite extensive surgery disappeared under the influence of ATT. Fellander, Hodgson, Mukopadhaya and others advocated universal surgical extirpation in all patients under the cover of drugs on the pretext that antitubercular drugs do not penetrate well into osseous tubercular lesions. However, later studies (using radioactive isotopes of streptomycin and isoniazide among others) have shown that antitubercular drugs effectively penetrate into osseous lesions including cavities, abscesses and even dry caseous lesions. Isoniazid, rifampicin and pyrazinamide have been found in foci inside the sclerotic wall. Konstam, Kaplan, Stevenson and many others showed excellent results with chemotherapy and rest alone. Spinal tuberculosis patients are usually anemic and have poor nutrition. While waiting for fitness for surgical decompression, some of the patients may show neural recovery and ulcer and sinuses may start healing. This observation formed the basis for "middle-path regimen" advocated by Tuli' which consistes of rest, antitubercular drugs, regular supervision, gradual mobilization after 6–9 months using spinal braces for the next 18–24 months and minor surgical procedures in certain cases, e.g. aspiration of abscess and instillation of streptomycin in cavity, excision of sinus tract.

ANTITUBERCULAR CHEMOTHERAPY

Even ATT regimens have undergone changes over the years. The mainstay of treatment is prolonged, uninterrupted multi-drug antitubercular chemotherapy for 12–18 months. It started as injection streptomycin (1 gram per day for 3 months), isoniazid 300 mg/day for 18–24 months, PAS 12 gm per day for 18 months. Later on ethambutol was added into the list of ATT. With the introduction of pyrazinamide, the short course regimen were introduced. WHO introduced intermittent (thrice a week) regimen. The current index TB guidelines for extra-pulmonary TB advocates the daily regimen with 2 monthly intensive phase (RHZE) followed by continuation phase (RHE) for 10 to 16 months. The duration of ATT remained undecided due to absence of well defined end point of treatment, i.e. healed status in osteoarticular tuberculosis. Current consenus is to give ATT varying from 12–18 months depending on the achievement of the healed status.

The treatment of tuberculosis of spine can be discussed in two groups:
1. TB spine without neural deficit
2. TB spine with neural deficit.

TREATMENT OF TB SPINE WITHOUT NEURAL DEFICIT

The choice of treatment of uncomplicated (without neurological complication) tuberculosis of spine was controversial. The management varied from radical surgery on one hand to ambulant chemotherapy on the other hand. These controversies were resolved by multicenter trials conducted in Korea, Zimbabwe, South Africa and Hong Kong by British Medical Research Council (BMRC) working party on tuberculosis of spine. The trial was conducted on 750 patients in Hong Kong, Korea, Bulawayo, Rhodesia and South Africa with a follow-up of 3 to 10 years. The recommendations were:

1. The comparison of 2 and 3 antitubercular drugs combination showed no difference in results in achieving favorable status of tuberculous lesions.
2. Comparison of effect of bed rest in one group and ambulant chemotherapy in other group showed no difference in cure rate.
3. Comparison of results after radical clearance of lesion and conservative treatment showed no improvement in results by surgery.
4. Comparison of Hong Kong method of anterior debridement and fusion with anterior spinal debridement alone also showed the same results. However, fusion has improved overall results and resulted in prevention of further deformity and collapse. The cure rate for conservative treatment was 85% and Hong Kong method 89.9%.

When the results of ambulant chemotherapy (rest in bed followed by mobilization with braces and complete ATT) are comparable, then it is advocated that all tuberculosis spine without neural complications should be treated by non-operative methods. These cases should be operated only in following conditions.

1. **Doubtful diagnosis** (Cases 1, 2; pages 311–317): The tissue must be procured by open surgery or percutaneous method for histological diagnosis.

2. **Panvertebral lesions** (Cases 8, 9, 11; pages 329–340): Here both the vertebral body and posterior complex are diseased. Such lesions are potentially unstable and spinal cord is at great risk to develop neurological complications even on treatment by nonoperative method. Such cases should be undertaken for instrumented posterior stabilization to reduce the risk of developing neurological complications.

3. **Tuberculosis spine with severe kyphosis** (pretreatment kyphosis of 60° or more or those who are going to achieve healed kyphosis of 60° or more) should be considered for anterior debridement and fusion with kyphotic deformity correction.

4. **Failure of conservative treatment (presumptive drug resistance)** (Cases 27, 28, 30; pages 372–380): The drug resistance is suspected when the patient does not show adequate clinicoradiological healing inspite of adequate nonoperative treatment, paravertebral shadow is increasing or abscesses are not reducing despite repeated drainage. The sinus fails to heel and wound dehiscence occurs after surgery. Surgical debridement is done in such cases to procure tissue for histology and *Mycobacterium* culture and drug sensitivity testing.

Ancillary Treatment in Adults and Children

A. Braces (Fig. 5.10)

1. *Cervical spine*: Ambulant chemotherapy with four post-collar.
2. *Dorsal and dorsolumbar spine*: Ambulant chemotherapy supported by anterior spinal hyperextension (ASH) brace or Taylor's brace with or without four post-collar.
3. *Lumbar and lumbosacral spine*: Ambulant chemotherapy with Taylor's or ASH brace for upper lumbar spine and lumbosacral frame for lower lumbar spine.

In children, a PVC body brace (Boston scoliosis brace) or a plaster jacket may substitute ASH brace.

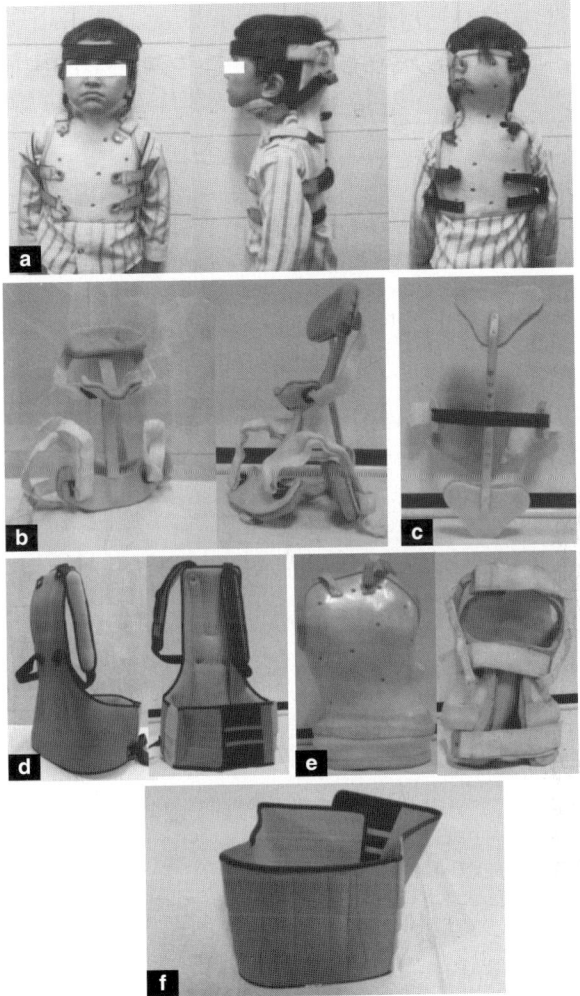

Fig. 5.10: Braces for ancillary treatment of spinal TB:

a. PVC modified SOMI brace for upper cervical spine disease.
b. Four post-collar for cervical spine and upper dorsal spine disease.
c. ASH brace for dorsolumbar disease.
d. Taylor's brace for dorsolumbar disease.
e. PVC thoracolumbar jacket for pediatric dorsolumbar disease. Alternatively, a plaster of Paris (POP) jacket can also be applied.
f. Lumbosacral corset for lower lumbar spine and lumbosacral junction disease.

B. Vitamin D Supplementation

Few studies have reported clinical improvement following additional vitamin D supplementation in pulmonary TB while single systematic review reported no effect.

Generally, the patients are undernourished, hence it is recommended that daily recommended dietary allowance of vitamin D (400–600 IU) should be given to patients undergoing antitubercular therapy. Therapeutic dosage to be restricted to those with documented vitamin D deficiency.

C. Protein Supplementation

Malnutrition can lead to secondary immunodeficiency that increases the host's susceptibility to infection. High protein diet is generally recommended by clinicians during the treatment of TB. It is thought to counteract the chronic wasting associated with the disease. However, there is no study where the role of high protein diet in treating spinal TB is evaluated.

Monitoring the Treatment Response of Patients

All cases of spinal TB should be monitored every 2 months.

a. *Clinical*: For general improvement in well-being, weight gain and an increase in appetite.
b. *Hematological*:
   1. *Increased Hb and RBC count*: The resolution of chronic inflammatory state results in decreased circulating proinflammatory cytokines which in turn leads to improvement in the persisting anemia of chronic disease.
   2. *Decreasing trend in ESR*: This is again due to resolution of inflammation with healing of disease.
c. *Radiological*: X-rays of spine showing appearance of remineralization of vertebral body, sharpening of disk margin. The healing of the disease is heralded by appearance of osseous or fibro-osseous fusion of involved vertebrae (Fig. 5.11).
d. *Imaging*: MRI with/without contrast at 9, 12 and 18 months to look for resolving collections, reduction in bone marrow edema and replacement of marrow by fat seen as bright signal in T1WI and T2WI.

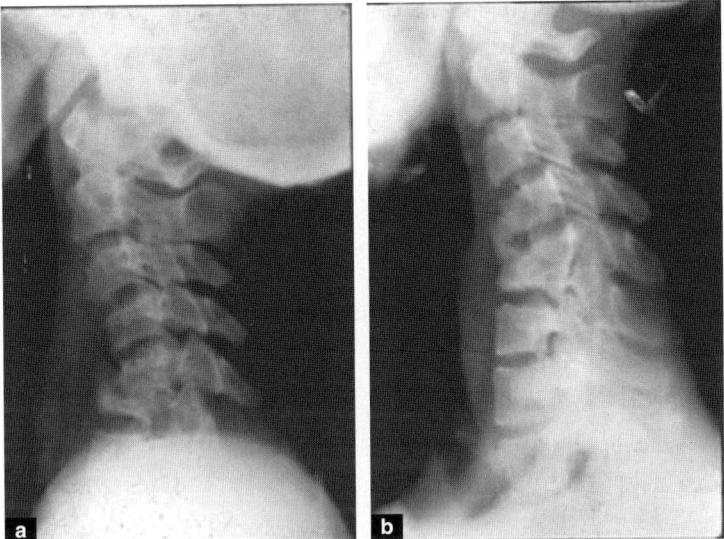

Fig. 5.11: Features of healing visible on X-rays: a. Pre-treatment X-ray, b. X-ray after 12 months of ATT showing remineralization of diseased bones, bony margins appear well defined and bony fusion between diseased vertebral bodies.

e. The patients on ambulant chemotherapy should be instructed to report immediately, if the signs of neural deficit appear and same should be documented at clinical examination.

Failure of Conservative Treatment

Drug resistance has a recorded history as old as the development of antibiotics. The bacteria undergo mutation when exposed to newer antibiotics and it occurs more if the drugs are exposed in subclinical doses. Drug resistance to antitubercular drugs has also been reported as early as 1948. When a patient of TB developed resistance to many drugs, it posed a serious health threat. 50% of the patients with multidrug resistant TB die within one year as used to happen with all spinal TB in the preantibiotic era.

The patient may show a poor response to treatment due to non-compliance or a faulty drug regimen in drug combination, dosage duration, or spurious drugs. Drug resistance is one of the causes of failure of treatment. It could be because of infection by an atypical organism in an immunocompromised patient or may be acquired. When an organism develops resistance to one drug, it is called monoresistance, while resistance to two or more drugs is described as polyresistance. If a patient develops resistance to **rifampicin and isoniazid,** it is defined as multi-drug resistance **(MDR-TB). Extensive drug resistance** is labeled when organisms are resistant to Rcin and INH (MDR-TB) and also to an injectable aminoglycoside (other than streptomycin) and a fluoroquinolone.

The most common cause of drug resistance is inappropriate treatment or by exposure to a case with pulmonary MDR-TB case or due to coinfection with HIV or in an immuno-compromised state due to socioeconomic deprivation or in a patient on anticancer therapy or in patients with comorbidities such as diabetes.

The diagnosis of drug resistant tuberculosis is a micro-biological diagnosis where drug resistance is proved on culture and sensitivity. In pulmonary TB, the drug resistance is suspected if sputum positive for AFB does not convert to sputum negative inspite of 5 months CAT I treatment or 4 months of CAT 2 treatment. In spinal TB, the suspicion has to be clinical. Spinal TB is paucibacillary disease, hence demonstration of drug resistance even after obtaining the tissue may not be possible in all cases.

The criteria to suspect drug resistance are listed below.

If a patient on conservative treatment does not show any improvement at 5 months:

a. *Clinical*: Persistent or worsening localized tenderness, fever
b. *Hematological*: Persistently raised ESR showing rising trend
c. MRI shows deterioration of lesion at 5–6 months
d. Appearance of new lesion
e. Failure to show healing of ulcer/sinus
f. New cold abscess/lymph node appears
g. Would dehiscence in a postoperative case.

In all such cases, drug resistance should be suspected and the lesion should be debrided to procure tissue for histology, smear for AFB, GeneXpert and Line Probe Assay (LPA) and culture and sensitivity.

Paradoxical Response

It is defined as a patient with confirmed or probable skeletal TB **on ATT** who initially improves and then subsequently reports with worsening of constitutional symptoms or signs of tuberculosis **in the absence of another diagnosis.** The presenting features may include increased size of lesion, appearance of new lesion, persistent fever and night sweats, or development of another form of TB.

In cases of suspected drug resistance, patient continues to remain stationary or worsens on treatment from the beginning whereas in case of paradoxical response, patient initially improves and then shows deterioration.

Drug sensitivity shall show a sensitive and susceptible organism. The continuation of standard ATT is all that is required in case of paradoxical response.

CT-guided aspiration of pus/tissue biopsy should be first attempted. Failing which the lesion should be surgically debrided to procure tissue.

The diagnosis has to be ascertained by procuring tissue and samples to be sent for:

1. Histopathology, cytopathology
2. Gram's stain
3. AFB staining
4. Culture and drug sensitivity testing (conventional LJ medium/BACTEC) for *Mycobacterium* (rule out fungal/brucellar infections)
5. *Molecular tests*:
   a. PCR.
   b. Line probe assay/CB-NAAT/GeneXpert for rapid drug sensitivity testing where available.

Immunocomptence should be confirmed by testing for diabetes mellitus, HIV, liver/kidney disease. Complete and differential blood counts are indicated. The therapy should be tailored as per drug sensitivity pattern in cases of confirmed laboratory drug resistance.

TREATMENT OF TB SPINE WITH NEURAL DEFICIT

The prevention of development of para-/quadriplegia is the best treatment of neurological complications in tuberculous spine. With the clinical awareness of condition and its complications and with advent of modern imaging techniques, one can diagnose tuberculous spine early in predestructive stage/preclassical stage well before classical clinical picture and radiological signs develop. It is neccessary that before the disease can be treated it must be recognized and before it can be recognized, it must be suspected and considered a diagnostic possibility. However, once tuberculous spine is complicated by neurological complications, early clinical diagnosis, confirmed by radiography, and MRI and early effective treatment can reverse paralysis and avert or minimize the potentially devastating effects of Pott's paraplegia.

Early Onset Paraplegia (Paraplegia with Active Disease)

Tuberculosis of spine with neurological complications warrants urgent and meticulous care. The early diagnosis and appropriate treatment is a major contributory factor to prevent incomplete neural recovery, reduceded morbidity and even mortality. The three definite methodologies have evolved about the treatment of TB spine with neurological deficit.

a. **Absolute non-operative:** Dabsen (1951) reported that 48% of paraplegia improved neurologically by traditional conservative care in preantibiotic era. This percentage would have further improved, if these patient would have received modern chemotherapy.

MRC trials (1978) considering early disease (limited disease with little kyphosis and mild to moderate paraparesis) have concluded that Pott's paraplegia from active disease could be managed by conservative methods on ATT only. This suggests compression is usually from increasing tension of the abscess and inflammatory edema. Drugs along with rest arrest the pathological process and reduces tension edema and relieves the compression. Until the end of 1970, most surgeons preferred nonoperative treatment and rarely performed surgery for fear of worsening the already existing neural deficit. The discrepancy in recovery rate in various series attributed to difference in the chronicity of disease, neural complications, general physical condition of the patients, bacterial drug sensitivity, and improper selection of patient for nonoperative treatment.

b. **Universal surgical extirpation** in all cases of tuberculous paraplegia was performed by second group of surgeons. Hodgson and Stock (1967), Kohli (1967), Goel (1967), Gurgius (1967), Martin (1971), Lifeso (1985) performed anterior decompression with or without fusion and reported neurological recovery varying from 37–94%.

Universal surgical extirpation was preferred because of the following advantages:

1. Diagnosis was established beyond doubt.
2. The quality and speed of neural recovery was good. The neural recovery time after surgical decompression had been quoted as less than 2 months, while nonoperative treatment took 2 to 6 months.
3. Surgical decompression removes fibrous barrier to drugs. The opinion in developed countries goes for surgical extirpation. We feel both methodologies of management are extreme.

c. Tuli had advocated **Middle Path Regimen** (1969). His observation was based on his experience in treating TB spine in india where most of his patients with paraplegia were from very low socioeconomic state with poor general health, anemia and many of them having associated pulmonary tuberculosis and were unfit for major surgery. While waiting for their turn for surgery/fitness for surgery, 38% started showing neurological recovery on antitubercular therapy, bed rest and nutritious diet in 4 to 6 weeks time.

Thus he concluded that every patient with paraplegia neither will be cured by orthodox conservative treatment nor all patients do need surgical intervention. A judicious combination of conservative therapy and operative decompression when needed should form a comprehensive integrated course of treatment for tuberculosis of the spine with neurological complications. Tubercular liquid pus, granulation tissue, caseous tissue causing compression and inflammatory edema are amiable to nonoperative treatment. In middle path regimen, 3 to 4 weeks delay will give a chance, for above mentioned reasons, of neural deficit to subside and patient may show neural recovery. Thus surgical decompression could be avoided in cases which would otherwise show neural improvement. Jain *et al.* demonstrated in a prospective study on MRI that the patient showing relatively preserved cord with evidence of edema/myelitis with predominantly fluid collection in extradural space will resolve well on nonoperative treatment provided panvertebral disease/unstable spine is excluded. This observation supports the philosophy of middle path regimen. By proper imaging (X-ray, CT and MRI), we can select the cases who are likely to be benefitted by nonoperative methods.

Indications of Surgery in Tuberculous Para-/Quadriplegia

Following indications of surgery are adapted from Griffith, Seddon, Tuli and Jain *et al.*

Treatment factors

1. Neurological complications developing during conservative treatment with rest and antitubercular drugs.
2. Neural complications not showing signs of improvement to a satisfactory functional level after a fair trial of conservative treatment (3–4 weeks).
3. Neural deficit getting worse on nonoperative treatment.

Clinical factors

1. *Paraplegia with rapid onset:* Generally, rapid onset neurological complications occur in TB spine due to mechanical accident such as pathological subluxation/dislocation or sudden loss of anterior bony height secondary to mechanical insult. It may also result from vascular thrombosis/endarteritis which cannot be proved/disproved. It remains an explanation for nonrecovery despite demonstrable adequate surgical decompression.
2. *Severe paraplegia*: Flaccid paraplegia, paraplegia in flexion, complete sensory loss, complete loss of motor power for more than 6 months.
3. *Spinal tumor syndrome*: Although not a common cause but surgical decompression is indicated to establish the diagnosis and relieve the spinal cord compression.

4. Paraplegia with neural arch affection.
5. Recurrent paraplegia.
6. Paraplegia accompanied by uncontrolled spasticity of such severity that reasonable rest and immobilization are impossible.
7. *Patient with massive prevertebral abscess*: Neurological signs are associated with difficulty of deglutition/respiration.

Imaging factors

1. *Paraplegia with panvertebral involvement*: It can be appreciated on plain radiographs with associated scoliosis and/or severe kyphosis in a case of TB spine. CT/MRI shows disease of anterior and posterior column of vertebral body (VB). The cause of paraplegia is instability, cord compression and inflammation. Hence in such cases instrumented stabilization of the spine is indicated besides decompression.
2. The cases of TB spine with paraplegia where MRI shows extradural compression consisting of granulation/caseous tissue with little fluid component, compressing spinal cord circumferentially and constricting the spinal cord with the features suggestive of cord edema/myelitis or myelomalacia, should be undertaken for surgical decompression.
3. Paraplegia with compression by sequestra or disk.

Patient factors

1. *Painful paraplegia*: Pain resulting from severe spasm or root compression.
2. Paraplegia with onset in old age because of hazards of immobilization.

Surgical Decompression

Vertebral body is affected in almost 98% cases of tuberculous spine. Surgical decompression should include full exposure of the front of the dura mater at the apex of kyphosis. Anterior decompression allows direct access to the focus of disease. The abscesses can be evacuated and all avascular material can be excised and kyphosis can be corrected to some extent.

Laminectomy for decompression in anterior disease is to be condemned. It removes the only healthy component of vertebrae in anterior disease, thus, rendering the spine unstable as found in panvertebral involvement. Many reports are available where patients with vertebral body disease were operated by laminectomy and shown appreciable deterioration in neural deficit, increase in kyphosis, pathological dislocation. Laminectomy as surgical decompression is indicated in isolated neural arch affection and in the compressive myelopathy due to spinal tumor syndrome (extradural granuloma).

Radical Surgery vs Debridement Surgery

These terms are used interchangeably in literature.

Debridement surgery: Debridement of spinal focus involves removal of all pus, caseous tissue, sequestra but without removal of unaffected or viable bone except to provide adequate access to the focus and to decompress the spinal cord.

Radical surgery: This technique is developed by Hodgson and Stock. Here radical excision of tuberculous focus is performed with repair of resultant gap with autologous bone grafting.

The excision of bone is carried out upward and downward until healthy, bleeding cancellous bone was exposed with surfaces suitable for reception of bone graft and the dura mater is uncovered. If the affected bodies were so extensively diseased that a healthy bleeding cancellous surface cannot be fashioned in the bodies themselves at one or both end of resection, the whole of upper and/or lower parts of affected bodies were removed. This involves the removal of intervertebral disks at the limit (or limits) of the resection and of the end plate of the vertebrae immediately above and/or below the diseased area. The healthy cancellous surfaces being cut in the vertebral bodies above and/or below the obviously affected one.

In every skeletal lesion, there are areas of bone which are infiltrated with tubercular disease but which are not necrosed and will recover and reconstitute under the influence of ATT. There are also areas of ischemic and infarcted bone and these will also recover and reconstitute without operation as the disease subsides and the circulation improves. Finally there are areas of necrosis which are past recovery and which harbor tubercular bacilli, and for these areas surgery in addition to

ATT is necessary. While performing surgical decompression, we should remove that part of viable bone which allows us to remove all pus, caseous tissue and sequestra, to decompress spinal cord. Whatever gap thus created should be bridged by 2 to 3 rib grafts/tricortical iliac crest strut graft to correct whatever maximum correction of kyphosis is possible.

Excision of too much bone up to healthy bleeding bone will leave a large gap to be bridged by a long graft. If this graft which is only a fraction of mass and strength of vertebral body slips or breaks will result in a unstable situation and may lead to neurological nonrecovery or deterioration. However, debridement where entire body is not excised leave a more stable spine. Upadhyay (1994) repeated a mean 15.3 years follow-up of 112 patients who were operated by radical or debridement surgery. The neurologic recovery in both radical and debridement surgeries was equally good and no patient had pain. At 6 months, radical surgery group showed marginal correction of deformity while the debridement group had detrioration of kyphotic deformity. The deformity angle had improved by 5° or more after radical surgery at 6 months follow-up in 45% patients. While deteriorated after debridement surgery in 53% patients. The patients of lumbar spine tuberculosis treated with radical surgery reported normal lordosis at final follow-up compared with only 63% after debridement. The correction of kyphotic deformity achieved after surgery at 6 months evaluation was practically maintained up to final evaluation.

Surgery of tuberculous paraplegia/quadriplegia poses certain difficulties and anxiety for surgeons:

1. The operation may be technically most difficult, and result may be most unpredictable as far as the neurological outcome is concerned.
2. Anesthetist should be ready to deal with instant blood loss from intercostal or extradural vessels or in the sinusoidal vessels of cancellous bone.
3. The personnel dealing with a patient of tuberculous spine with neurological complications must be conversant with problems of paralytic patients suffering from chronic

infective pathology who is debilitated and might even have concomitant pulmonary tuberculosis, thus a bad risk patient to manage post-surgery.

SURGICAL APPROACHES TO TUBERCULOUS SPINE

The approach to the spine in tuberculosis depends on the availability of appropriate facilities, trained personnel and also on the nature of the case. In cervical and lumbar spine, the approach is well defined and has to be anterior. In dorsal spine, however, there are two approaches: (i) Thoracotomy, (ii) extrapleural (anterolateral) approach.

The spinal cord can be decompressed by anterior approach where the vertebral body is accessed directly. The anterior approach does not require removal of any healthy part of vertebral body. The disease focus can be reached directly and debridement/resection of disease, can be performed to decompress the spinal cord. The posterior approach (laminectomy) for an anterior disease requires removal of healthy posterior column to decompress the spinal cord and reach anterior diseased vertebral bodies. The instrumented stabilization of spine by pedicle screw fixation system is a must for stabilization of spine, if posterior approach is preferred.

Upper Cervical Spine (Occiput to C3)

The anterior decompression can be performed through transoral or retropharyngeal approach. The exposure from C1 to C3 can be made by incising the posterior wall of the pharynx. The anterior decompression and fusion can then be performed. The anterior retropharyngeal approach allows extramucosal exposure, anterior debridement, and fusion of upper cervical spine. Since this entails extramucosal exposure of diseased vertebrae, hence less risk of secondary infection.

Lower Cervical Spine (C3–C7)

For a cervical spine tuberculosis from C3 to C7, the anterior approach is used to reach the disease focus and decompress the spinal cord anteriorly. Through a transverse or longitudinal incision, a plane is developed between the sternocleidomastoid, carotid sheath laterally and trachea, esophagus and thyroid medially to expose the vertebral bodies between two longus colli. This gives adequate exposure anteriorly up to the uncovertebral joint for anterior decompression, anterior fusion with or without an anterior cervical locking plate fixation. Generally, this approach is sufficient to expose cervical vertebrae from C2 to C7/T1 and to decompress the spinal cord, reconstruct the bone defect by tricortical graft/cages, and instrument it by plate osteosynthesis. Rarely in a severe kyphotic deformity of cervical spine with a long segment disease one may have to resort to two stage surgery where posterior instrumentation is followed by anterior decompression and bone grafting (Case 18; page 354). Cervicodorsal junction is a transition area where cervical lordosis abruptly changes into thoracic kyphosis. Low anterior cervical approach allows limited exposure up to first thoracic vertebra. A high transthoracic approach allows exposure from C6 to T4 where the thoracic cavity is accessed through the bed of the second or third rib in the presence of kyphosis. Sternum splitting approach of Hodgson gives exposure from C4 to T4 anteriorly. Later on, this approach is modified where full sternotomy is modified with a trans-upper-sternal approach.

Dorsal Spine

The evolution of surgical approaches took place for a dorsal or dorsolumbar spine. Initially, the anterior decompression was advocated by **extrapleural anterolateral approach** which was initiated by Menard (1895) and refined by Seddon (1935), Griffith (1952), and Roaf (1958). Alexander developed an operation with Dott of Edinburgh in which he opened the paravertebral abscess and decompressed it from the front after removal of the posterior end of three or more ribs, their corresponding transverse process, and pedicles and an adjacent portion of vertebral bodies. Capner described the lateral rachotomy in which the purpose was to deal directly with the cause of cord compression. Menard as quoted by Capner used 5–7 cm long transverse incision over the rib which seemed to correspond with the apex of kyphus. Tuli, Dott,

Capener, and Seddon described semicircular incision concave medially for extrapleural anterolateral approach. Once thick fasciocutaneous flap was lifted, the 6–8 cm posterior part of the ribs at the apex of the lesion was removed. The transverse process of the vertebra, the pedicle, and the anterolateral surface of the vertebral body are exposed and removed. The removal of 2–3 intercostal nerves allows adequate exposure of the lateral and anterior surface of the vertebral body. The presence of paraspinal abscess allows the placing of spatula anterior to the vertebral body. The spinal canal can be decompressed adequately.

Jain *et al.* (2004) modified the incision to a T-incision where a 14–15 cm midline incision was given centering the apex of kyphosis and a connecting transverse incision of about 8 cm from the midline and perpendicular to it at the apex of kyphosis on left side was added (Fig. 5.12). The two triangular fasciocutaneous flaps were held with stay sutures. The rest of the anterolateral decompression was same as described above.

The advantage of "T" approach is that a simultaneous exposure of anterior as well as posterior column is possible where anterior corpectomy and bone grafting with simultaneous posterior Hartshill fixation is the intended procedure. This obviated the need for second stage posterior instrumentations. The posterior column shortening can also be performed, if kyphus correction is the intended objective of surgery. This approach has been reported for thoracolumbar lesions

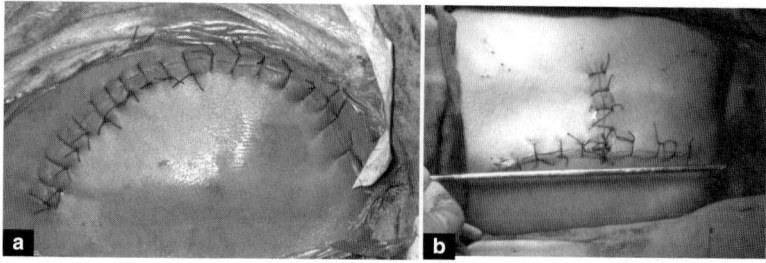

Fig. 5.12: (a) Classical semicircular incision described for extrapleural anterolateral decompression and (b) T shaped modification of incision by Jain *et al.*

also,where the D12 VB was exposed after removal of the 12th rib and intercostal nerve (Fig. 5.13). The tip of transverse processes of L1 and L2 identified. The subperiosteal dissection of transverse process is done. The L1 and L2 nerve roots are protected using an infant feeding tube. The quadratus lumborum and psoas muscle are reflected over D12 L1 and L1 L2 disk. The segmental lumbar arteries are identified and ligated. The spatula is placed over the anterolateral surface of L1 and L2 VB. The disease focus is curetted and decompressed. Since the patient is in lateral position only Hartshill instrumentation can be applied. However, if pedicle screw system is a preferred fixation, then the patient can be placed in prone position to stabilize the spine first and then turned in lateral position to perform anterior decompression and bone grafting by extrapleural and retroperitoneal exposure.

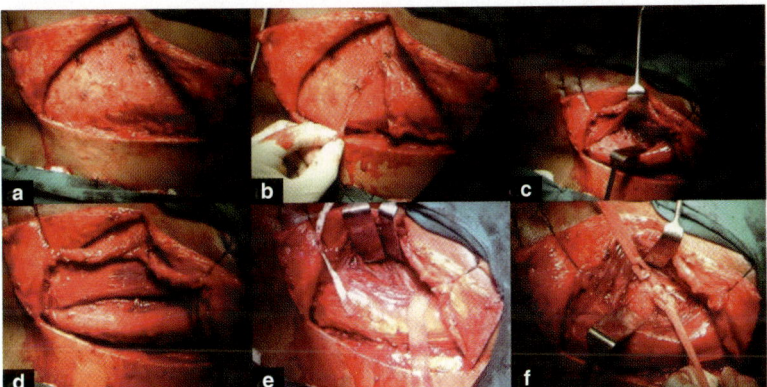

Fig. 5.13A: Showing intraoperative photograph of the extrapleural retroperitoneal approach/exposure showing (a) "T" incision with full thickness fasciocutaneous flap lifted up, (b) thoracolumbar fascia incised in the line of incision, (c) a plane between iliocostalis and longissimus muscle made, (d) skin and muscle flap were reflected and held by stay suture with split in paraspinal muscles seen, (e) posterior 6 cm of the 11th and 12th rib was exposed, (f) 12th rib was subperiosteally removed. (Adapted from Jain AK, Dhammi IK, Jain S, Kumar J. Simultaneously anterior decompression and posterior instrumentation by extrapleural retroperitoneal approach in thoracolumbar lesions. *Indian J Orthop* 2010 Oct;44(4):409–16).

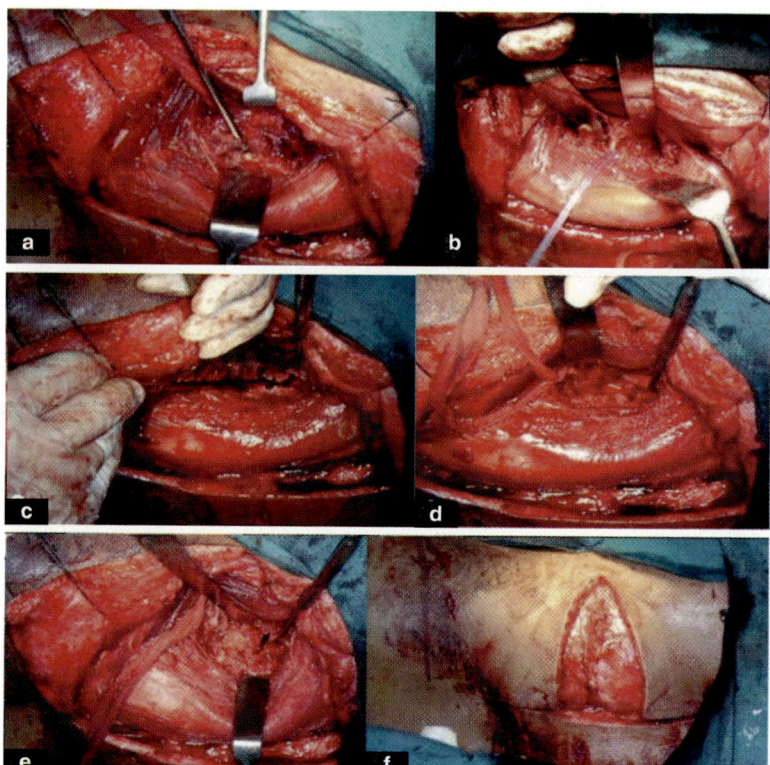

Fig. 5.13B: Intraoperative photograph of extrapleural retroperitoneal approach/exposure shows (a) blunt dissection done in front of transverse process creating an anterior flap of muscle of psoas, quadratus lumborum, (b) lumbar nerves identified, protected, (c) a spatula was placed under reflected psoas muscle exposing anterolateral surface of fractured vertebral body, (d) spinal cord decompression done by corpectomy of fractured vertebra and removal of adjacent disk and bed for graft created, (e) tricortical strut graft from ipsilateral iliac crest, placed between fractured vertebral body and proximal intact vertebral body, (f) wound closed in layers. (*Courtesy:* Adapted from Jain AK, Dhammi IK, Jain S, Kumar J. Simultaneously anterior decompression and posterior instrumentation by extrapleural retroperitoneal approach in thoracolumbar lesions. *Indian J Orthop* 2010 Oct;44(4):409–16)

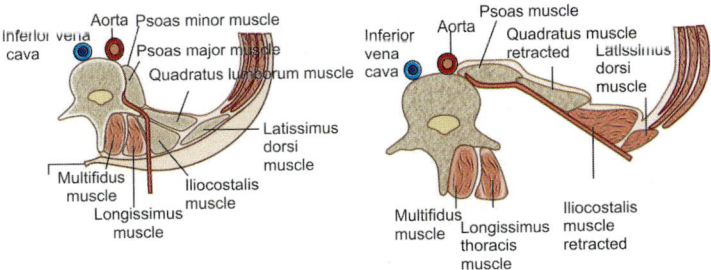

Fig. 5.13C: Line diagram of horizontal section of abdomen through thoraco-lumbar junction showing (a) L1 vertebra with musculature and abdominal wall layers. Thick line denotes the proposed entry from the posterior to anterior underneath quadratus lumborum and psoas major muscle to reach lateral surface to the vertebral body, (b) exposure of the lateral surface of body, pedicle and anterior transverse process once psoas major and quadratus lumborum retracted by spatula. (*Courtesy*: Adapted from Jain AK, Dhammi IK, Jain S, Kumar J. Simultaneously anterior decompression and posterior instrumentation by extrapleural retroperitoneal approach in thoracolumbar lesions. *Indian J Orthop* 2010 Oct;44(4):409–16)

The advantages of this approach are:

a. Patient is stable in lateral position.

b. Span of posterior instrumentation and exposure can be increased, if needed.

c. The plane of surgery is extrapleural and retroperitoneal, without opening chest cavity and cutting diaphragm, hence less morbid and reduces/avoids pulmonary sequelae. Simultaneous sequential anterior decompression and posterior instrumentation with or without posterior column shortening can be performed.

Transthoracic transpleural approach: Hodgson and stock described and propagated this approach to perform anterior clearance of lesion, and reconstruction by bone grafting for dorsal and dorsolumbar spine. The patient is placed in lateral position. Thoracic cavity is entered through the bed of a rib corresponding to the involved vertebrae. Once the thoracic cavity is entered and the lung is deflated on a double lumen endotracheal tube, the lesion is identified. The pleural adhesions from an old healed pleural tubercular lesion if observed, are gradually cleared of lung to achieve deflation of lung. The segmental vessels over the vertebral body are identified and ligated. The intercostal nerve is a useful guide to intervertebral foramina. The lesion is debrided to achieve anterior decompression of the spinal canal. The exposure of lower thoracic and upper lumbar vertebrae for thoracolumbar lesion is difficult because of the presence of the diaphragm and it is incised to expose chest cavity and retroperitoneal space.

Thoracolumbar region: The 10th rib is resected to provide adequate exposure of T10–L2. First thoracic cavity is entered. The diaphragm is incised to join the thoracic cavity with the abdominal cavity to expose the thoracolumbar vertebrae. Hodgson always advocated excision of diseased vertebral body up to healthy vertebral body. The good results of Hodgson and Stock could not be replicated in all other series.

The transthoracic approach had extensive morbidity particularly with the patients who have poor pulmonary function, due to concomitant active or healed lung disease, paretic intercostal muscles, prolonged surgery, and huge anterior bone defect requiring long bone grafts. Patients with TB spine are usually anemic, have paretic or paralyzed intercostal muscles with compromised pulmonary function, and may have evidence of healing/healed pulmonary TB. It does require trained spine surgeons and intensive care unit facilities. The usual outcome reported was healing of the lesion with residual kyphotic deformity. The usual complications were graft slippage/breakage and neural deterioration. With transthoracic, transpleural approach, if concomitant posterior instrumented stabilization is indicated, one may have to resort to same stage/or second stage posterior instrumentation.

On the contrary, the **extrapleural anterolateral decompression** can still be performed in cases where patient has compromised pulmonary reserve, as it is:

   i. Simpler and safe technique.
  ii. Skilled team in open chest surgery is not required.
 iii. Debilitated patient could be operated.
  iv. Does not require care of chest tube so pulmonary complication can be reduced.
   v. It allows an easier exposure of spinal cord in severely kyphotic spine which is technically difficult by transthoracic approach.

vi. It reduces the postoperative morbidity. It can even be performed in those cases where the entry to the space between lungs and pleura cannot be achieved due to pleural adhesions secondary to old pulmonary disease.

Limitations of extrapleural (anterolateral) approach

1. This has a long learning curve to master the technique of adequate decompression.
2. It provides limited exposure and limited space for bone grafting as described by various authors but has not been our experience and of other authors. It provides adequate exposure of spinal cord, and we can excise even total vertebral body and make a suitable bed for gap grafting.

Out of two approaches, the determining factor for particular approach are preference and technical skills of surgeon, availability of surgical facilities and general and pulmonary reserve of patient. If everything is good, one can perform decompression by either approach. However, if any one is wanting, lateral extrapleural (anterolateral) approach gives adequate exposure to perform adequate decompression of the spinal cord.

Posterior only approach: This approach has been popularized in the recent past. The spine is exposed by midline posterior approach. The disadvantage of this approach in TB spine is that it necessitates resection of the lamina (post-complex) which is the only healthy segment of vertebra in an anterior disease which will render spine grossly unstable. The spine is temporarily stabilized by pedicle screw fixation of proximal and distal spine for 2–3 levels. The posterior column of the apex vertebral body is excised. The disease focus could be approached through the pedicles (transpedicular route). The anterior decompression can also be performed after removal of posterior part of 2–3 ribs on both sides at affected level. The anterior aspect of vertebral lesion can be exposed after removal of transverse process and pedicles on both side. The advantage of this procedure is that decompression and deformity correction can be performed in single stage. It is a good approach when 2–3 vertebral bodies are diseased. It is less morbid as compared to thoracotomy or thoracoabdominal approach and has shorter hospital stay.

The disadvantages are:

a. Pedicle screw system as a temporary stabilization is a must before the posterior column shortening is performed.

b. The availability of pedicle screw size for small children is an issue.

c. In a long segment tubercular spinal lesion when pedicle probe is inserted, the pus starts pouring out through pedicle which makes it unsuitable for pedicle screw purchase in diseased vertebral body particularly in children, hence the span of instrumentation is increased up to 2–3 healthy vertebral bodies proximally and distally.

d. The decompression anterior to spinal cord is difficult to perform and has a long learning curve.

e. It is a highly skilled procedure and cannot be performed unless state of art facilities for spinal surgery are available.

f. Potential risk of vascular insult to major blood vessels while performing the procedure is an issue and if it occurs is difficult to manage posteriorly.

Lumbar Spine

The retroperitoneal anterior approach allows exposure of lumbar vertebral body to achieve decompression with or without anterior instrumentation. The patient is placed in the lateral position. The incision may vary depending on the level of the lumbar vertebrae involved. It is a modification of the lumbar sympathectomy approach. The oblique incision is made over the 12th rib from the lateral border of quadratus lumborum to the lateral border of the rectus abdominis. Abdominal muscles are cut in line with skin incision. The retroperitoneal space is reached. The lumbar vertebrae are palpated and the lumbar vessels are ligated over the affected level. The psoas muscle is lifted from the anterior border and the pedicle and intervertebral foramina are identified. The anterior decompression can now be perfomed. If the disease is limited to one or two vertebrae, the anterior instrumentation can be added. Whenever concomitant posterior instrumentation is indicated one has to resort to separate posterior approach.

Recently, only posterior approach is advocated for lumbar spine where posterior pedicle screw fixation is performed. The laminectomy of the apex vertebrae is performed. The anterior vertebral body is approached through pedicles of apex vertebrae.

Indications of Instrumented Stabilization

1. *Panvertebral disease*: The spine is potentially unstable in TB lesions of all three columns. The instrumented stabilization should be performed to prevent on the treatment subluxation/dislocation of the spine. However, if pathological sub-luxation/dislocation of the spine has already occurred, then besides posterior instrumentation, anterior decompression is also indicated.

2. *Long segment disease*: Instrumented stabilization is indicated to provide mechanical stability to anterior bone graft follow-ing anterior decompression in a spinal TB lesion with disease of four or more vertebral bodies (length of bone graft >4–5 cm).

3. *In lumbar and cervical spine*: There are no costotransverse and costovertebral articulations that provide extrastability as in the dorsal spine, hence instrumentation is indicated when these sites are subjected to decompression and fusion.

4. *When kyphosis correction surgery is contemplated*: Kyphosis correction in active disease can be performed by anterior corpectomy, posterior column shortening, anterior fusion, posterior fusion and posterior instrumentation.

5. TB spine in junctional area such as CD spine and DL spine.

Implant Choice

Implant choice should be individualized according to the case. The anterior plate or rods and screws can be used in short-segment disease. Regional osteopenia is the essential feature of the TB lesion. Hence, the screw should be placed in the healthy vertebral bodies above and below the diseased segment to acquire purchase and provide mechanical stability. This system can be used in mild to moderate kyphosis only. Anterior instrumentation can only be used when disease affects the anterior and middle columns only and the posterior column is healthy. In panvertebral disease, anterior instrumentation alone does not provide mechanical stability. Hence, stabiliza-tion by posterior instrumentation and anterior bone grafting is indicated.

Anterior instrumentation appears to be more advantageous than posterior instrumentation, as both instrumentation and bone grafting are done as single-stage surgery through the same incision, minimizing total blood loss and surgery time with no risk of the graft slippage. The problems with anterior instrumentation in tubercular lesions are: (a) Lack of adequate space to insert the anterior implants, (b) possible problem of prominent hardware impaling the great vessels, particularly in the thoracic spine. (c) The retrieval of dislodged anterior implant is more risky in cases of implant failure, due to adjacent major vessels.

Hartshill instrumentation can be applied, gaining purchase against a healthy posterior complex. It should be spanned to at least 6 levels with one healthy vertebral body on either side of the lesion. Isolated insertion of cages should be avoided; it should be supported by anterior or posterior instrumentation.

PROGNOSIS IN TUBERCULOUS PARA-/QUADRIPLEGIA

The neurological recovery in tuberculous para-/qudriplegia is not predictable and depends on many factors.

The advanced/aggressive disease shows delayed neural recovery. Such patients also tolerate surgery poorly. The spinal canal at cervicodorsal junction and upper dorsal spine is narrowest, hence show poor/delayed neural recovery as compared to other segments of spine. The patients of neurological complication with active disease show better neurological recovery as compared to the patients of healed disease. The patients having severe kyphosis show poor neural recovery. The neurological complications of shorter duration show better neurological recovery than of longer duration as spinal cord develops some permanent changes in long-standing paraplegia, thus leading to nonrecovery or poor recovery. Neurological complications rapidly developing to severe deficit (in a few hours/a few days) show the worst prognosis. It may be either due to mechanical insult or due to a pressure from disk/ sequestra or pathological subluxation/dislocation or vascular endarteritis. Patients presenting with severe paraplegia (stage IV paraplegia or paraplegia with flexor spasm or with sphincter involvement or with complete sensory loss) show poor neural improvement, while less severe grade of neural deficit shows a partial card involvement thus better chances of neural recovery. The cases who had only anterior vertebral body affection (paraplegia due to compression alone) show a better prognosis as compared to panvertebral destruction having gross instability which may damage spinal cord. Extradural compression of fluid nature resolves well on treatment, and patients show a good neural recovery while the patients with extradural compression of mixed or granulomatous (dry) nature showing constriction of cord show delayed/poor neural improvement. Preserved cord with edema/myelitis of cord on MRI would show a good neural recovery while spinal cord showing myelomalacia with reduction in cord volume may show a poor neural recovery. The cord showing syringomyelia with reduction in cord volume/cord atrophy would show very poor neural recovery. On surgical decompression, if pus is drained out (wet lesion) along with extradural compression of granulation tissue and bony sequestra, the patient is likely to show better neural recovery in comparison to thick inspissated pus, caseous tissue, fibrous tissue, bony sequestra and disk (dry lesion).

COMPLICATIONS OF TB SPINE: SPINAL DEFORMITY

Pathology of Kyphotic Deformity (Fig. 5.14)

The tuberculous lesion starts as a paradiscal inflammation in 98% cases. As the disease progresses, the vertebral end plates become structurally weak and intervertebral disk starts ballooning/herniating into the diseased vertebral body. Since the line of weight transmission in thoracic spine is in the anterior half of vertebral bodies, the vertebral body loses more anterior height than posterior. Thoracic kyphosis increases and gradually an angular kyphosis appears. The severity of kyphosis depends on the number of vertebral bodies affected, severity of loss of anterior vertebral body height and segment of the spine affected. A case of dorsal spine or dorsolumbar spinal tuberculosis with three or more vertebral body affection is more likely to develop moderate to severe kyphotic deformity. In cervical and lumbar spine, the line of weight transmission is

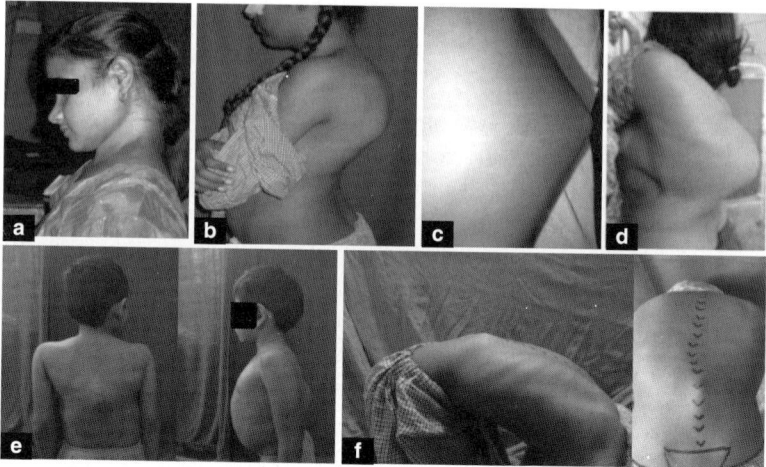

Fig. 5.14: Patients with deformities in spine at all levels due to tuberculosis. (a) Kyphotic deformity in cervical spine, (b) rounded kyphus in dorsal spine, (c) classical severe angular deformity in thoracic spine, (d) rounded kyphus (Gibbus) in dorsal spine, (e) angular kyphus in dorsolumbar spine, (f) kyphoscoliotic deformity in upper lumbar spine

in posterior half of vertebral bodies hence it causes first obliteration of natural cervical and/or lumbar lordosis and later on kyphosis starts appearing. By the time a kyphosis appears in the spine, the disease is already in about three to four months of pathogenesis of the disease. About 95% cases show a clinically detectable kyphosis or reversal of normal lordosis, when patient reports for specialized treatment in developing countries.

Behavior of Kyphosis in Adults

The observations of behavior of kyphotic deformity are as under:

1. The kyphosis continues to grow while being treated. However, the progression of kyphosis can be minimized by prescribing suitable braces.
2. Patients treated non-operatively have an average increase of 15° in deformity and 3 to 5% end up with a deformity greater than 60°.
3. Kyphotic deformity increases more following surgical decompression in comparison to non-operative treatment.

4. Kyphosis also continues to grow in a TB spine lesion which is surgically decompressed and bridged by bone graft. The bone graft is most weak on the day it is implanted. As a result, graft-related complications such as graft slippage and breakage will give rise to progression of kyphosis.
5. The increase in deformity is more in patients who have a long segment disease necessitating a long bone graft after surgical decompression in a dorsal or dorsolumbar spine.
6. Kyphosis, once healed, with osseous fusion does not grow alarmingly in adults in later life. However, when the lesion heals with fibrous or fibro-osseous healing it may still progress.

Sequelae of Severe Kyphosis

Severe kyphosis on a long follow-up affects the biomechanics of the spine and body. The proximal and distal segments of the spine compensate by creating reverse deformity. The consequent degenerative process will produce back pain and/or radiculopathies. If a dorsal kyphosis is more than 60°, the spinal cord undergoes cord insult as a result of repeated stretching over internal salient and may develop clinical signs of upper motor neuron deficit, which has worse prognosis in comparison to paraplegia with active disease. The lumbar or lumbosacral kyphosis may produce a compensatory hyperlordosis proximally and distal to healed lesion. On a long follow-up, they develop evidence of severe lumbar canal stenosis. These morphological changes occur in both fusion mass and uninvolved level. The capacity of chest cavity and in turn vital capacity is also reduced. The costal margins come closer to iliac crest and diaphragm gets pushed into the chest cavity, reducing the vital capacity further. Ventilatory failure may develop after a gap of many years in patients with a severe thoracic kyphosis due to tuberculosis. Gradual impingement of costal margins over iliac crest may become painful.

Treatment of Spinal Tuberculosis with Kyphosis

The development of severe kyphosis and its sequelae can be prevented by: (a) Diagnosing TB spine early before a kyphosis develops, (b) identifying those TB spines which are likely to have severe kyphosis at the end of the treatment and likely to progress with growth. These patients with angular kyphosis should be undertaken for correction of kyphosis in active stage of disease.

1. Diagnosis of TB Spine in Predestructive (Well Before Deformity Develops) Stage

In TB spine, it takes 3–4 months in pathogenesis before kyphosis starts appearing. These patients continue to report with persistent low back pain with or without constitutional symptoms. Initially X-rays of these patients, may not have radiological finding. Such patients should be kept under observation in an endemic region for tuberculosis and if on sequential X-rays, with a gap of 6–8 weeks, show reduction of disk height they should be subjected to MRI. On MRI, they can be confidently labeled as TB spine, if the vertebrae show low signal in T1WI and hyperintense signal in T2WI, suggestive of inflammation with a septate pre- and paravertebral abscess, contiguous vertebral body involvement with preserved intervertebral disk. In the absence of such finding, a CT-guided needle biopsy will help reach an early diagnosis. The TB spine lesions, when diagnosed in predestructive stage of disease (inflammatory stage), may heal by uninterrupted ambulatory antitubercular chemotherapy with no or minimal sequelae of kyphosis.

2. Patients Report with Established Kyphotic Deformity

The objective of treatment in these patient is to ensure that kyphosis does not progress while on treatment. The pan-vertebral involvement should be ruled out on imaging, and if present such cases should be operated for instrumented stabilization. The kyphosis which is likely to progress on treatment needs to be kept under observation and for the need for surgical correction in active disease. The progression of kyphosis depends on number of vertebral body involvement, initial vertebral body loss and segment of spine affected.

One vertebral body height loss produces about 30°–35° kyphosis. The acceptable kyphosis may vary with different segment of spine. Tuli was of the opinion that if patients developed 60° or more kyphosis at dorsal or dorsolumbar spine they are likely to develop late onset paraplegia. With the increased life expectancy, these patients are likely to live longer and a localized kyphosis of 50°–60° may be disabling due to biomechanical stresses on proximal and distal segments of spine even though late onset paraplegia may not develop.

The kyphosis continues to increase on non-operative treatment. Rajasekaran and Soundarapandian suggested a formula to predict final kyphotic deformity in adult patients of TB spine; $Y = a + bx$, where Y is the final angle, "a" and "b" are the constant 5.5 and 30.5 respectively and x is the initial loss of height of vertebral body. Jain *et al.* observed the behavior of kyphotic angle in the spinal tuberculosis in 70 adult cases and observed that prediction of kyphosis is possible with this formula. However, the angle could be predicted by ±10°, hence any patient with initial vertebral body loss of 1.5 vertebral body height in dorsal and dorsolumbar spine will develop kyphosis of 50°±10°.

The kyphosis progresses more after surgical decompression. Rajasekaran *et al.* observed that anterior bone graft is able to provide sufficient stability and structural support in only 41% of patients with a short defect. Graft related complications occur when length of bone graft spans two vertebral body heights (4–5 cm). In all such instances, additional support in the form of extended bed rest, plaster jacket or instrumented stabilization is indicated.

All patients of TB spine, likely to heal with more than 50° kyphosis need a closer observation or kyphus correction surgery. Keeping that in mind any adult patients with three or more vertebral body affection with initial vertebral body loss of 1 to 1.5 vertebral body height in a dorsal or dorsolumbar spine, need to be taken up for kyphosis correction.

3. Kyphosis Correction in Active Disease

The outcome of treatment in TB spine is described with emphasis on kyphosis. Most of the studies describe one stage or two stage surgery to decompress the spinal cord and stabilize the spine with the objective to prevent post-treatment deterioration of kyphosis. Many studies have described anterior or posterior instrumentations to correct kyphosis or prevent on treatment deterioration of kyphosis. Unfortunately the variables to analyze kyphosis were not described by most of them. Jain and Dhammi analysed all series of TB spine where spinal instrumentation was performed and were published from 1986–2005. In cumulative cases with anterior instrumenta-tion (n = 635), mean 25° kyphosis was brought to 9° post-operatively and final kyphosis remained 11° while in posterior instrumented group (n = 369) mean kyphosis of 40° was corrected to 18° and which finally healed by 22°. It seems these surgeries were primarily done for stabilization of spine to prevent progression of kyphosis and not for correction of kyphosis. Very few studies cover the broad principles of kyphosis correction in spinal tuberculosis.

Angular kyphosis in spinal TB lesion has 3 or more vertebral body affection with loss of anterior body height but a few more may be inflamed. The spinal cord may be compressed anteriorly, with disk, granulation tissue and pus and meninges may be inflamed, hence more vulnerable for neural deterioration. Epidural blood vessels and intercostal and anterior spinal arteries may be thrombosed. The issues involved in kyphosis correction surgery include:

a. **Intraspinal compression** by retropulsion of disk, granulation tissue and bony sequestrum. Correction of the kyphosis without opening the anterior disease area and without anterior decompression will correct soft deformity in active disease but will produce more prominent spinal cord compression by retropulsed fragment (internal salient) and consequently neural deficit. Hence internal salient should be removed by anterior debridement and corpectomy.

b. Moderate to severe kyphosis warranting deformity correc-tion is a long-standing problem. The vertebral column is shortened anteriorly and spinal cord has adjusted to a shortened length. The abrupt correction of kyphosis will produce lengthening of anterior column. This will stretch the spinal cord with consequent neural deficit. Thus it is desirable to shorten the vertebral column posteriorly.

c. The anterior corpectomy and posterior column shortening leave the the spine grossly unstable. Hence posterior instrumented stabilization with anterior gap grafting and posterior fusion need to be performed.

The anterior implant may not stabilize the spine in view of anterior corpectomy and posterior column shortening hence posterior instrumentation is desirable.

Final steps of the kyphosis correction in TB spine involves anterior corpectomy to achieve anterior decompression, shortening of posterior column, posterior instrumentation and anterior and posterior bone grafting. Ideally both steps should be undertaken in the same sitting and sequentialy. In whole procedure, the spinal cord should be kept under vision and correction of kyphosis should be so gradual that the spinal cord is not damaged.

The surgical approaches for kyphosis correction in spinal TB are:

1. Single stage transpedicular approach
2. Single or two-staged anterior decompression with bone grafting
3. Single stage kyphosis correction by extrapleural anterolateral approach.

a. Single Stage Transpedicular Approach

Guven *et al.* (1994) described anterior decompression by posterior midline exposure. The vertebral column was stabilized by posterior stabilization with two vertebrae on either side of dorsal spine and one in lumbar spine by pedicle screw fixation. This procedure was performed to prevent postsurgery progression of kyphosis. The author reported only 3.4° loss of correction till complete healing of disease where seven cases had two vertebral body disease and three had one vertebral body disease. Laheri *et al.* reported 28 patients of post-tubercular kyphosis (mean 64.3°) where the patients were operated in prone position. Posterolateral retropleural approach was used. A midline incision was made centering at kyphosis. A costotransversectomy and excision of pedicle was carried out at the apex of the kyphosis. The abscess was drained, granulation tissue and bony sequestrum were debrided and spinal cord was decompressed. All bony tissues and soft tissues preventing the correction of kyphosis were removed. Segmental spinal instrumentation using Hartshill rectangle with sublaminar wiring or pedicle instrumentation was done and kyphosis is gradually corrected. The author was careful in achieving gradual kyphosis correction to avoid the streching of the spinal cord. The anterior defect was subsequently grafted.

Lee *et al*. reported single stage transpedicular decompression and posterior instrumentation in active TB spine lesion where bone distruction was less (n = 10) and compared with anterior decompression fusion and anterior instrumentation (n = 7). This was not aimed at kyphosis correction and mean preoperative kyphosis was corrected from 18°–20° to 14°–16°. Gokce *et al*. reported correction of sagittal balance in 12 TB spine cases with kyphosis by posterior closing wedge osteotomy with posterior instrumented fusion. The patients were taken in prone position and posterior approach was used. The level to be instrumented were exposed to the tips of transverse process at lumbar and to costal attachment at thoracic region. The pedicle screws are inserted and temporary stabilization was done. Laminectomy and posterior decompression of the apex vertebrae was performed. At the apex of the deformity, soft tissue on the lateral wall of the pedicle and vertebral body to be removed are dissected bluntly and elevated on both sides. The cancellous bones were curetted until only the residual bony cortex remained. The adjacent end plates and posterior part of the vertebral body attached to the posterior longitudinal ligament were removed. The wedge-shaped portion of the cortical bone at the vertebral body was removed. Gradual closure of the spine was done with closing dorsally based osteotomy site. The author reports correction of kyphosis from 51.1° to 23° in lower dorsal and dorsolumbar spine.

b. Single or Two-Staged Anterior and Posterior Surgery

The correction of kyphosis could be achieved by anterior decompression followed by posterior instrumentation. After anterior decompression by transthoracic transpleural or retroperitoneal approach, the gap may be filled by the bone graft. 2–3 weeks later the posterior instrumentation can be performed.

Moon performed posterior instrumentation first followed by transthoracic decompression and anterior bone grafting two weeks later in earlier part of the study. However, later on he performed both in the same sitting. The mean preoperative, immediate postoperative kyphosis and final kyphosis were 37°, 16° and 18°, respectively. These cases did not have severe kyphosis. He primarily aimed at prevention of deterioration of kyphosis and not for kyphosis correction.

Louw reported a series of 19 patients of TB spine of dorsal and dorsolumbar region with neural deficit. He performed transthoracic transpleural anterior decompression and vascularized rib grafting, during the same procedure (n = 13) or 2 weeks later (n = 6) by shortening of posterior column by multilevel posterior osteotomy, instrumentation and fusion. Thus overall anterior column length was not altered and kyphosis was corrected with anterior graft acting as a pivot. The mean preoperative kyphosis could be corrected from 56 to 27°.

c. Single Stage Kyphosis Correction by Extrapleural Anterolateral Approach

The author believes that procedure for kyphus correction in spinal tuberculosis is anterior decompression/corpectomy followed by posterior column shortening, instrumented stabilization and reconstruction of anterior gap by bone graft sequentially in one stage. The patient is placed in a lateral position and a T-shaped posterior incision of about 14–15 cm is made with the center of lesion in the apex of the kyphosis and the transverse incision about 8 cm from the midline and perpendicular to it at the apex of kyphosis on left side. Standard extrapleural anterolateral decompression is performed after removing posterior 6–8 cm of 3 ribs at the apex of the lesion. The diseased apex vertebral body is removed as far as possible to the opposite side. The anterior wound is now packed. The posterior paraspinal exposure is done to expose three segments on either side of apex vertebrae. The space for passing sublaminar wire is created and sublaminar wires are passed. Now Hartshill rectangle is selected and a prebend shape is given. The spinous process, laminae, pedicles of the vertebrae at apex of kyphosis are removed. The posterior part of the rib attached at the apex vertebrae on right side is also removed. At this stage, the spinal cord has no bone around it. The sublaminar wires are tightened first distally and then proximally to gradually correct the kyphosis. At all times, spinal cord is kept under vision and correction is carefully achieved to ensure that spinal cord is not elongated. Once correction is achieved, the anterior grafting is performed from iliac crest graft. The ribs are used as bone graft for posterior spinal fusion. The wakeup test should be done for all those who have no neural deficit.

The advantages of this procedure are:
1. Patient is in lateral position; hence remains stable all the time to obviate the need of temporary stabilization.
2. Chest cavity and retroperitoneal exposure is not required, hence it is less morbid.
3. It provides simultaneous exposure of anterior and posterior columns of the spine, thereby allowing opportunity to perform anterior and posterior procedure simultaneously.
4. Kyphosis from D2 to L2 can be corrected by this approach.

Kyphosis Correction in Healed Lesion

Severe kyphosis produces progressive restriction of pulmonary functions. In one study, out of 23 patients of severe kyphosis, 11 had more than 50% restriction of pulmonary functions, while 10 had between 25 and 50% and 2 had mild restriction of pulmonary functions. Correction of such severe kyphosis of long standing is a technically demanding surgery with higher risk of neurologic injury. Yau has performed a multi-staged surgery where anterior osteotomy and decompression was performed after fitting a halo pelvic distractor. In second stage, posterior osteotomy and fusion was done. As a third stage, again anterior fusion was done. The patient was maintained in halo pelvic distractor till sound fusion was achieved. The mean preoperative kyphosis in this series was 115.5° and the correction obtained was 28.3°. Three patients out of 29 died. The author concluded that it may be a relatively small reward for such a major undertaking. Such treatment should be instituted where deformity is severe with active disease and paraplegia or death from chest complication is imminent. Yau and many other authors later on also believed that for patients with healed disease in whom danger of paraplegia and rapid progression of deformity are less, the hazard of deformity correction outweighs the gain hence it should not be carried out for cosmetic reasons only. Even for late onset paraplegia, the surgeon should not be too ambitious to correct deformity and the patient should be forewarned about the risk of neural deterioration and life risk.

Transpedicular decancellation osteotomy has also been described for correction of healed post-tubercular kyphosis at dorsolumbar spine. Here again pedicle screws are placed two to three vertebrae above and below. Temporary rod stabilization on one side is done. The laminectomy of the apex vertebra is done. The egg shell decancellation of the vertebral body (kyphotic mass) was performed through pedicle preserving medial wall of pedicle. Once decancellation is done or adjacent disks are removed from the adjacent side of the vertebral bodies, the rods are contoured and placed bilaterally. The reduction is carried out via sequential compression on the rods until posterior elements start touching. The thecal sac is constantly kept under observation during the reduction.

This method has been reported with a successful correction of kyphosis in dorsolumbar and lumbar kyphosis with mean preoperative kyphosis correction from 29.9° to 12.2° and mean preoperative kyphosis from 58.8° to 13.7° respectively in two series.

Late Onset Paraplegia or Paraplegia with Healed Disease (Fig. 5.15)

These patients report with long-standing severe kyphosis with a history of being treated for spinal TB, 10 or more years ago and now present with signs of upper motor neuron paraparesis/paraplegia. The cause may be a reactivation of old healed lesion at kyphus or intrinsic changes in spinal cord due to continued stretch on the internal salient. Anterior decompression and fusion is advocated in all such cases. The internal salient is

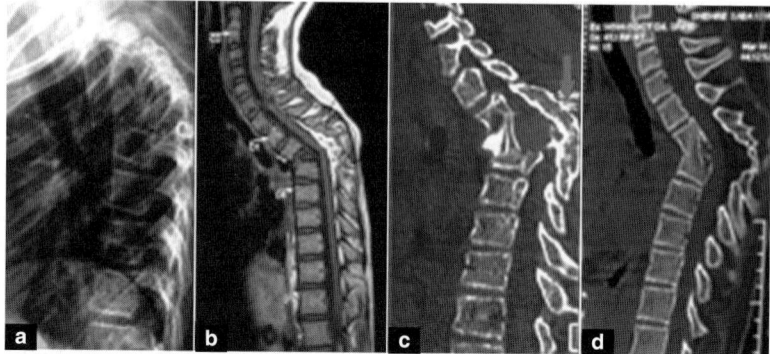

Fig. 5.15: Showing preoperative (a) X-ray lateral view, (b) sagittal T1WI MRI shows kyphus deformity internal gibbus at D3 in an 11-year-old girl following old childhood diseases. The lesion has no activity. (c) Immediate postoperative sagittal reconstruction image shows internal kyphectomy and anterior transposition of the spinal cord, (d) same image at one year follow-up shows incorporated bone graft (Adapted from Jain AK, Sreenivasan R, Mukunth R, Dhammi IK. Tubercular spondylitis in children. *Indian J Orthop* 2014 Mar;48(2):136–44)

removed either by transthoracic transpleural anterior approach or by the extrapleural anterolateral approach. The internal kyphectomy allows spinal cord to transpose anteriorly. The response to anterior decompression is faster, better and safe in patients with active disease. While in patients with healed disease the anterior decompression is technically more difficult and the recovery less satisfactory. Complications, such as neural deterioration (transient or permanent) and CSF fistula, have been reported and patient should be warned before the surgery about the possibility of neural deterioration.

Since these patients already have a compromised pulmonary function extrapleural anterolateral or costotransversectomy approach is advocated. It also allows direct exposure of internal salient and it does not jeopardize the already compromised pulmonary function. Here the posterior 5 cm of three crowded ribs at apex are removed along with the transverse processes. Care is needed to remain extrapleural or retroperitoneal. Segmental intercostal nerves serve as a guide to intervertebral foramina. Two or three pedicles at apex are removed and dura is seen. One or more intercostal vessels are ligated. The pleura is elevated at the apex of kyphosis. The removal of posterior half of the collapsed vertebrae is done with a high-speed burr leaving behind posterior rim until last to avoid forward migration of dural sac. This allows spinal cord to be transposed anteriorly and adequate length of anterior dura is exposed. Cortical strut grafting is performed as far anteriorly as possible after exposing the proximal and distal limits of angular kyphus. Generally, these patients develop spontaneous posterior spinal fusion hence remain relatively stable inspite of internal kyphectomy.

TB SPINE IN CHILDREN: ONSET OF DEFORMITY

TB spine is reported in infants as latent tuberculosis. The spinal tuberculosis in children is a different disease entity than in adults. The vertebral bodies in children are cartilaginous. Younger the child, larger is the cartilage volume in each vertebral body. Hence, whenever a tubercular infection affects the vertebral bodies, the cartilage loss occurs rapidly and severe deformities occur within a short span of time (Fig. 5.16). Younger is the child, more severe is the expected deformity (Fig. 5.17). The spinal deformities once developed as a result of TB progresses with growth. The growth potential is also damaged due to the disease and secondary to surgical

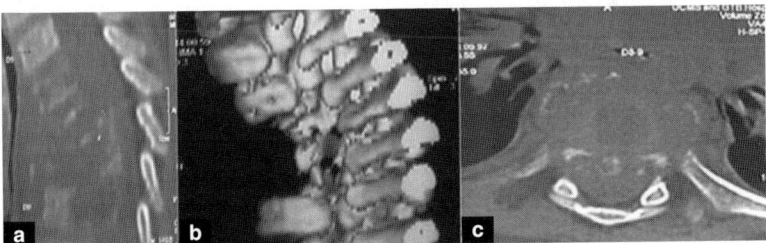

Fig. 5.16: (a) Computed tomography (CT) scan (sagittal section) of upper dorsal spine in a 3-year-old child shows 5 vertebral body disease. The vertebral body almost disappeared, (b) on 3D reconstruction and (c) axial CT shows no trace of bone in VB. (Adapted from Jain AK, Sreenivasan R, Mukunth R, Dhammi IK. Tubercular spondylitis in children. *Indian J Orthop.* 2014 Mar;48(2):136–44)

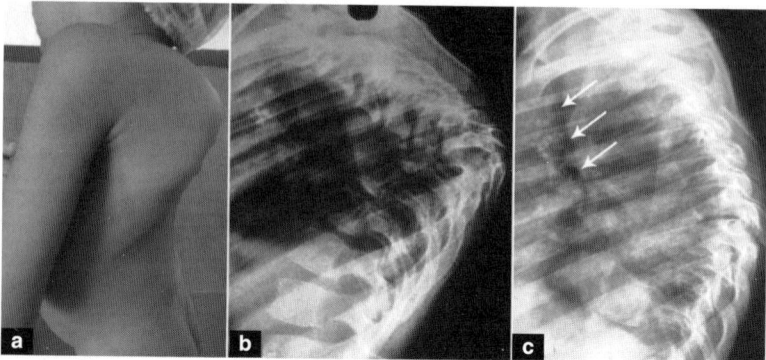

Fig. 5.17: (a) Clinical photograph of a 6-year-old child reported with severe kyphosis following long segment tuberculosis of spine, (b) lateral X-ray shows severe kyphosis with destruction of D5-9 vertebral bodies, (c) the lateral X-ray of the same patient taken 3 months before (which patient was carrying) also shows widening of prevertebral soft tissue shadow seen as deviation of tracheal shadow infront of upper dorsal spine (white arrows). The diagnosis was missed at this stage. (Adapted from Jain AK, Sreenivasan R, Mukunth R, Dhammi IK. Tubercular spondylitis in children. *Indian J Orthop* 2014 Mar;48(2):136–44)

intervention. The growth potential is lost when anterior corpectomy is performed.

The Dimeglio "formula" states that for each vertebral segment 0.7 mm per year of longitudinal growth is lost after posterior arthrodesis. The progression of kyphosis in a solidly fused kyphotic block was studied by Schultz (1997). He compared the kyphosis progression in a group of children where (a) only anterior debridment was performed, (b) anterior radical resection was performed, (c) anterior radical resection and posterior fusion was performed.When posterior fusion is added to the anterior radical resection and fusion, the progression of deformity was not severe as the posterior growth was also retarded. Where only anterior debridement was done, the progression of the deformity was the least because the anterior growth potential is retained partially. The authors concluded that the radical anterior surgery destroys the anterior growth and limits the capacity for spinal remodeling and posterior column does contribute to some growth. Upadhyay compared the observations in 2 groups of radical resection and debridement surgeries on a 15.3 years follow-up and concluded that there is no evidence to suggest that the disproportionate posterior growth contributes to progression of deformity after anterior spinal fusion in children. In another series, he compared a group of children (n = 29) with mean age of 4.3 years to a series of adult patients (n = 34) who were part of MRC series at Hong Kong and only debridement was performed without anterior bone grafting. A 6 months, one year and final mean follow up of 15.6 years observed no progress in kyphotic deformity in children and adults and that the deformity corrected at dorsolumbar junction to a small extent to suggest a preserved growth potential even after debridement surgery. Rajasekaran reported in a series of TB spine in children with long follow up (a natural history of kyphotic deformity progression with growth) and reported that in 44% cases of TB spine kyphosis does not progress, 17% remains stationary and in 39% deformity progresses.

Diagnosis of TB Spine in Children

The clinical presentation is almost similar to adults. The children report with persistent localized back pain, loss of appetite, and inability to walk. The child is pale, listless and anemic. They have a cautious gait and tend to walk keeping both hands at thigh to support the trunk. If the cervical spine is involved, they walk supporting the head with both hands. On clinical examination, one may find a knuckle/angular spinal deformity with or without a local/distant palpable cold abscess. They may present with variable severity of the kyphosis on first presentation (Fig. 5.18) TB spine in children is suspected clinically and the diagnosis can be confidently made on plain X-rays and other imaging (MRI) observations supported by raised ESR and positive Mantoux test.

Treatment

The drug therapy is similar to adults except that we need to prescribe the drugs as per weight of the child.

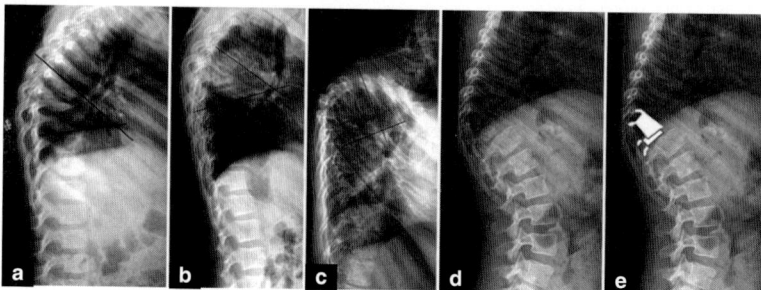

Fig. 5.18: Lateral X-rays of spine in 3 children show (a, b) moderate kyphotic deformity, (c) severe kyphotic deformity following TB of spine. (d, e) Lateral X-rays and two bodies shown in white showing the proximal vertebrae resting on anterior surface on to distal vertebrae. (Adapted from Jain AK, Sreenivasan R, Mukunth R, Dhammi IK. Tubercular spondylitis in children. *Indian J Orthop* 2014 Mar;48(2):136–44)

Precautions while prescribing ATT in children:

1. Avoid underdosing of individual drugs in children
2. Modification of drug dosage when child gains weight on treatment. Hence, ATT dosage should be adjusted by weight on every follow-up visit.
3. Avoid inappropriate formulations particularly for infants.

The drugs which are toxic to children, such as streptomycin and ethambutol, are given with due care to avoid the development of toxicity.

Generally uncomplicated spinal tuberculosis is to be treated with ATT and suitable orthoses. Once they develop neural deficit, the spinal lesion is to be evaluated for instability in term of panvertebral disease. Such lesions should be stabilized. The spinal deformity in TB spine has a serious consideration and clinical presentation. We need to be watchful for kyphosis. The patient may repair will varying grades of kyphotic deformity on presentation. There are 2 scenarios of clinical presentation in TB spine with active disease:

1. Patients with active disease and no clinical kyphosis
2. Patients with active disease and kyphosis.

Patients with Active Disease and No Clinical Kyphosis

In patients with TB spine with no or minimal kyphosis, the treatment principle, diagnosis, drug therapy are the same as for adults. TB spine without neural deficit is treated by ambulant chemotherapy. Surgery is indicated for neural deficit which appears during course of treatment and/or associated with unstable spine. The patients should be kept under observation while on treatment for appearance/progression of kyphosis. The patient should be evaluated once a year for the appearance/progression of the kyphosis till skeletal maturity after ATT is stopped and patient has achieved a healed status.

Patients with Active Disease and Kyphosis

These patients already have kyphotic deformity of some severity when they report first for the treatment of spinal TB. The disease heals under the influence of ATT but kyphosis either will remain stationary or progresses/reduces while on treatment and thereafter in growth phase. Rajasekaran has reported the natural history of kyphosis in children (n = 63). The deformity of spine continues to increase in active phase and even after healing of disease (Fig. 5.19). The progression of deformity depends on severity of angle before treatment, level of lesion and age of the patients. In children less than 7 years of age, with 3 or more vertebral body affection in dorsal

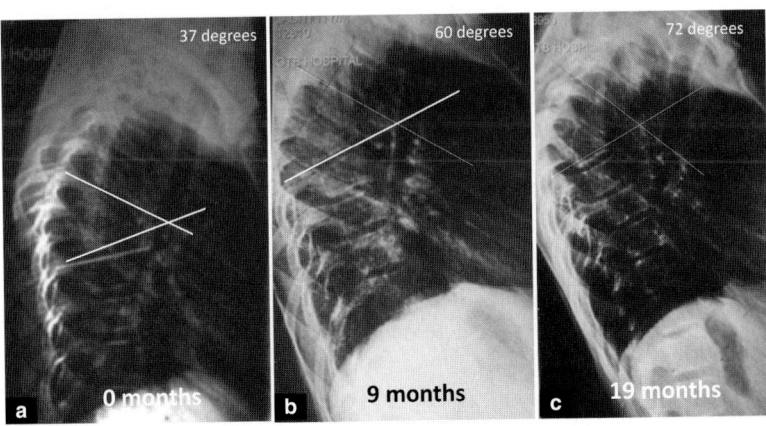

Fig. 5.19: Progression of kyphotic angle on serial radiographs of 12-year-old female child after completion of ATT. (a) X-rays at the time of completion of ATT, (b) 9 months post-completion of ATT, (c) 19 months post-completion of ATT

or dorsolumbar spine, the deformity produced is severe and it progresses further, and the patients continue to live with severely deformed spine.

These patients, on long follow-up, are likely to develop severe lumbar canal stenosis and/or late onset paraplegia. They develop cardiorespiratory embarrassment with painful costo-pelvic impingement. They are a bad risk case for major surgical undertaking. The correction of such severe kyphosis is hazardous and fraught with complications as most of the systems/organs have adapted to the long-standing deformed spine. Once they develop late onset paraplegia, the prognosis becomes further poor. The spinal cord undergoes atrophic or myelomalacic/syringomyelic changes, as a result of movement of spinal cord over angular internal salient like the strings of a violin. Since the degree of vascular or intrinsic damage of the spinal cord is not known, any inadvertent handling of the spinal cord while excising hard internal salient would have a risk of neural deterioration and consequent delayed or poor neural recovery.

The best treatment of all such sequelae is prevention by early diagnosis well before a deformity develop to achieve healing with no or minimal deformity or correction of kyphotic deformity in active stage of the disease.

The progression of the kyphosis occurs as a result of anterior growth loss and continuing posterior column growth. The summation of number of vertebral affection also decides the progression of kyphosis. When a spine lesion heals, it either heals with a bone block formation or fibro-osseous or fibrous healing. The lesion heals primarily with fibrous and fibro-osseous healing till eventually an anterior fusion mass is formed. If the disease segment does not heal with bone block, the proximal segment of the spine keeps on collapsing on distal spine till it stabilizes and thus kyphosis eventually increases. This progressive kyphosis leads to facet subluxation, toppling at some stage and eventually the deformity becomes fixed.

Progression of Kyphosis in Children

The kyphotic spine produces asymmetric loading on the disease segment. As a result, some part of kyphotic block grows faster

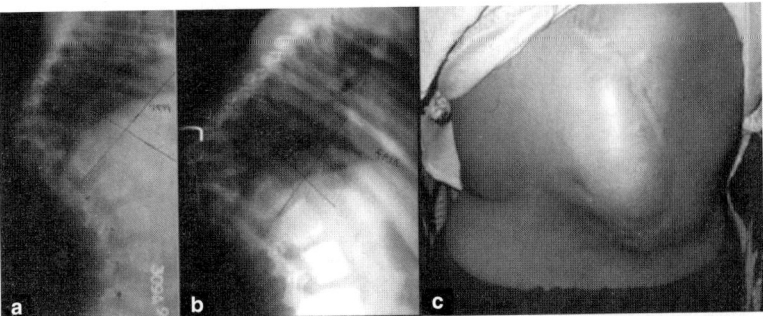

Fig. 5.20: Lateral X-ray of a dorsolumbar spine (a) shows a severe kyphosis secondary to childhood tuberculosis spine with complete destruction of D9-11. This kyphosis is expected to grow with growth. Lateral X-ray of the same patients, (b) 2½ years later shows progression of kyphosis in spite of successful posterior spinal fusion. Clinical photograph, (c) of the same patient shows deformity and scar of posterior fusion (Adapted from Jain AK, Dhammi IK, Jain S, Mishra P. Kyphosis in spinal tuberculosis – Prevention and correction. *Indian J Orthop* 2010 Apr;44(2):127–36)

than others and this asymmetric growth of vertebral body produces progression of kyphosis. The internal salient is off loaded and grows faster ending uncontrolled growth of internal salient to produce cord compression. The segment of growing kyphotic block which is not loaded grows faster and is added to apex of kyphosis and consequently the indentation of the spinal cord by internal salient also increases. The kyphosis continues to increase even if posterior spinal fusion alone is performed (Fig. 5.20).

Rajasekaran (2001) suggested 4 **spine at risk signs** (Fig. 5.21). They are **facet subluxation, retropulsion, toppling and, lateral translation**. The presence of 2 or more signs are indicative of a progressive kyphosis. Lateral translation can only occur in a panvertebral lesion when posterior complex is also destroyed along with the vertebral body disease. This is a potentially unstable spine, hence considered a bad prognostic sign for neural loss and progression of kyphotic deformity. Retropulsion, facet subluxation or toppling signs are usually observed in severe kyphosis. The intervertebral disk is ballooned and well hydrated in children. It retains its shape

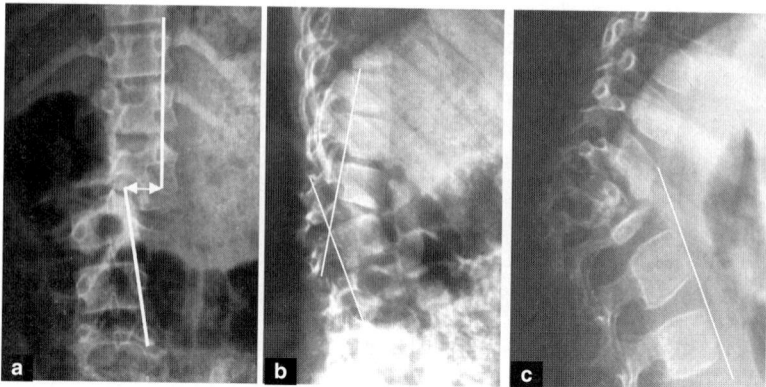

Fig. 5.21: X-rays with 'spine at risk signs': (a) Lateral translation, (b) retropulsion and facetal separation, (c) toppling, facetal separation and retropulsion (only toppling shown for clarity)

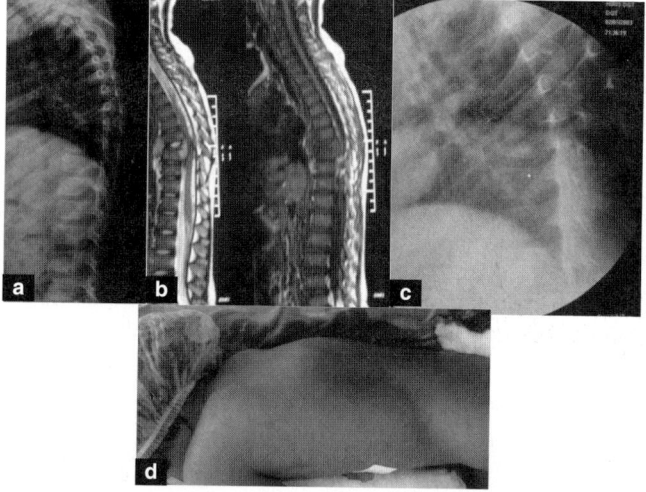

Fig. 5.22: A plain X-ray (a) lateral view of dorsolumbar spine of a 5-year-old child shows paradiscal tubercular lesion at D6–D8. MRI, (b) (T1WI and T2WI sagittal sections) shows all classical findings of infective lesion. Patient was treated with ambulatory chemotherapy. At 5-month follow-up, mother of the child noticed that the deformity increases on standing while reduces on lying down, (d) X-ray under fluoroscopy, (c) shows a cleavage (arrow) between D6 and D8 vertebral body. Child was taken for anterior bone grafting and posterior Hartshill fixation using extrapleural anterolateral approach

and size in children when the disease heals under the influence of ATT. The disk still continues to maintain its shape and does not allow proximal spine to stabilize on distal segment. Consequently, the children have an unstable spine and deformity progresses on vertical loading (Fig. 5.22).

We have to identify those kyphotic deformities which are likely to show progression of kyphosis during the treatment and subsequently in healed stage of disease (Fig. 5.19). The posterior spinal fusion used to be advocated as a method to halt posterior column growth to stop progression of the kyphosis. It was observed that all spines have features of progressive kyphosis. The kyphosis continues to increase in spite of successful posterior spinal fusion (Fig. 5.20). The posterior spinal fusion can only succeed in preventing progression of kyphosis if patients do not have features suggestive of progressive kyphosis which even otherwise will not show significant progression of kyphosis. In all such instances, it is better to correct these kyphotic deformities in active stage of disease (Fig. 5.23).

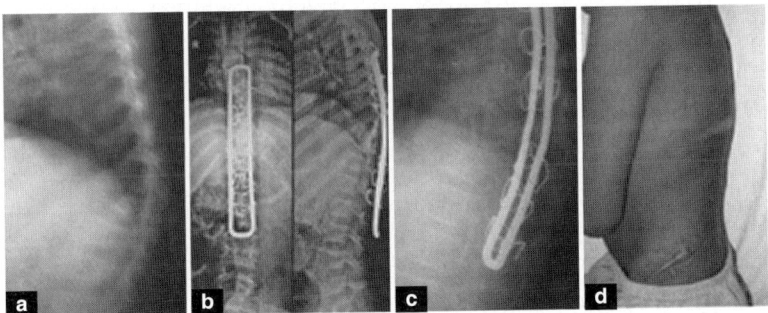

Fig. 5.23: A 5-year-old child with TB of spine on antitubercular treatment for 6 months presented with a radiological signs of progressive kyphotic deformity (a) Standard extrapleural anterolateral decompression was done with stabilization using a closed Hartshill (b and c) was done (d) clinical photograph showing the surgical scar over iliac crest and healed posterior T-incision (Adapted from Jain AK, Sreenivasan R, Mukunth R, Dhammi IK. Tubercular spondylitis in children. *Indian J Orthop* 2014 Mar;48(2): 136–44)

Summarily, all these children who are younger and have 3 or more vertebral body affection in a dorsal or dorsolumbar spine are likely to have progression of kyphosis and hence are indicated for surgical correction of spinal deformity (Fig. 5.23).

INSTRUMENTATION IN CHILDREN

The vertebral bodies in children are smaller. As a result of kyphotic deformity and active disease, the paraspinal muscles are thinner. It is difficult to procure adequate size pedicle screw in very young children (less than 5 years). The profile of pedicle screw is likely to produce ischemia of skin and consequent wound dehiscence or ulcer. In a very young child, the Hartshill rectangle which is open at distal end becomes a good implant. However, it should be bent properly and seated in soft tissue. The children should be placed in a Minerva jacket for 3–4 months till such time anterior and posterior fusion is achieved. In immediate postoperative period, it is advised to keep the child is lateral positions to prevent ischemic insult to skin between matress and metallic implement and may lead to consequent wound dehiscence. The parents should be advised not to take children on shoulder least the anterior graft/cage collapse, if fusion is not achieved anteriorly.

BIBLIOGRAPHY

1. Agarwal A, Arora A, Kumar S. A survey of prescribing pattern for osteoarticular tuberculosis: orthopaedic surgeons' and infectious disease experts' perspective. Indian J Tuberc 2009;56-4:201–5.

2. Arora A, Nadkarni B, Dev G, Chattopadhya D, Jain AK, Tuli SM, Kumar S. The use of immunomodulators as an adjunct to antituberculous chemotherapy in non-responsive patients with osteo-articular tuberculosis. J Bone Joint Surg Br 2006;88-2:264–9.

3. Breton G, Bourgarit A, Pavy S, Bonnet D, Martinez V, Duval X, Longuet P, Abgrall S, Simon A, Leport C. Treatment for tuberculosis-associated immune reconstitution inflammatory syndrome in 34 HIV-infected patients. Int J Tuberc Lung Dis 2012;16-10:1365–70.

4. Bhojraj S, Nene A. Lumbar and lumbosacral tuberculous spondylodiscitis in adults. Redefining the indications for surgery. J Bone Joint Surg Br 2002;84-4:530–4.

5. Bezer M, Kucukdurmaz F, Guven O. Transpedicular decancellation osteotomy in the treatment of posttuberculous kyphosis. J Spinal Disord Tech 2007;20-3:209–15.

6. Barclay WR, Ebert RH, Le Roy GV, Manthei RW, Roth LJ. Distribution and excretion of radioactive isoniazid in tuberculous patients. J Am Med Assoc 1953;151-16:1384–8.

7. Crofton J, Mitchison DA. Streptomycin resistance in pulmonary tuberculosis. Br Med J 1948;2-4588:1009–15.

8. Comroe JH, Jr. Pay dirt: the story of streptomycin. Part I. From Waksman to Waksman. Am Rev Respir Dis 1978;117-4:773–81.

9. Cameron JA, Robinson CL, Robertson DE. The radical treatment of Pott's disease and Pott's paraplegia by extirpation of the diseased area and anterior spinal fusion. Am Rev Respir Dis 1962;86:76–80.

10. Chahal AS, Jyoti SP. The radical treatment of tuberculosis of the spine. Int Orthop 1980;4-2:93–9.

11. Cheung WY, Luk KD. Clinical and radiological outcomes after conservative treatment of TB spondylitis: is the 15 years' follow-up in the MRC study long enough? Eur Spine J 2013;22 Suppl 4:594–602.

12. Chaisson RE. Treatment of chronic infections with rifamycins: is resistance likely to follow? Antimicrob Agents Chemother 2003;47-10:3037–9.

13. Crofton J, Mitchison DA. Streptomycin resistance in pulmonary tuberculosis. Br Med J 1948;2-4588:1009–15.

14. Cardoso RF, Cooksey RC, Morlock GP, Barco P, Cecon L, Forestiero F, Leite CQ, Sato DN, Shikama Mde L, Mamizuka EM, Hirata RD, Hirata MH. Screening and characterization of mutations in isoniazid-resistant Mycobacterium tuberculosis isolates obtained in Brazil. Antimicrob Agents Chemother 2004;48-9:3373–81.

15. Chen WJ, Wu CC, Jung CH, Chen LH, Niu CC, Lai PL. Combined anterior and posterior surgeries in the treatment of spinal tuberculous spondylitis. Clin Orthop Relat Res 2002-398:50–9.

16. Crenshaw AH. Surgical techniques and approaches. In: Canale ST Beaty J, ed. Campbell's Operative Orthopaedics, 11th ed. Pennsylvania, USA: Mosby Elsevier, 2008.

17. Capener N. The evolution of lateral rhachotomy. J Bone Joint Surg Br 1954;36-B-2:173–9.

18. Consigilieri G, Kakarla UK, Theodore N. Pott disease in a 13-month-old: case report. Neurosurgery 2011;68-5:E1485-90; discussion E90.

19. Controlled clinical trial of four short-course regimens of chemotherapy for two durations in the treatment of pulmonary tuberculosis: first report: Third East African/British Medical Research Councils study. Am Rev Respir Dis 1978;118-1:39–48.

20. Controlled clinical trial of four short-course regimens of chemotherapy for two durations in the treatment of pulmonary tuberculosis. Second report. Third East African/British Medical Research Council Study. Tubercle 1980;61-2:59–69.

21. de Bruyn G, Garner P. Mycobacterium vaccae immunotherapy for treating tuberculosis. Cochrane Database Syst Rev 2003-1:CD001166.

22. Dott NM. Skeletal traction and anterior decompression in the management of Pott's paraplegia. Edinb Med J 1947;54-11-12:620–7.

23. Dlugovitzky D, Fiorenza G, Farroni M, Bogue C, Stanford C, Stanford J. Immunological consequences of three doses of heat-killed Mycobacterium vaccae in the immunotherapy of tuberculosis. Respir Med 2006;100-6:1079–87.

24. Dlugovitzky D, Notario R, Martinel-Lamas D, Fiorenza G, Farroni M, Bogue C, Stanford C, Stanford J. Immunotherapy with oral, heat-killed, Mycobacterium vaccae in patients with moderate to advanced pulmonary tuberculosis. Immunotherapy 2010;2-2:159–69. Dlugovitzky D, Stanford C, Stanford J. Immunological basis for the introduction of immunotherapy with Mycobacterium vaccae into the routine treatment of TB. Immunotherapy 2011;3-4:557–68.

25. Dooley S, Simone M. The extent and management of drug-resistant tuberculosis: the American experience. Clinical Tuberculosis. In: Davis PDO, ed. London: Chapman and Hall 1994:171–89.

26. David HL. Probability distribution of drug-resistant mutants in unselected populations of Mycobacterium tuberculosis. Appl Microbiol 1970;20-5:810–4.

27. Desai SS. Early diagnosis of spinal tuberculosis by MRI. J Bone Joint Surg Br 1994;76-6:863–9.

28. Dureja S, Sen IB, Acharya S. Potential role of F18 FDG PET-CT as an imaging biomarker for the noninvasive evaluation in uncomplicated skeletal tuberculosis: a prospective clinical observational study. Eur Spine J 2014;23-11:2449–54.

29. Dickinson JM, Mitchison DA. In vitro studies on the choice of drugs for intermittent chemotherapy of tuberculosis. Tubercle 1966;47-4:370–80.

30. Dickinson JM, Ellard GA, Mitchison DA. Suitability of isoniazid and ethambutol for intermittent administration in the treatment of tuberculosis. Tubercle 1968;49-4:351–66.

31. Dickinson JM, Mitchison DA. Suitability of rifampicin for intermittent administration in the treatment of tuberculosis. Tubercle 1970;51-1:82–94.

32. Dimeglio A, Ferran JL. [Three-dimensional analysis of the hip during growth]. Acta Orthop Belg 1990;56-1 Pt A:111–4.

33. Eighth Report of the Medical Research Council Working Party on Tuberculosis of the Spine. A 10-year assessment of a controlled trial comparing debridement and anterior spinal fusion in the management of tuberculosis of the spine in patients on standard chemotherapy in Hong Kong. J Bone Joint Surg Br 1982;64-4:393–8.

34. East African/British Medical Research C. Controlled clinical trial of four short-course (6-month) regimens of chemotherapy for treatment of pulmonary tuberculosis. The Lancet 1973;301-7816:1331–9.

35. Fine PEM, Carneiro, I.A.M., Milstein, J.B., Clements, C.J Issues relating to the use of BCG in immunization programs. Geneva: DEPARTMENT OF VACCINES AND BIOLOGICALS, WHO, 1999.

36. Fellander M. Radical operation in tuberculosis of the spine. Acta Orthop Scand Suppl 1955;19:1–117.

37. Francis IM, Das DK, Luthra UK, Sheikh Z, Sheikh M, Bashir M. Value of radiologically guided fine needle aspiration cytology (FNAC) in the diagnosis of spinal tuberculosis: a study of 29 cases. Cytopathology 1999;10-6:390–401.

38. Fellander M, Hiertonn T, Wallmark G. Studies on the concentration of streptomycin the treatment of bone and joint tuberculosis. Acta Tuberc Scand 1952;27-3-5:176–89.

39. Friedman B. Chemotherapy of tuberculosis of the spine. J Bone Joint Surg Am 1966;48-3:451–74.

40. Fourteenth report of the Medical Research Council Working Party on Tuberculosis of the Spine. Five-year assessment of controlled trials of short-course chemotherapy regimens of 6, 9 or 18 months' duration for spinal tuberculosis in patients ambulatory from the start or undergoing radical surgery. Int Orthop 1999;23-2:73–81.

41. Ge Z, Wang Z, Wei M. Measurement of the concentration of three antituberculosis drugs in the focus of spinal tuberculosis. Eur Spine J 2008;17-11:1482–7.

42. Goel MK. Treatment of Pott's paraplegia by operation. J Bone Joint Surg Br 1967;49-4:674–81.

43. Guven O, Kumano K, Yalcin S, Karahan M, Tsuji S. A single stage posterior approach and rigid fixation for preventing kyphosis in the treatment of spinal tuberculosis. Spine (Phila Pa 1976) 1994;19-9:1039–43.

44. Gokce A, Ozturkmen Y, Mutlu S, Caniklioglu M. Spinal osteotomy: correcting sagittal balance in tuberculous spondylitis. J Spinal Disord Tech 2008;21-7:484–8.

45. Hodgson AR, Stock FE. Anterior spinal fusion a preliminary communication on the radical treatment of Pott's disease and Pott's paraplegia. Br J Surg 1956;44-185:266–75.

46. HJ S. Pott's paraplegia-prognosis and treatment. Br J Surg 1935;22:769–99

47. Hever E, Risko T. Studies on streptomycin levels of blood and abscess. Acta Tuberc Scand 1960;38:40–50.

48. Heym B, Alzari PM, Honore N, Cole ST. Missense mutations in the catalase-peroxidase gene, katG, are associated with isoniazid resistance in Mycobacterium tuberculosis. Mol Microbiol 1995;15-2:235–45.

49. Held M, Laubscher M, Zar HJ, Dunn RN. GeneXpert polymerase chain reaction for spinal tuberculosis: an accurate and rapid diagnostic test. Bone Joint J 2014;96-b-10:1366–9.

50. Hodgson AR, Stock FE, Fang HS, Ong GB. Anterior spinal fusion. The operative approach and pathological findings in 412 patients with Pott's disease of the spine. Br J Surg 1960;48:172–8.

51. Hodgson AR, Skinsnes OK, Leong CY. The pathogenesis of Pott's paraplegia. J Bone Joint Surg Am 1967;49-6:1147–56.

52. Hoffman EB, Crosier JH, Cremin BJ. Imaging in children with spinal tuberculosis. A comparison of radiography, computed tomography and magnetic resonance imaging. J Bone Joint Surg Br 1993;75-2:233–9.

53. Hsu LC, Cheng CL, Leong JC. Pott's paraplegia of late onset. The cause of compression and results after anterior decompression. J Bone Joint Surg Br 1988;70-4:534–8.

54. Jain AK. Tuberculosis of the spine: a fresh look at an old disease. J Bone Joint Surg Br 2010;92-7:905–13.

55. Jain AK, Jain S. Instrumented stabilization in spinal tuberculosis. Int Orthop 2012;36-2:285–92.

56. Jain AK, Sethi A, Sethi R, S K. Atypical Presentation of Spinal Tuberculosis. Indian J Orthop 1997;31-3:164–70.

57. Jain AK. Treatment of tuberculosis of the spine with neurologic complications. Clin Orthop Relat Res 2002-398:75–84.

58. Jain AK, Aggarwal A, Mehrotra G. Correlation of canal encroachment with neurological deficit in tuberculosis of the spine. Int Orthop 1999;23-2:85–6.

59. Jain AK, Jena A, Dhammi IK. Correlation of clinical course with magnetic resonance imaging in tuberculous myelopathy. Neurol India 2000;48-2:132–9.

60. Jain AK, Jena SK, Singh MP, Dhammi IK, Ramachadran VG, Dev G. Evaluation of clinico-radiological, bacteriological, serological, molecular and histological diagnosis of osteoarticular tuberculosis. Indian J Orthop 2008;42-2:173–7.

61. Jain R, Sawhney S, Berry M. Computed tomography of vertebral tuberculosis: patterns of bone destruction. Clin Radiol 1993;47-3:196–9.

62. Jain AK, Sreenivasan R, Saini NS, Kumar S, Jain S, Dhammi IK. Magnetic resonance evaluation of tubercular lesion in spine. Int Orthop 2012;36-2:261–9.

63. Jain AK, Sinha S. Evaluation of systems of grading of neurological deficit in tuberculosis of spine. Spinal Cord 2005;43-6:375–80.

64. Jain AK, Aggarwal A, Dhammi IK, Aggarwal PK, Singh S. Extrapleural anterolateral decompression in tuberculosis of the dorsal spine. J Bone Joint Surg Br 2004;86-7:1027–31.

65. Jain AK, Dhammi IK, Prashad B, Sinha S, Mishra P. Simultaneous anterior decompression and posterior instrumentation of the tuberculous spine using an anterolateral extrapleural approach. J Bone Joint Surg Br 2008;90-11:1477–81.

66. Jain AK, Dhammi IK, Jain S, Kumar J. Simultaneously anterior decompression and posterior instrumentation by extrapleural retroperitoneal approach in thoracolumbar lesions. Indian J Orthop 2010;44-4:409–16.

67. Jain AK, Maheshwari AV, Jena S. Kyphus correction in spinal tuberculosis. Clin Orthop Relat Res 2007;460:117–23.

68. Jain AK, Kumar S, Tuli SM. Tuberculosis of spine (C1 to D4). Spinal Cord 1999;37-5:362–9.

69. Jain AK, Kumar J. Tuberculosis of spine: neurological deficit. Eur Spine J 2013;22 Suppl 4:624–33.

70. Jain A, Jena A, Dhammi I, Kumar S. Fate of intervertebral disc space in paradiscal tuberculous lesions. Indian J Orthop 1999;33:90–4.

71. Jain AK, Aggarwal PK, Arora A, Singh S. Behaviour of the kyphotic angle in spinal tuberculosis. Int Orthop 2004;28-2:110–4.

72. Jain AK. Tuberculosis of the spine. Clin Orthop Relat Res 2007;460:2–3.

73. Jain AK, Dhammi IK. Tuberculosis of the spine: a review. Clin Orthop Relat Res 2007;460:39–49.

74. Jain AK, Dhammi IK, Jain S, Mishra P. Kyphosis in spinal tuber-culosis – Prevention and correction. Indian J Orthop 2010;44-2:127–36.

75. Jain AK, Dhammi IK, Modi P, Kumar J, Sreenivasan R, Saini NS. Tuberculosis spine: Therapeutically refractory disease. Indian J Orthop 2012;46-2:171–8.

76. Kim SJ, Kim IJ, Suh KT, Kim YK, Lee JS. Prediction of residual disease of spine infection using F-18 FDG PET/CT. Spine (Phila Pa 1976) 2009;34-22:2424–30.

77. Kang M, Gupta S, Khandelwal N, Shankar S, Gulati M, Suri S. CT-guided fine-needle aspiration biopsy of spinal lesions. Acta Radiol 1999;40-5:474–8.

78. Konstam PG, Konstam ST. Spinal tuberculosis in Southern Nigeria with special reference to ambulant treatment of thoracolumbar disease. J Bone Joint Surg Br 1958;40-B-1:26–32.

79. Kaplan CJ. Conservative therapy in skeletal tuberculosis: an appraisal based on experience in South Africa. Tubercle 1959;40:355–68.

80. Kohli SB. Radical surgical approach to spinal tuberculosis. J Bone Joint Surg Br 1967;49-4:668–73.

81. Kumar K. The penetration of drugs into the lesions of spinal tuberculosis. Int Orthop 1992;16-1:67–8.

82. Khoo LT, Mikawa K, Fessler RG. A surgical revisitation of Pott distemper of the spine. Spine J 2003;3-2:130–45.

83. Kotil K, Alan MS, Bilge T. Medical management of Pott disease in the thoracic and lumbar spine: a prospective clinical study. J Neurosurg Spine 2007;6-3:222–8.

84. Kalra KP, Dhar SB, Shetty G, Dhariwal Q. Pedicle subtraction osteotomy for rigid post-tuberculous kyphosis. J Bone Joint Surg Br 2006;88-7:925–7.

85. Louw JA. Spinal tuberculosis with neurological deficit. Treatment with anterior vascularised rib grafts, posterior osteotomies and fusion. J Bone Joint Surg Br 1990;72-4:686–93.

86. Luk KD, Krishna M. Spinal stenosis above a healed tuberculous kyphosis. A case report. Spine (Phila Pa 1976) 1996;21-9:1098–101.

87. Laheri VJ, Badhe NP, Dewnany GT. Single stage decompression, anterior interbody fusion and posterior instrumentation for tuberculous kyphosis of the dorso-lumbar spine. Spinal Cord 2001;39-8:429–36.

88. Lee SH, Sung JK, Park YM. Single-stage transpedicular decompression and posterior instrumentation in treatment of thoracic and thoracolumbar spinal tuberculosis: a retrospective case series. J Spinal Disord Tech 2006;19-8:595–602.

89. Lee IC, Quek YW, Tsao SM, Chang IC, Sheu JN, Chen JY. Unusual spinal tuberculosis with cord compression in an infant. J Child Neurol 2010;25-10:1284–7.

90. Lodha R, Menon PR, Kabra SK. Concerns on the dosing of antitubercular drugs for children in RNTCP. Indian Pediatr 2008;45-10:852–4.

91. Lee IS, Lee JS, Kim SJ, Jun S, Suh KT. Fluorine-18-fluorodeoxyglucose positron emission tomography/computed tomography imaging in pyogenic and tuberculous spondylitis: preliminary study. J Comput Assist Tomogr 2009;33-4:587–92.

92. Loddenkemper R, Sagebiel D, Brendel A. Strategies against multidrug-resistant tuberculosis. Eur Respir J Suppl 2002;36:66s-77s.

93. Liu YL, Hao YJ, Li T, Song YM, Wang LM. Trans-upper-sternal approach to the cervicothoracic junction. Clin Orthop Relat Res 2009;467-8:2018–24.

94. Mukopadhaya B. The role of excisional surgery in the treatment of bone and joint tuberculosis. Ann R Coll Surg Engl 1956;18-5:288–313.

95. Mondal A, Misra DK. CT-guided needle aspiration cytology (FNAC) of 112 vertebral lesions. Indian J Pathol Microbiol 1994;37-3:255–61.

96. Mishra S, Tuli SM. Penetration Of Antitubercular Drugs In Cold Abscesses Of Skeletal Tuberculosis And In Tuberculous Joint Aspirates. Indian J Orthop 1983;17-1:14–8.

97. Meintjes G, Skolimowska KH, Wilkinson KA, Matthews K, Tadokera R, Conesa-Botella A, Seldon R, Rangaka MX, Rebe K, Pepper DJ, Morroni C, Colebunders R, Maartens G, Wilkinson RJ. Corticosteroid-modulated immune activation in the tuberculosis immune reconstitution inflammatory syndrome. Am J Respir Crit Care Med 2012;186-4:369–77.

98. Mohan K, Rawall S, Pawar UM, Sadani M, Nagad P, Nene A, Nene A. Drug resistance patterns in 111 cases of drug-resistant tuberculosis spine. Eur Spine J 2013;22 Suppl 4:647–52.

99. Mehta JS, Bhojraj SY. Tuberculosis of the thoracic spine. A classification based on the selection of surgical strategies. J Bone Joint Surg Br 2001;83-6:859–63.

100. Moon MS, Woo YK, Lee KS, Ha KY, Kim SS, Sun DH. Posterior instrumentation and anterior interbody fusion for tuberculous kyphosis of dorsal and lumbar spines. Spine (Phila Pa 1976) 1995;20-17:1910–6.

101. Mukhtar AM, Farghaly MM, Ahmed SH. Surgical treatment of thoracic and lumbar tuberculosis by anterior interbody fusion and posterior instrumentation. Med Princ Pract 2003;12-2:92–6.

102. Moon MS. Tuberculosis of the spine. Controversies and a new challenge. Spine (Phila Pa 1976) 1997;22-15:1791–7.

103. Moon MS, Kim SS, Lee BJ, Moon JL. Spinal tuberculosis in children: Retrospective analysis of 124 patients. Indian J Orthop 2012;46-2:150–8.

104. Ninth report of the Medical Research Council Working Party on Tuberculosis of the Spine. A 10-year assessment of controlled trials of inpatient and outpatient treatment and of plaster-of-Paris jackets for tuberculosis of the spine in children on standard chemotherapy. Studies in Masan and Pusan, Korea. J Bone Joint Surg Br 1985;67-1:103–10.

105. Negi SS, Khan SF, Gupta S, Pasha ST, Khare S, Lal S. Comparison of the conventional diagnostic modalities, bactec culture and polymerase chain reaction test for diagnosis of tuberculosis. Indian J Med Microbiol 2005;23-1:29–33.

106. Pyle MM. Relative numbers of resistant tubercle bacilli in sputa of patients before and during treatment with streptomycin. Proc Staff Meet Mayo Clin 1947;22-21:465–73.

107. Parthasarathy R, Sriram K, Santha T, Prabhakar R, Somasundaram PR, Sivasubramanian S. Short-course chemotherapy for tuberculosis of the spine. A comparison between ambulant treatment and radical surgery—ten-year report. J Bone Joint Surg Br 1999;81-3:464–71.

108. Pande KC, Pande SK, Babhulkar SS. An atypical presentation of tuberculosis of the spine. Spinal Cord 1996;34-12:716–9.

109. Risko T, Novasazel, T. Experience with radical operations in tuberculosis of the spine. J Bone Joint Surg Am 1963;45:53–68.

110. Raja A. Immunology of tuberculosis. Indian J Med Res 2004;120-4:213–32.

111. Rivas-Garcia A, Sarria-Estrada S, Torrents-Odin C, Casas-Gomila L, Franquet E. Imaging findings of Pott's disease. Eur Spine J 2013;22 Suppl 4:567–78.

112. Rajeswari R, Balasubramanian R, Venkatesan P, Sivasubramanian S, Soundarapandian S, Shanmugasundaram TK, Prabhakar R. Short-course chemotherapy in the treatment of Pott's paraplegia: report on five year follow-up. Int J Tuberc Lung Dis 1997;1-2:152–8.

113. Rajasekaran S, Soundarapandian S. Progression of kyphosis in tuberculosis of the spine treated by anterior arthrodesis. J Bone Joint Surg Am 1989;71-9:1314–23.

114. Rajasekaran S. The problem of deformity in spinal tuberculosis. Clin Orthop Relat Res 2002-398:85–92.

115. Rajasekaran S, Shanmugasundaram TK. Prediction of the angle of gibbus deformity in tuberculosis of the spine. J Bone Joint Surg Am 1987;69-4:503–9.

116. Rajasekaran S. The natural history of post-tubercular kyphosis in children. Radiological signs which predict late increase in deformity. J Bone Joint Surg Br 2001;83-7:954–62.

117. Rajasekaran S. Buckling collapse of the spine in childhood spinal tuberculosis. Clin Orthop Relat Res 2007;460:86–92.

118. Rajeswari R, Balasubramanian R, Venkatesan P, Sivasubramanian S, Soundarapandian S, Shanmugasundaram TK, Prabhakar R. Short-course chemotherapy in the treatment of Pott's paraplegia: report on five year follow-up. Int J Tuberc Lung Dis 1997;1-2:152–8.

119. Standring S. Gray's Anatomy: The Anatomical Basis of Clinical Practice. Elsevier Health Sciences UK, 2008.

120. Study of historic tuberculosis. Am J Phys Anthropol 2005;126-1:32–47.

121. Stevenson FH, Manning CW. Tuberculosis of the spine treated conservatively with chemotherapy: series of 72 patients collected 1949-1954 and followed to 1961. Tubercle 1962;43:406–11.

122. Study of chemotherapy regimens of 5 and 7 months' duration and the role of corticosteroids in the treatment of sputum-positive patients with pulmonary tuberculosis in South India. Tubercle 1983;64-2:73–91.

123. Sundararaj GD, Behera S, Ravi V, Venkatesh K, Cherian VM, Lee V. Role of posterior stabilisation in the management of tuberculosis of the dorsal and lumbar spine. J Bone Joint Surg Br 2003;85-1:100–6.

124. Schulitz KP, Kothe R, Leong JC, Wehling P. Growth changes of solidly fused kyphotic bloc after surgery for tuberculosis. Comparison of four procedures. Spine (Phila Pa 1976) 1997;22-10:1150–5.

125. Stanford J, Stanford C, Grange J. Immunotherapy with Mycobacterium vaccae in the treatment of tuberculosis. Front Biosci 2004;9:1701–19.

126. Taylor GM, Murphy E, Hopkins R, Rutland P, Chistov Y. First report of Mycobacterium bovis DNA in human remains from the Iron Age. Microbiology 2007;153-Pt 4:1243–9.

127. Tuli SM. Tuberculosis of the Skeletal System: Bones, Joints, Spine and Bursal Sheaths. 3rd ed. New Delhi: Jaypee Brothers, 2004.

128. Tuli SM. Tuberculosis of the spine: a historical review. Clin Orthop Relat Res 2007;460:29–38.

129. Thirteenth Report of the Medical Research Council Working Party on Tuberculosis of the Spine. A 15-year assessment of controlled trials of the management of tuberculosis of the spine in Korea and Hong Kong. J Bone Joint Surg Br 1998;80-3:456–62.

130. Tuli SM. Results of treatment of spinal tuberculosis by "middle-path" regime. J Bone Joint Surg Br 1975;57-1:13–23.

131. Tuli SM, Kumar K, Sen PC. Penetration of antitubercular drugs in clinical osteoarticular tubercular lesions. Acta Orthop Scand 1977;48-4:362–8.

132. Talu U, Gogus A, Ozturk C, Hamzaoglu A, Domanic U. The role of posterior instrumentation and fusion after anterior radical debridement and fusion in the surgical treatment of spinal tuberculosis: experience of 127 cases. J Spinal Disord Tech 2006;19-8:554–9.

133. Tuli SM. Severe kyphotic deformity in tuberculosis of the spine. Int Orthop 1995;19-5:327–31.

134. Upadhyay SS, Saji MJ, Yau AC. Duration of antituberculosis chemotherapy in conjunction with radical surgery in the management of spinal tuberculosis. Spine (Phila Pa 1976) 1996;21-16:1898–903.

135. Upadhyay SS, Saji MJ, Sell P, Sell B, Hsu LC. Spinal deformity after childhood surgery for tuberculosis of the spine. A comparison of radical surgery and debridement. J Bone Joint Surg Br 1994;76-1:91–8.

136. Upadhyay SS, Saji MJ, Sell P, Yau AC. The effect of age on the change in deformity after radical resection and anterior arthrodesis for tuberculosis of the spine. J Bone Joint Surg Am 1994;76-5:701–8.

137. Upadhyay SS, Saji MJ, Sell P, Hsu LC, Yau AC. The effect of age on the change in deformity after anterior debridement surgery for tuberculosis of the spine. Spine (Phila Pa 1976) 1996;21-20:2356–62.

138. Von Groll A, Martin A, Jureen P, Hoffner S, Vandamme P, Portaels F, Palomino JC, da Silva PA. Fluoroquinolone resistance in Mycobacterium tuberculosis and mutations in gyrA and gyrB. Antimicrob Agents Chemother 2009;53-10:4498–500.

139. WHO. Tuberculosis diagnostics: Xpert MTB/RIF Test 2014.

140. WHO. Global Tuberculosis Control 2010. Geneva: WHO Press, 2010.

141. WHO. Treatment of tuberculosis: GUIDELINES. 4th ed. Geneva, Switzerland. WHO Press, World Health Organization, 2010.

142. WHO. Multidrug and extensively drug-resistant TB (M/XDR-TB): 2010 global report on surveillance and response. Geneva: WHO Press, 2010

143. Wong YW, Leong JC, Luk KD. Direct internal kyphectomy for severe angular tuberculous kyphosis. Clin Orthop Relat Res 2007;460:124–9.

144. Yang L, Liu Z. Analysis and therapeutic schedule of the postoperative recurrence of bone tuberculosis. J Orthop Surg Res 2013;8:47.

145. Yau AC, Hsu LC, O'Brien JP, Hodgson AR. Tuberculous kyphosis: correction with spinal osteotomy, halo-pelvic distraction, and anterior and posterior fusion. J Bone Joint Surg Am 1974;56-7:1419–34.

146. Yang XY, Chen QF, Li YP, Wu SM. Mycobacterium vaccae as adjuvant therapy to anti-tuberculosis chemotherapy in never-treated tuberculosis patients: a meta-analysis. PLoS One 2011;6-9:e23826.

147. Zink AR, Grabner W, Nerlich AG. Molecular identification of human tuberculosis in recent and historic bone tissue samples: The role of molecular techniques for the

148. Ziganshina LE, Squire SB. Fluoroquinolones for treating tuberculosis. Cochrane Database Syst Rev 2008-1:CD004795.

Chapter 6

Evidence Based Management Guide (EBMG)

SPINE

Q. 1. How do you clinically diagnose spinal TB in early and advanced stage of disease?

TB spine can occur at any age and to either sex. It is more common in patients with immunocompromised state (like HIV/AIDS), severe malnutrition (hypoproteinemia), following acute viral infection/exanthematous infection, following steroid therapy and in extremes of age. TB spine has been reported to get activated/flared up during pregnancy. Tubercular spine can be difficult to diagnose (especially in early stages) as it can mimic other propitious as well other ominous pathologies. Clinically, there are some sign and symptoms which indicate this disease, however, presence of all is not mandatory.

Clinical features/indicators of early stage of disease
1. Localized persistent back pain for more than 6 weeks
2. Tenderness over paraspinal region or spinous process (direct/or on rotational stress)
3. Fever (low grade, evening rise of temperature, night sweats)
4. Weight loss, anorexia
5. Rarely upper motor neuron signs (increased muscle tone, ill sustained clonus at ankle and/or extensor plantar reflex) may be the first presentation.

In advanced stage of disease
1. Persistent localized back pain increased with activity
   - Rest pain—pain persistent during rest;

- Night cries—pain occurring usually after 2–3 hr of onset of sleep (REM sleep), as loss of muscle tone in REM sleep allows inflamed bony surfaces to rub against each other generating pain and muscle spasm.
2. Palpable spinal deformity [knuckle, kyphus, gibbus (angular/rounded)]
3. Paraspinal swelling (due to cold abscess)
4. Wasting of paraspinal muscles
5. Neurological deficit (ranges from increased tone, ankle/ patellar clonus to complete paraplegia with bladder/bowel involvement and/or flexor spasms)
6. Bed sores

---

1. Tuli SM. Tuberculosis of the Spine. In: Tuli SM, ed. Tuberculosis of the skeletal system. 3rd edn. New Delhi, India: Jaypee Brothers Medical Publishers (P) Ltd.; 2004:191–345.

Q. 2. How do you investigate a case of spinal TB?

These patients are investigated hematologically and on imaging using plain roentgenograms, CT/MRI scans as indicated.

1. *Hematological*
    a. *Complete and differential blood counts*: Patient may have anemia of chronic disease (normocytic normochromic to microcytic hypochromic) with associated lymphocytosis.
    b. *Erythrocyte sedimentation rate*: Usually increased.
    c. *Baseline liver and kidney function tests*: May or may not be deranged. They are also needed 'to detect antitubercular drugs induced hepatic toxicity, if taken earlier'.
2. X-rays (anteroposterior and lateral views) of the concerned area of spine (findings described in the next question). A chest radiograph may show features of active/old pulmonary tuberculosis.
3. MRI (CT scan, if MRI is not available and surgery is anticipated).
4. *Tuberculin skin test (Mantoux)*: Limited role in adults, significant clinical role in pediatric cases. This test is not diagnostic of tuberculosis. The patient may show positive

reaction in a long-standing disease. Negative test in a healthy patient rules out the TB. This test may be negative in presence of active disease in an immunocompromised state (HIV), severe malnutrition/hypoproteinemia, following viral infection/exanthematous infection, following steroid therapy and at extremes of age.

5. *IGRA (interferon gamma release assay)/gold quantiferon (banned in India)/immunological test*: It has no clinical/ therapeutic implication. Negative IGRA test makes the diagnosis of tuberculosis unlikely.

---

2. Colmenero JD, Ruiz-Mesa JD, Sanjuan-Jimenez R, Sobrino B, Morata P. Establishing the diagnosis of tuberculous vertebral osteomyelitis. Eur Spine J 2013 Jun; 22 Suppl 4:579–86.

"The usefulness of the TSTC (tuberculin sensitivity test) in the diagnosis of tuberculosis has been questioned due to inter-reader variability, cross-reactivity with non-tuberculous mycobacteria and false positive results in patients vaccinated with BCG. Furthermore, TST also has a low sensitivity in immunosuppressed patients. Recently, IGRAs for tuberculosis have overcome most of these limitations. These immunoassays detect in vitro interferon-c secreted by peripheral blood mononuclear cells in response to specific antigens of M. tuberculosis. Currently, multiple data show that IGRA tests are equally sensitive but more specific than TST in diagnosing latent tuberculosis infection and active tuberculosis.

*In countries with a high prevalence of tuberculosis, the usefulness of TST and IGRA in the diagnosis is very limited, as these tests cannot differentiate between latent infection and active disease. However, their negative predictive value is very high, regardless of the prevalence of tuberculosis. For these reasons, it seems advisable to perform an IGRA test in any patient suspected as having tuberculous vertebral osteomyelitis, because, regardless of the prevalence of tuberculosis, **a negative IGRA test makes the diagnosis of spinal tuberculosis very unlikely,** and thus requires other causes of vertebral osteomyelitis to be ruled out".*

Q. 3. How and when do you diagnose spinal TB with only X-ray findings?

X-ray changes take approximately 3–4 months to show up after disease onset. The patient may remain symptomatic with persistent localized back pain with or without clinical localization signs for 6–12 weeks before an early radiological sign appears (30–40% reduction in mineral content can only be appreciated as regional osteopenia).

A. *Early disease*

1. *Regional osteoporosis*: In an early disease, regional osteoporosis may be observed in symptomatic region of the spine.
2. *Reduction of disk height*: Slight reduction of disk space/height may be the earliest radiological sign of tuberculosis. In a normal person, the disk height at all levels is either same or slightly more than disk height above except L5–S1 and D12–L1. At a symptomatic level, reduction of disc height is considered to be a sign for tuberculosis and MRI is indicated to ascertain the diagnosis.

B. *Established lesion*: In established lesion, following radiological signs are observed in tubercular spine.

On lateral view

1. Regional osteoporosis with fuzzy disk margin
2. Reduction/obliteration of disk space
3. Loss of anterior body height
4. Kyphotic deformity (as measured by Konstam angle) (Fig. 5.4)
5. Increase in the prevertebral soft tissue shadow for cervical spine disease
6. Increase in the paravertebral shadow in anteroposterior view of spine.

Diagnosis only on basis of radiograph is tough in early stages of disease. A patient who belongs to an endemic region, having history of persistent localized back pain and supportive classical radiological findings can be presumed to be having tuberculosis of the spine and patient can be treated for the same.

3. WY Cheung, Keith DK Luk. Clinical and radiological outcomes after conservative treatment of TB spondylitis: Is the 15 years' follow-up in the MRC study long enough? Eur Spine J (2013) 22 (Suppl 4):S594–S602.
4. Jain AK. Tuberculosis of the spine: A fresh look at an old disease. J Bone Joint Surg Br. 2010 Jul; 92(7):905–13.

Q. 4. What are imaging correlates on: MRI/contrast MRI/CT/ PET-CT?

The advents of modern imaging techniques have helped in diagnosis and management of Pott's spine much like in other diseases. Knowledge about these techniques and their clinical application is a must for a modern day clinician.

MRI (Magnetic Resonance Imaging)

MR scan will show following findings in a case of TB spine:

1. Marrow edema (low signal on T1WI and high signal on T2WI, bright signal on STIR images)
2. Subligamentous and epidural extension of collection
3. Paravertebral collections (with or without septations)
4. Endplate erosions
5. Discitis
6. Epidural extension of intraosseous abscess
7. Uniform enhancement/rim enhancement on administration of contrast (Chapter 7; Case 30; Fig. f, g)
8. In a tubercular lesion, the shadow imparted by the aorta and vena cava is lifted from vertebral bodies while in lesions due to malignancy, the aorta and vena cava rests on vertebral bodies (Fig. 5.7).
9. Spinal cord may also show observations like edema, thinning of the spinal cord, myelomalacia, syringohydromelia, clumping of roots (arachnoiditis) in cases with paraplegia.

No. 1, 2 and 3: The constellation of these MRI signs is observed consistently in TB spine lesion consistently.

Eighty-three percent of patients in a series (n = 49) reported by Jain *et al* had a constellation of paravertebral collections, marrow edema, subligamentous and epidural extension, endplate erosions and discitis occurring together.

CT Scan (Computed Tomography Scan)

CT scan is inferior in assessment of early spinal diseases. It is more reliable in detection of calcific foci, bone destruction and guide for interventional biopsy/procedures.

1. *Four types of vertebral body destruction*:
   a. Fragmentary, predominantly consists of numerous residual bony fragments which frequently migrate into soft tissue masses. It is strongly suggestive of TB
   b. Osteolytic
   c. Subperiosteal
   d. Localized

2. *Intravenous contrast administration clearly shows*:
   a. The multiloculated cystic paraspinal masses
   b. Enhancement of the granulomatous tissue and the walls of abscess located in both bone and soft tissues.

PET-CT (Positron Emission Tomography/Computed Tomography Scan)

PET scan on the basis of differential uptake of radioactive glucose is able to detect and grade the activity of the suspected lesion, while a CT scan gives the anatomical detail. Hence, a combined scan tells both about the morphology and activity of the lesion. Following observations have been seen in studies using PET/CT in tuberculosis of spine:

1. SUV_{max} (maximum standardized uptake value) of the early phase on 18F FDG PET-CT scanning is statistically significant in differentiating tuberculous from pyogenic spondylitis.

2. High sensitivity and specificity for detecting and identifying the process of inflammatory activity in spondylitis.

But, these observations and their definite clinical relevance in active/undertreatment/treated vertebral disease is still a matter under study.

5. Jain AK, Sreenivasan R, Saini NS, Kumar S, Jain S, Dhammi IK. Magnetic resonance evaluation of tubercular lesion in spine. Int Orthop. 2012 Feb; 36(2):261–9.

6. Rivas-Garcia A, Sarria-Estrada S, Torrents-Odin C, Casas-Gomila L, Franquet E. Imaging findings of Pott's disease. Eur Spine J. 2013 Jun; 22 Suppl 4:567–78.

7. Lee IS, Lee JS, Kim SJ, Jun S, Suh KT. Fluorine-18-fluorodeoxyglucose positron emission tomography/computed tomography imaging in pyogenic and tuberculous spondylitis: preliminary study. J Comput Assist Tomogr. 2009 Jul-Aug;33(4):587–92.

8. Kim SJ, Kim IJ, Suh KT, Kim YK, Lee JS. Prediction of residual disease of spine infection using F-18 FDG PET/CT. Spine (Phila Pa 1976). 2009 Oct 15;34(22):2424–30.

1. *"All (100%) cases had a combination of marrow edema and paravertebral collections. A total of 92% had marrow edema and subligamentous spread of disease; 98% of cases had marrow edema, paravertebral collections and endplate erosions. Endplate erosions, subligamentous spread, marrow edema and paravertebral collections were seen in 91.8%. A total of 83% had subligamentous spread and epidural components suggestive of spread anterior and posterior to the VB; 83% had paravertebral collections, marrow edema, subligamentous and epidural extension, endplate erosions and discitis".*

2. *"In comparison with radiography, CT better evaluates radiographic findings and the lesion extent, due to its high contrast resolution and its tomographic nature. The new multi-detector computed tomography technology provides excellent multiplanar reconstruction imaging for the assessment of bone and soft tissue infection, essential for presurgical planning. Intravenous contrast administration clearly shows the multiloculated cystic paraspinal masses, enhancing the granulomatous tissue and the walls of abscesses located in both bone and soft tissues. Among the four types of body destruction described (fragmentary, osteolytic, subperiosteal and localized), the fragmentary type predominates and consists of numerous residual bony fragments which frequently migrate into soft tissue masses. It is strongly suggestive of TB. Paraspinal mass and abscess formation are found early in the disease, being reported in 45–100% of spinal TB. This lesion lies anterolateral to vertebral bodies and expands with tendency for distant spread along the tissue planes and epidural space. An abscess rarely occurs in the absence of observable vertebral infection. Secondary extension of TB into the posterior elements is not infrequent. Isolated involvement of the vertebral arch or the extradural space is found in 2–10% of cases being common in nonwhite patients and patients who have AIDS. The advantages of CT over MRI are a more reliable detection of calcified foci and it also provides a guide to interventional procedures. However, CT is inferior to MR imaging in the early assessment of the spinal canal disease".*

3. *"The maximum SUVs of early phase PET-CT may be complemen-tary to MRI for differentiating pyogenic and tuberculous spondylitis and reflecting the activity of infectious spondylitis".*

"F-18 FDG PET-CT is useful for discrimination of residual and nonresidual SI after treatment. Among the various quantitative indexes, % SUV$_{max}$ is a potent predictor of residual SI in the current study".

Q. 5. When we can start antitubercular therapy (ATT) without biopsy in a case of TB spine?

If a patient has clinical and radiological findings consistent with tuberculosis with corroborating MRI features [contiguous vertebral involvement (low signal T1WI and bright in T2WI), septate paravertebral abscess, intraosseous abscess and subligamentous and epidural extension with discitis] we can start anti-tubercular therapy (ATT) without biopsy (presumptive diagnosis). In the remaining cases (diagnostic dilemma), we must obtain percutaneous/CT guided biopsy or open biopsy to establish the diagnosis before starting ATT.

---

4. Jain AK. Tuberculosis of the spine: a fresh look at an old disease. J Bone Joint Surg Br. 2010 Jul;92(7):905–13.

9. S. Bhojraj, A. Nene. Lumbar and lumbosacral tuberculous spondylodiscitis in adults: Redefining the indications for surgery. J Bone Joint Surg [Br] 2002;84-B:530–4.

Q. 6. How to take biopsy/tissue from spinal lesions/cold abscess?

Biopsy from vertebral lesions can be obtained by:

- Percutaneous biopsy/CT-guided biopsy
- Open biopsy

Percutaneous (where accessible or using ultrasound where available) or CT-guided biopsy is indicated prior to considering a formal open biopsy in all cases where an immediate surgery is not indicated. The approach depends on level of lesion and the expertise of the radiologist/chest physician/spinal/ orthopedician/neurosurgeon doing the procedure. The fluctuant cold abscess may be aspirated by a thick bore needle. The landmarks depend on the location of the abscess.

---

9. S. Bhojraj, A. Nene. Lumbar and lumbosacral tuberculous spondylodiscitis in adults: Redefining the indications for surgery. J Bone Joint Surg [Br] 2002;84-B:530–4.

10. E. Oguz, A. Sehirlioglu, M. Altinmakas, C. Ozturk, M. Komurcu, C. Solakoglu, A. R. Vaccaro. A new classification and guide for surgical treatment of spinal tuberculosis. Int Orthop. 2008 Feb; 32(1): 127–133.

11. Sucu HK, Ciçek C, Rezanko T, Bezircioðlu H, Erþahin Y, Tunakan M, Minoðlu M. Percutaneous computed tomography-guided biopsy of the spine: 229 procedures. Joint Bone Spine. 2006 Oct;73(5):532–7.

Q. 7. What investigations are to be done once tissue and fluid is procured?

The tissue samples obtained should be sent for:

1. Histopathology and cytopathology
2. Gram's stain
3. Ziehl-Neelsen (ZN) staining for AFB
4. Fungal cultures
5. Drug sensitivity testing for tuberculosis may not be done in an untreated case of spinal TB, however, if patient is already on ATT then culture (LJ medium, BACTEC) and drug sensitivity testing is indicated.
6. *Molecular tests*
   a. *TB-PCR*: It denotes the presence of genome of Mycobacterium, which may be dead/alive. But the presence of a positive test of TB-PCR for *Mycobacterium tuberculosis* in a clinical disease suggests tuberculosis.
   b. *Line probe assay/CB-NAAT/GeneXpert* for rapid drug sensitivity testing where available.

Q. 8. What ATT should be prescribed once a patient is diagnosed to be suffering from TB spine?

The rational of drug therapy is described in the initial chapter. The present consensus as evolved in INDEX bone and joint TB guidelines is to start ATT with intensive phase (HRZE) for 2 months includes 4 drugs [isoniazid (H), rifampicin (R), pyrazinamide (Z) and ethambutol (E)] followed by 3-drug continuation phase (HRE) for 10 to 16 months. The drugs can be given as daily dosage regimen or intermittent dosage regimen as suggested by DOTS (direct observed treatment short-course chemotherapy). The current consensus is to give

ATT on daily basis. The dosage of each drug is to be calculated individually according to patient's weight; hence, weight of the patient should be checked monthly. After starting ATT, liver function tests of the patient should be done after every 2 weeks initially, followed by after every 2 months. The patients on ATT should be monitored by clinically (every 2 months), serial hematological (every 2 months) and by MRI at 12 and 18 months.

---

*Index TB Guidelines: Guidelines on extrapulmonary tuberculosis for India, Ministry of health and family welfare, Govt. of India 2016.

12. Donald PR. The chemotherapy of osteoarticular tuberculosis with recommendations for treatment of children. J Infect 2011;62:411–39.

13. Jain AK, Srivastava A, Saini NS, Dhammi IK, Sreenivasan R, Kumar S. Efficacy of extended DOTS category I chemotherapy in spinal tuberculosis based on MRI-based healed status. Indian J Orthop. 2012 Nov;46(6):633–9.

14. Watts HG, Lifeso RM. Current concepts review: tuberculosis of bone and joints. J Bone Joint Surg [Am] 1996;78-A:288–98.

Ref 13: *"35.2% patients demonstrate MRI based healed vertebral lesion at the end of 8 months of extended category 1 DOTS regimen. It is unscientific to stop the ATT by fixed time frame and MRI evaluation of the patients is required after 8 months of ATT and subsequently to decide for the continuation stoppage of treatment".*

Q. 9. Besides ATT, what is the ancillary treatment prescribed in adults and children (ambulation, braces, etc.) of cervical spine TB, dorsal spine TB, dorsolumbar spine TB, lumbar spine TB?

In ambulant chemotherapy, patients are treated by ATT and mobilization on braces/orthosis. The patient is advised to apply suitable orthosis while lying down and then made to sit to mobilize. Since the vertebral bodies are diseased and structurally weak, the patients are discouraged to travel using scooter, bikes and bicycles. They may travel in a train or in a car in lying down posture. Orthoses (Fig. 5.10) used depending upon region involved are:

1. *Cervical spine*: Four post-collar (Fig. 5.10a).

2. *Cervicodorsal spine*: A combination of Taylor's brace and four post-collar (Fig. 5.10b).

3. *Dorsal and dorsolumbar spine TB*: ASH (anterior spinal hyperextension) brace/Taylor's brace (Fig. 5.10c, d).

4. *Lumbar and lumbosacral spine*: Taylor's or ASH brace for upper lumbar spine and lumbar corset for lumbosacral spine.

However, in children, a PVC body brace (Boston scoliosis brace) or a plaster jacket may substitute ASH brace.

Q. 10. What should be the protocol for follow-up evaluation of spinal TB patient (with/without neural deficit)?

All cases of tuberculosis of spine should be asked to report to the hospital to look for any improvement or any drug related complication after 2 weeks of starting ATT (for drug related complications) and at one month then every 2 months. The patients without any neurological deficit and on ambulant chemotherapy should be examined for the signs of appearance of neural deficit, particularly in first 2–3 months of treatment.

a. *Clinical*: The general improvement in well-being, weight gain and an improved appetite is appreciated on treatment.

b. *Hematological*: Increased Hb, reduced ESR is documented.

c. *Radiological*: The remineralization of vertebral body, sharpening of disk margin in comparison to pre-treatment X-rays is appreciated in early post-treatment follow-up (2 months onwards). At the end of treatment, 70% lesions heal with osseous or fibro-ossoeus fusion. The improvement on treatment is better appreciated on plain X-rays during first 6 months of treatment, hence it is imperative to have a good quality pre-treatment radiographs for comparison at 2nd, 4th and 6th months post-treatment and subsequently. It is a common observation that patient are advised MRI for initial diagnosis and follow-up; while X-rays are important to document treatment response in first 6 months.

d. *Imaging*: MRI is useful investigation to assess healing changes at 9, 12, 18 months of treatment. MRI should preferably not be done for first 6 months after starting ATT. The MRI findings generally do not change (rather may worsen) in first 3–4 months after starting ATT.

In cases of TB spine with neural deficit, in addition to the above:

1. The staging of neural deficit should be performed by Jain and Sinha staging/Tuli and Kumar's grading.

2. The patient with neural deficit should be evaluated for neural charting once a week to document early evidence of neural recovery or deterioration (cases of stationary or deteriorating neural deficit should be considered for surgical decompression).

Once the lesion heals and ATT is stopped, these patients should be followed up every 6 months post-healing (for at least 2 years) and yearly thereafter for 15 years, to look out for any recurrence/relapse of disease, progression of kyphotic deformity and late onset paraplegia.

15. Jain AK, Sinha S. Evaluation of systems of grading of neurological deficit in tuberculosis of spine. Spinal Cord 2005 Jun;43(6):375–80.

4. Jain AK. Tuberculosis of the spine: a fresh look at an old disease. J Bone Joint Surg Br 2010 Jul;92(7):905–13.

3. WY Cheung, Keith DK Luk. Clinical and radiological outcomes after conservative treatment of TB spondylitis: is the 15 years' follow-up in the MRC study long enough? Eur Spine J (2013) 22 (Suppl 4): S594–S602.

1. Tuli SM. Tuberculosis of the Spine. In: Tuli SM, ed. Tuberculosis of the skeletal system. 3rd ed. New Delhi, India: Jaypee Brothers Medical Publishers (P) Ltd.; 2004:191–345.

Q. 11. When should we therapeutically aspirate the cold abscess?

The palpable psoas abscess, iliopsoas abscess (pseudo-hip flexion deformity) or fluctuant swelling palpable posteriorly on both side of spinous process or along the chest wall may be aspirated. The retropharyngeal abscess causing dysphagia/difficulty in breathing also needs aspiration. There is no defined role of instilling streptomycin in the abscess cavity after aspiration.

10. Oguz E, Sehirlioglu A, Altinmakas M, Ozturk C, Komurcu M, Solakoglu C, Vaccaro AR. A new classification and guide for surgical treatment of spinal tuberculosis. Int Orthop 2008 Feb; 32(1):127–133.

Q. 12. What are the indications of surgery in cases of spinal TB without neural deficit?

The surgery is indicated when:

a. *Diagnostic dilemma:* When the destructive lesion of vertebrae does not show the imaging signs characteristic of tuberculosis of spine, as described above (Chap. 7; Cases 1 and 2). The biopsy is indicated which may be an open biopsy or percutaneous biopsy to obtain tissue for diagnosis. There is **no role of empirical treatment by ATT** in destructive lesions of the vertebrae.

b. *Panvertebral disease:* Simultaneous affection of vertebral body and posterior complex is described as panvertebral lesion (Chap. 7; Cases 8–12). Such lesions are potentially unstable and instrumented stabilization is indicated in order to prevent pathological subluxation/dislocations of spine and neurological complications.

c. *Failure of conservative management (presumptive drug resistance):* Patients who are already on treatment for tuberculosis of spine and do not show adequate clinico-radiological improvement and/or a new lesion develops and/or ulcer/sinus fail to heal and/or wound dehiscence occurs (Chap. 7; Cases 28–30). In such cases, drug resistance is suspected and lesions may be debrided to procure tissue for histology/cytology, AFB smear, BACTEC culture, GeneXpert and Line Probe Assay.

d. *Spinal deformity:* Surgical correction of spinal deformity is indicated in patients who report with TB spine with severe kyphotic deformity or whose kyphotic deformity is likely to progress and end in a final kyphus of 60°or more (Chap. 7; Cases 16–25, 26, 27, 31–33).

---

16. Jain AK, Kumar S, Tuli SM. Tuberculosis of spine (C1 to D4). Spinal Cord 1999; 37:362–369.

4. Jain AK. Tuberculosis of t spine: A fresh look at an old disease. J Bone Joint Surg Br 2010 July; 92(7):905–13.

Q. 13. How do we decide the type of surgery in patients of TB spine without neural deficit?

a. *Diagnostic biopsy:* The biopsy may be performed by CT guided biopsy or transpedicular biopsy (percutaneous method) or open biopsy. The approach will vary with the segment of spine affected.

b. *Suspected drug resistance*: The diseased vertebral body is to be debrided and tissue procured should be subjected for histology molecular diagnosis and tubercular culture and sensitivity. The surgical approach will vary with the segment of spine.

c. *Panvertebral lesion*: Instrumented stabilization is indicated with or without decompression of the spinal cord.

d. *Kyphotic deformity correction*: Surgery needs meticulous planning, and the steps of deformity correction include anterior corpectomy, posterior column shortening, posterior instrumented stabilization as well as anterior and posterior bone grafting. They are performed in a single stage sequentially/simultaneously.

16. Jain AK, Kumar S, Tuli SM. Tuberculosis of spine (C1 to D4). Spinal Cord 1999; 37:362–369.

17. Jain AK, Jain S. Instrumented stabilization in spinal tuberculosis. Int Orthop. 2012; 36(2):285–92.

18. Khoo LT, Mikawa K, Fessler RG. A surgical revisitation of Pott distemper of the spine. Spine J 2003; 3(2):130–45.

Q. 14. What are the indications of kyphotic deformity correction in tuberculosis of spine. Which deformity is to be surgically corrected? Timing of deformity correction in active disease?

Any spinal deformity in adult which is likely to heal with severe deformity (60° or more) need to be surgically corrected. In children, the deformity is progressive with the growth of the child in 44% cases. A pretreatment vertebral body loss of 1.5 VB height in the dorsal and dorsolumbar regions and 1.0 in lumbar region is described as an indication for surgery. No such parameters are defined for cervical spine.

The deformity correction should be preferably performed in active disease.

19. Kotil K, Alan MS, Bilge T. Medical management of Pott disease in the thoracic and lumbar spine: a prospective clinical study. J Neurosurg Spine 2007 Mar; 6(3):222–8.

20. Rajasekaran S: The problem of deformity in spinal tuberculosis. Clin Orthop Relat Res 398:85–92, 2002.

18. Khoo LT, Mikawa K, Fessler RG.A surgical revisitation of Pott distemper of the spine. Spine J. 2003 Mar-Apr; 3(2):130–45.

21. Jain AK, Dhammi IK, Jain S, Mishra P.Kyphosis in spinal tuberculosis – Prevention and correction. Indian J Orthop. 2010 Apr; 44(2):127–36.

22. Jain AK, Agarwal PK, Aroa A, Singh S. Behaviour of kyphotic angle in spinal orthopaedics 2004; 28: 110–14.

23. Jain AK, Sreenivasan R, Mukunth, Dhammi IK. Tubercular spondylities in children. Indian J Orthop. 2014; 48:136–44.

Ref 20: *"Rajasekaran reported that the progress of deformity occurs in two distinct phases: Phase I includes the changes in the active phase, and Phase II includes changes after the disease is cured. The deformity progression is influenced by the severity of the angle before treatment, the level of the lesion, and the age of the patient. Adults have an increase of the kyphotic angle of less than 30° during the active phase with no additional treatment. There is an average increase of 15° deformity in all patients who are treated conservatively, and 3 to 5% of patients may end up with a deformity that is greater than 60°. Children, in contrast, have significant changes even in the healed phase of the disease."*

Rajasekaran suggested a formula where final kyphosis can be predicted before starting the treatment. From the formula

$Y = 5.5 + 30.5X$

(Y = final angle of the deformity, X = initial loss of vertebral body height), Patients with an excessive predicted Y value were surgically reconstructed. Cases with multiple levels of vertebral involvement, thoracic lesions, active growth and skeletal immaturity were also predictive of an increased amount of post-treatment kyphosis. Based on these considerations, an attempt should be made to estimate the amount of kyphosis expected after medical treatment alone. When this figure is excessively high or there is evidence of significant progression during medical treatment, surgical intervention to correct and prevent deformity is reasonable. Absolute criteria of the degree of acceptable deformity will vary tremendously from case to case. Whereas a 20-degree deformity may be considered acceptable to patients in developing nations with limited medical resources, few patients in Western countries would be willing to accept such a severe long-term cosmetic deformity. However, operative correction of severe kyphosis is extremely technically demanding and carries a high risk of neurological injury. Reduction of significant chronic fixed deformities for cosmetic reasons should be performed sparingly and with great caution. In such cases, it is best to operate earlier on while the kyphosis is still mobile and not excessive."

Q. 15. How do you grade severity of neural deficit?

The neural deficit is to be graded by:

a. Kumar and Tuli's classification (Table 6.1)

Table 6.1: Classification of tubercular paraplegia/quadriplegia*

Stage	Clinical features
I	Negligible patient unaware of neural deficit, physician detects plantar extensor and/or ankle clonus
II	Mild patient aware of deficit but manages to walk with support
III	Moderate nonambulatory because of paralysis (in extension), sensory deficit less than 50%
IV	Severe III + Flexor spasms/paralysis in flexion/flaccid/sensory deficit more than 50%/sphincters involved

*Applicable to compression of cord and not cauda equina.

"An ideal classification system should assess the functional status of the tetra-/paraplegic patient and should reflect the severity of cord compression. Classification suggested by Tuli and modified by Jain seems most rational which classifies all cases of paraplegia and reflects the severity of cord compression as score for sensory and motor deficit is added. The neurological deficit could be categorized into 5 stages as by,

b. Jain and Sinha's classification

Stage I. Patient unaware of neural deficit, clinician detects plantar extensor and/or ankle clonus.

Stage II. The patient has spasticity with motor deficit but is a walker. The anticipated motor score in tetraparesis is between 60 and 100. In paraparesis, it is between 80 and 100. The sensory impairment is of the lateral column sensation, i.e. pain and temperature and crude touch.

Stage III. Bedridden spastic patient. Anticipated motor score for quadriplegic is 0–30, and for paraplegic it is 50–80. Sensory scoring is the same as in Stage II.

Stage IV. Bedridden patient with severe sensory loss, and/or pressure sores. Anticipated motor score in tetraplegia is 0 and in paraplegia it is 50. There is impairment of both lateral and posterior column sensations, i.e. pain, temprature touch (fine and crude), vibration and position sense.

Stage V. Same as stage IV and/or bladder and bowel involvement, and/or flexor spasms/flaccid tetraplegia/paraplegia.

Almost in 95% of all cases, tetraplegia/paraplegia at level of spinal cord in tuberculosis could be classified. However, the lesions around conus and cauda equina present with sphincter involvement very early in the disease process and also have UMN/LMN mixed paraparesis/plegia with more sensory loss (bizarre neural deficit). Neural deficit association with intraspinal granulomas and atypical locations of the lesions may not always fit in the classification."

---

24. Jain AK, Sinha S Evaluation of systems of grading of neurological deficit in tuberculosis of spine. Spinal Cord 2005 Jun; 43(6):375–80.

1. Tuli SM. Tuberculosis of the skeletal system. 3rd ed. New Delhi, India: Jaypee Brothers Medical Publishers; 2004.

25. Kumar K. A clinical study and classification of posterior spinal tuberculosis. Int Orthop 1985;9(3):147–52.

26. Goel MK. Treatment of Pott's paraplegia by operation. J Bone Joint Surg Br 1967 Nov; 49(4):674–81.

Q. 16. Can we prognosticate the neural recovery in TB spine? Are there imaging correlates for TB spine with neural deficit?

In general paraplegia of active disease (or early onset paraplegia) has a better prognosis than that of healed disease (or late onset paraplegia).

Factors influencing a good prognosis include:
1. *Young age*: Younger the patient, better is the prognosis.
2. Lower dorsal/lumbar level of lesion (wide canal) shows better neural recovery.
3. *On MRI*:
   - Extradural collection of fluid, pus which has hypointense (grey) signal on T1WI and hyperintense (bright) signal on T2WI (as opposed to dry granuloma showing a heterogeneous signal) has better chances of recovery.
   - Preserved spinal cord volume (as opposed to thinning of spinal cord seen in long-standing cases) on MRI is a good prognostic indicator for neural recovery.

- Preserved spinal cord morphology (as opposed to syringohydromelia or myelomalacia seen in long-standing cases) with cord edema have better chances of recovery.

4. *Intraoperatively*: If during surgical decompression the presence of fluid, pus and soft granulation tissue (wet lesion) have a better chances of neural recovery in comparison to thick inspissated pus, caseous tissue, fibrous tissue, bony sequestrae or bony salient and disk (dry lesion). Wet lesions has a better chances of neural recovery.

27. Jain AK. Treatment of Tuberculosis of the spine with neurologic complications. Clin Orthop Relat Res 2002 May; (398):75–8.

28. Jain AK, Jena A, Tuli SM. Correlation of clinical course with magnetic resonance imaging in tuberculous myelopathy. Neurology India 2000; 48(2):132–139.

Ref 28: *"Jain et al. studied MRI observations in 43 patients with tuberculosis of the spine with neurologic complications sequentially and correlated them with the clinical behavior of the disease. Extradural compression attributable to fluid on MRI scans resolves well with treatment and patients have a good neural recovery in comparison with extradural compression of mixed or granulomatous (dry) nature showing constriction of the cord. Patients with preserved cord volume with edema or myelitis of the cord on MRI scans have a good neural recovery. Myelomalacia of the spinal cord was found to be a poor prognostic sign of neural recovery.[8] The magnitude of thinning of the spinal cord did not always correlate with severity of neural deficit; however, thinning of the cord in association with myelomalacia, syrinx, or both carries a bad prognosis. The patient is likely to have better neural recovery if, on surgical decompression, pus and granulation tissue are drained (wet lesion) in comparison with thick inspissated pus, caseous tissue, fibrous tissue, bony sequestrae or bony salient and disk (dry lesion).*

Q. 17. What are the indications of surgery in TB spine with neural deficit?

Indications of surgery in TB spine with neural deficit:

1. Neural complications developing or neurological deficit getting worse or remaining stationary during the course of non-operative treatment (3–4 weeks).

2. *Paraplegia of rapid onset*: The paraplegia developing and progressing rapidly, indicating mechanical instability.

3. *Intraspinal tubercular granulomas*: These patients may present as spinal tumour syndrome, i.e. compressive myelopathy

with clinical localization and without radiological diagnosis (normal X-ray) of TB spine. MRI is useful for diagnosis. Wide surgical decompression with removal of intraspinal granulomas is advocated.

4. *Neural arch disease with neural complications*: In these patients, excision of neural arch and decompression is performed.

5. The patients of TB spine with severe paraplegia (flaccid paraplegia, paraplegia in flexion, complete sensory loss, and complete loss of motor power for more than 6 months) should be undertaken for early surgical decompression.

6. Painful paraplegia in elderly patient.

7. Large symptomatic abscess, for example, a large prevertebral abscess in cervical region causing dysphagia.

29. Jain AK, Kumar J. Tuberculosis of spine: neurological deficit. Eur Spine J (2013) 22 (Suppl 4):S624–S633.

16. Jain AK, Kumar S, Tuli SM. Tuberculosis of spine (C1 to D4). Spinal Cord 1999; 37:362–369.

18. Khoo LT, Mikawa K, Fessler RG. A surgical revisitation of Pott distemper of the spine. Spine J 2003; 3(2):130–45.

30. Louw JA. Spinal tuberculosis with neurological deficit. Treatment with anterior vascularised rib grafts, posterior osteotomies and fusion. J Bone Joint Surg Br 1990; 72(4):686–93.

Ref 29: *The early surgical decompression is indicated when neural complication has developed during conservative treatment or remaining stationary with no neural improvement after fair trial of conservative treatment (3–4 weeks) or neural deficit getting worse on non-operative treatment. The patients who have pretreatment long segment (4 or more vertebral disease) disease with kyphosis are likely to progress with final kyphosis of 60⁰ or more or already have 60 kyphosis should be undertaken for decompression and kyphosis correction. The rapid onset paraplegia indicates mechanical accident (pathological subluxation/ dislocation), hence the patient needs to be evaluated for instability. The patients with severe paraplegia (flaccid paraplegia, paraplegia in flexion, complete sensory loss, and complete loss of motor power for more than 6 months) should be undertaken for decompression. The patient of spinal tumor syndrome is to be decompressed to establish the diagnosis. The paraplegia with neural arch affection, recurrent paraplegia and paraplegia accompanied by uncontrolled spasticity of such severity that reasonable rest and immobilization are impossible and massive prevertebral abscess at upper cervical spine causing difficult deglutition/respiration in the patient are other clinical indications for* *surgical decompression. The paraplegia with panvertebral involvement (disease of both anterior and posterior column) as observed on plain radiograph with associated scoliosis and/or severe kyphosis or showing destruction of all components of VB should be undertaken for instrumented stabilization besides anterior decompression, since instability besides mechanical compression is the contributing factor for paraplegias. Patient of TB paraplegia with MRI observation of extradural compression consisting of granulation/caseous tissue with little fluid component compressing spinal cord circumferentially and constricting the cord or compression with sequestrated disk with the features suggestive of cord edema/myelitis or myelomalacia should be undertaken for early surgical decompression.*

Q. 18. Should instrumented stabilization be done in TB spine. What are the indications of instrumented stabilization?

The instrumentation can be safely performed in tuberculosis, as there is very low/negligible risk of biofilm formation. However, the instrumentation is indicated in cases of:

1. Panvertebral disease, due to it is being potentially unstable.
2. Long segment disease, where a >4–5 cm long graft is required to bridge the gap after surgical decompression in dorsal spine. The graft is most unstable on the day of surgery, it may get displaced or break, consequently producing neural complications.
3. *In lumbar and cervical spine*: Any deformity correction would require instrumented stabilization.
4. When kyphosis correction surgery is contemplated.
5. TB spine in junctional area such as cervicodorsal spine and dorsolumbar spine. These are junctions of mobile and relatively fixed segments of spine. Hence, after spinal decompression and fusion, instrumented stabilization is indicated to support and protect inserted graft to bridge the post-debridement defect.

17. Jain AK, Jain S. Instrumented stabilization in spinal tuberculosis. Int Orthop 2012 Feb; 36(2):285–92.

4. Jain AK. Tuberculosis of the spine: a fresh look at an old disease. J Bone Joint Surg Br 2010 Jul; 92(7):905–13.

31. Sundararaj GD, Behera S, Ravi V, Venkatesh K, Cherian VM, Lee V. Role of posterior stabilisation in the management of tuberculosis of the dorsal and lumbar spine. J Bone Joint Surg Br 2003 Jan; 85(1):100–6.

32. Talu U, Gogus A, Ozturk C, Hamzaoglu A, Domanic U. The role of posterior instrumentation and fusion after anterior radical debridement and fusion in the surgical treatment of spinal tuberculosis: experience of 127 cases. J Spinal Disord Tech 2006 Dec; 19(8):554–9.

33. Mehta JS, Bhojraj SY. Tuberculosis of thoracic spine a classification based on the selection of surgical strategies. J Bone Joint Surg Br 2001; 83B:859–863.

34. Wen-Jer C, Chi-Chuan W, Chi-Hsiung J, Lih-Huei C, Chi-ChienN, Po-Liang L. Combined anterior and posterior aurgeriesin the treatment of spinal tuberculous spondylitis. Clin Orthop Relat Res 2002; 398:50–59.

35. Moon MS, Woo YK, Lee KS, Ha KY, Kim SS, Sun DH. Posterior instrumentation and anterior interbody fusion for tuberculous kyphosis of dorsal and lumbar spines. Spine 1995; 20:1910–1916

Q. 19. How do we treat tuberculosis of craniovertebral junction (CVJ) and C1–C2 vertebrae?

All cases of suspected CVJ tuberculosis should be referred to a neurosurgeon/spinal/orthopedic surgeon or a tertiary level center. The treatment of CVJ tuberculosis cannot be standardized and has to be tailored to the condition of the patient and extent of the disease. The main features that dictate management protocol are neurological grade of the patient, extent of bony destruction and compression of spinal cord, associated atlantoaxial dislocation, and clinical response to antituberculous drug therapy. CT scan and MRI are mandatory to judge extent of disease and plan treatment. The first step is confirmation of diagnosis by CT-guided biopsy/transoral biopsy in cases of diagnostic dilemma.

The treatment includes:

1. *ATT and immobilization with traction/orthoses is advocated*: Patients with early disease and no demonstrable radiological instability with no significant compression of spinal cord should be treated by ATT and orthosis. Patient should be routinely assessed for instability and any incipient neural deficit. Generally most of the patients stablizes spontaneously on conservative treatment. The dynamic X-rays (X-rays of cervical spine in flexion and extension) should

be taken at 3 months follow-up. The translation of anterior arch of C1 over C2 suggests instability. In such cases, posterior occipitocervical fusion is indicated.

2. *ATT and transoral/anterior retropharyngeal decompression alone*: In patients with mild bony changes and no atlantoaxial dislocation, dynamic X-rays (cervical spine lateral view in flexion and extension) to be taken on X-ray table to ascertain the presence of instability at C1 and C2. If unstable, proceed for posterior fusion (instrumented/uninstrumented). However, in case of stridor and/or difficulty in deglutition, the anterior retropharyngeal decompression is performed.

3. *ATT and decompression with posterior occipitocervical fusion*: Patients with extensive bony changes at the start of treatment and those after extensive debridement show instability, those with dislocation/subluxation prior to surgery require posterior occipitocervical fusion.

The duration of ATT recommended in literature is at least for 18 months.

However, as per INDEX TB Guidelines, the lesion may evaluated by contrast MRI at 12 months to decide continuation of ATT for further 6 months, if lesion shows activity of disease.

16. Jain AK, Kumar S, Tuli SM. Tuberculosis of spine (C1 to D4). Spinal Cord 1999 May; 37(5):362–9.

36. Shukla D, Mongia S, Devi BI, Chandramouli BA, Das BS. Management of craniovertebral junction tuberculosis. Surg Neurol 2005 Feb; 63(2):101–6

37. Chadha M, Agarwal A, Singh AP. Craniovertebral tuberculosis: a retrospective review of 13 cases managed conservatively. Spine (Phila Pa 1976). 2007 Jul 1;32(15):1629–34.

38. Qureshi MA, Afzal W, Khalique AB, Pasha IF, Aebi M. Tuberculosis of the craniovertebral junction. Eur Spine J 2013 Jun; 22 Suppl 4:612–7.

39. Arora S, Sabat D, Maini L, Sural S, Kumar V, Gautam VK, Gupta A, Dhal A. The results of nonoperative treatment of craniovertebral junction tuberculosis: review of twenty-six cases. J Bone Joint Surg Am 2011 Mar 16;93(6):540–7.

40. Krishnan A(1), Patkar D, Patankar T, Shah J, Prasad S, Bunting T, Castillo M, Mukherji SK.Craniovertebral junction tuberculosis: a review of 29 cases. J Comput Assist Tomogr 2001 Mar-Apr; 25(2):171–6.

TB SPINE IN CHILDREN

Q. 20. How to suspect spinal TB in children?

Common findings:
1. Persistent localized back pain
2. Low grade fever/persistent malaise/loss of appetite
3. Failure to thrive

Additional findings:
1. Night cries
2. Inability to walk/cautious gait
3. Tendency to support trunk on thighs with both hands (dorsal spine involvement)—Cantilever sign
4. Tendency to support head with both hands (cervical spine involvement)
5. Palpable cold abscess
6. Visible/palpable kyphotic deformity

Lab parameters:
1. Raised ESR
2. Anemia
3. Low normal or decreased serum albumin
4. Relative lymphocytosis/monocytosis with near normal total leukocyte count
5. Positive Mantoux test

X-ray, CT and MRI features are similar to those in adults, though the involvement is often more extensive. Younger the child, more extensive and more rapid progression of lesions.

---

41. Jain AK, Sreenivasan R, Mukunth R, Dhammi IK. Tubercular spondylitis in children. Indian J Orthop 2014 Mar;48(2):136–44.
42. Eisen S, Honywood L, Shingadia D, Novelli V. Spinal tuberculosis in children. Arch Dis Child 2012 Aug; 97(8):724-9.

Ref 41: *"The children with TB spine usually present with persistent localized back pain, loss of appetite, weakness of both lower limb and inability to walk. The child is usually pale, listless and anemic. They also have a cautious gait and tend to walk keeping both hands at thigh to support the trunk. If the cervical spine is involved, they :valk supporting the head with both hands. Clinically, one may find a knuckle/angular spinal deformity with or without a local/distant palpable cold abscess."*

Q. 21. What are the indications of surgery in children?

The indications for surgery are same as in adults, which are:

1. *Diagnostic dilemma*—to confirm diagnosis
2. Cord compression and neurological complications
3. Large abscesses/dysphagia caused by large cervical pre-vertebral abscess
4. Spinal instability
5. *Spinal deformity correction*: In children, the kyphotic deformity may increase with growth, hence a low threshold is kept for deformity correction.
6. *Suspected drug resistance*—to obtain tissue for culture and sensitivity.

41. Jain AK, Sreenivasan R, Mukunth R, Dhammi IK. Tubercular spondylitis in children. Indian J Orthop 2014 Mar;48(2):136–44.

43. Seddon JA, Donald PR, Vlok GJ, Schaaf HS. Multidrug-resistant tuberculosis of the spine in children—characteristics from a high burden setting. J Trop Pediatr 2012 Oct;58(5):341–7.

44. Rajasekaran S. Natural history of Pott's kyphosis. Eur Spine J 2013 June; 22(Suppl 4): 634–640.

Ref 41: *...surgical intervention is indicated for spinal deformity, neurological complications, instability, large abscesses and to obtain tissue in a case of diagnostic dilemma and suspected MDR-TB.*

Q. 22. What is the follow-up protocol for a child with spinal TB?

Ans. The children treated for spinal tuberculosis should be followed up every one month for first 6 months followed by every 2 months till the lesion heals. Thereafter, once in a year to observe the behavior of kyphosis and document progression of kyphosis with growth till maturity. The spinal deformity continues to increase in children in view of growth alteration in children. Hence they need to be observed/follow-up till maturity for growth-related increase in deformity.

41. Jain AK, Sreenivasan R, Mukunth R, Dhammi IK. Tubercular spondylitis in children. Indian J Orthop 2014 Mar;48(2):136–44.

42. Eisen S, Honywood L, Shingadia D, Novelli V. Spinal tuberculosis in children. Arch Dis Child 2012 Aug;97(8):724–9.

44. Rajasekaran S. Natural history of Pott's kyphosis. Eur Spine J 2013 June; 22 (Suppl 4): 634–640.

Q. 23. What are the clinicoradiological risk factors to suspect progression of kyphotic deformity in a child with spinal TB?

The kyphotic deformity has increased risk of progression in cases of:

1. Age of less than 7 years at the time of the disease
2. Cervicothoracic and thoracolumbar junctional lesions
3. Affection of 3 or more vertebral bodies
4. The presence of radiographic spine-at-risk signs (Rajasekaran *et al.*).

41. Jain AK, Sreenivasan R, Mukunth R, Dhammi IK. Tubercular spondylitis in children. Indian J Orthop 2014 Mar;48(2):136–44.
44. Rajasekaran S. Natural history of Pott's kyphosis. Eur Spine J 2013 June; 22(Suppl 4): 634–640.

Ref 41, 44: *"The clinical risk factors for developing progressive kyphosis are age less than 7 years, more than three vertebral body affection and the disease at lower dorsal and dorsolumbar junctional area. The radiological "spine at risk" signs are facet subluxation, retropulsion, toppling and lateral translation. The kyphotic deformity progresses if 2 or more spine at risk signs are observed in the presence of the clinical risk factors."*

Q. 24. What are radiological 'spine at risk' signs? (Fig. 5.21)

Rajasekaran described four simple radiological signs which reliably predict and identify children who are at risk for progression of kyphotic deformity. These signs are observed on AP and lateral X-rays of the spine. These signs are:

a. **Subluxation of the facet joint:** The facet joint subluxates at the apex of the curve, causing instability and loss of alignment.

b. **Retropulsion:** The posterior retropulsion of the diseased vertebral segment is identified by drawing two lines on lateral X-rays of the spine first along the posterior surfaces of the first upper and second along lower normal vertebra. Any shadow posterior to the junction of these lines is considered retropulsion in the spinal canal.

c. **Lateral translation** is confirmed, when the line drawn through the middle of the pedicle of the lower vertebra does not touch the line drawn from the pedicle of the superior vertebra. This means the proximal spine has translated over the distal spine. In such instance, the vertebral bodies and posterior complex are diseased simultaneously.

d. **Toppling sign:** The line along the anterior surface of the lower normal vertebra is drawn and it intersects the inferior surface of the upper normal vertebra. Toppling has occurred when the line intersects above the middle of the anterior surface of the upper normal vertebra.

All these signs represent the presence of spinal instability due to dislocation of the facet joints. Each sign is given a score of 1 with a maximum possible score of 4. A spinal instability score of more than 2 is associated with a significantly larger final deformity. A score of 3 or more accurately predicts an increase in the angles of deformity and kyphosis of more than 30° and a final deformity of more than 60°.

44. Rajasekaran S. Natural history of Pott's kyphosis. Eur Spine J 2013; 22(Suppl 4): 634–640.

45. Rajasekaran S. The natural history of post-tubercular kyphosis in children: radiological signs which predict lateincrease in deformity. J Bone Joint Surg 2001; 83B:954–962.

46. Rajasekaran S. Buckling collapse of the spine in childhood spinal tuberculosis. Clin Orthop Relat Res 2007; 460:86–92.

47. Rajasekaran S, Shanmugasundaram TK. Prediction of the angle of gibbus deformity in tuberculosis of the spine. J Bone Joint Surg 1987; 69:503–509.

Q. 25. What should be the treatment guide, if progressive kyphosis is suspected?

A case of TB spine with clinicoradiological signs of progressive kyphosis should be surgically undertaken for surgical correction of kyphotic deformity in active or healed stage of disease.

In active disease: The deformity correction is easier in active disease than in healed disease. The principles of deformity correction is described in text. However, various surgical procedures described are:

1. Anterior decompression and pedicle screw fixation by a posterior only approach
2. Anterior decompression with posterior column shortening and pedicle screw fixation
3. Decompression and anterior column reconstruction with cortical strut graft/allograft/titanium cage with or without posterior instrumentation stablization
4. Anterolateral decompression and deformity correction by extrapleural anterolateral approach using Hartshill rectangle

In healed disease, decompression and deformity correction is described by:

1. Transpedicular decancellation osteotomy
   • to correct kyphotic deformity
2. Direct internal kyphectomy
   • to perform anterior decompression by removing internal salient in late onset paraplegia.
3. Pedicle subtraction osteotomy to correct angular kyphosis.
4. Closing/opening wedge osteotomy for deformity correction.

41. Jain AK, Sreenivasan R, Mukunth R, Dhammi IK. Tubercular spondylitis in children. Indian J Orthop 2014 Mar;48(2):136–44.
48. Rajasekaran S. Kyphotic deformity in spinal tuberculosis and its management. Int Orthop 2012; 36:359–365.
49. Jain AK, Maheshwari AV, Jena S. Kyphus correction in spinal tuberculosis. Clin Orthop Relat Res 2007 Jul;460:117–23.
50. Bezer M, Kucukdurmaz F, Guven O. Transpedicular decancellation osteotomy in the treatment of posttuberculous kyphosis. J Spinal Disord Tech 2007;20:209–15.
51. Kalra KP, Dhar SB, Shetty G, Dhariwal Q. Pedicle subtraction osteotomy for rigid posttuberculous kyphosis. J Bone Joint Surg Br 2006;88:9257.
52. Wong YW, Leong JC, Luk KD. Direct internal kyphectomy for severe angular tuberculous kyphosis. Clin Orthop Relat Res 2007 Jul;460:124–9.
53. Kawahara N, Tomita K, Hisatoshi B et al. Closing–opening wedge osteotomy to correct angular kyphotic deformity by a single posterior approach. Spine 2001; 26:391–402.

Ref 41: *"Those kyphotic deformities which are likely to show progression should be considered for correction of kyphosis in active disease or in early post-treatment stage as surgery is easier and associated with less risk in the active stage."*

"The principles of such correction are also the same with anterior corpectomy, posterior column shortening, closing/opening wedge osteotomy and instrumented stabilization. In such instances, since there is no active disease hence pedicle screw construct with posterior only multilevel modified vertebral column resection can allow good deformity correction."

"Transpedicular decancellation osteotomy', 'pedicle subtraction osteotomy', and 'direct internal kyphectomy' have been used to treat kyphosis in active as well as healed disease."

SEQUELAE OF TB SPINE

Q. 26. What is the definition of late onset paraplegia (Paraplegia with healed disease)?

Late onset paraplegia is defined as appearance of neural deficit after a disease/symptom free period of at least 2 years in any patient who was treated adequately for TB spine with or without neural deficit and achieved healed status and has a residual kyphotic deformity. [Adequate treatment implies completion of standard treatment (medical ± surgical) and complete resolution of disease on imaging as well as restoration of laboratory parameters]. In general terms, the paraplegia developing or progressive paraplegia secondary to long-standing kyphotic deformity after healing of the disease. Generally, these patients with severe healed kyphotic deformity report 10 years or later, after being treated for tuberculosis of spine. They complain of gradual onset and slowly progressive neurological deficit/deterioration of existing deficit.

54. Hsu LCS, Cheng CL, Leong JCY. Pott's paraplegia of late onset.The cause of compression and results after anterior decompression. J Bone Joint Surg [Br] 1988;70-B:534–8.

55. Bilsel N, Aydingoz O, Hanci M, Erdogĭan F. Late onset Pott's paraplegia. Spinal Cord (2000) 38, 669–674.

29. Jain AK, Kumar J. Tuberculosis of spine: neurological deficit. Eur Spine J 2013; 22 (Suppl 4):S624–S633.

27. Jain AK. Treatment of tuberculosis of the spine with neurologic complications. Clin Orthop Relat Res 2002 May;(398):75-84.

Ref 54&55: *"Seddon(1935), describing this variety (his Type III paraplegia) stated that the patient usually had fairly extensive spinal caries early in life but made an apparent recovery and remained symptomless apart from increasing kyphosis. Then, after a long period of "anything from four to 40 years", paraplegia set in, usually incomplete but sometimes severe. Seddon was uncertain whether this type of paraplegia was caused by reactivation or by a healing bony ridge."*

"Hodgson et al described two basic groups in preoperative evaluation of the lesion. Group A: paraplegia with active disease, which included two subtypes: (1) External pressure on the cord; (2) penetration of the dura by infection; Group B: paraplegia of healed disease, which included two subtypes: (1) Transection of the cord by a bony ridge; (2) constriction of the cord by granulation and

*fibrous tissue The distraction of the spinal cord in the kyphotic area may cause
ischemia and spinal tract atrophy and gliosis can be the outcome. Both the
effects of this distraction and the direct compression to the spinal cord may be
the cause of the paraplegia."*

Q. 27. What are clinical predictors of apparent/impending late onset paraplegia (paraplegia with healed disease)?

Predictors of late onset paraplegia in a patient with healed
kyphotic deformity include:

1. Reappearance of UMN signs after a minimum 2 years disease
   free period.
   a. Slowly progressing mild spasticity/weakness of lower
      limbs
   b. Unsteady spastic gait
   c. Extensor Babinski's plantar reflex
   d. Ankle clonus (which may disappear on 30 minutes rest).
2. Urinary incontinence
3. Numbness in lower limbs

Rapid development of the above signs indicates reactivation
of disease as opposed to the slow progression seen in healed
disease.

---

55. Bilsel N, Aydingoz O, Hanci M, Erdoğan F. Late onset Pott's
    paraplegia. Spinal Cord (2000) 38, 669–674.

29. Jain AK, Kumar J. Tuberculosis of spine: neurological deficit. Eur
    Spine J 2013; 22 (Suppl 4):S624–S633.

Ref 55: *"Clinically, paraplegia due to reactivation/recrudescence is severe and
has a relatively rapidly developing course as compared to late onset paraplegia
with healed lesion. Similarly, such paraplegia with reactivation/recrudescence
responds early and better to treatment than paraplegia with healed lesions."*

Ref 29: *"The severity of kyphotic deformity has not been correlated with
development of neural deficit. Tuli believed that chances of late onset paraplegia
is more if the initial lesion heals with kyphosis of 60° or more. This type of
paraplegia is usually seen in patients with severe kyphosis in dorsal and
dorsolumbar spine. It is attributed to the stretching of spinal cord over internal
salient. There may indeed be a very sharp ridge at the angle of kyphosis, and
the cord in its membrane may be found stretched across it like a violin string
across a fiddle bridge."*

Ref 55: *"The most common symptom in the middle-aged patients with kyphosis
is slowly progressing weakness and numbness of the lower extremities together*

with urinary incontinence and unsteady spastic gait. Luk reported that tuberculosis under control by chemotherapy could still recur many years later. Once the signs of neurological dysfunction appears, the treatment must be decompression and even if the adequate decompression can be achieved the results are not guaranteed."

Q. 28. How should a patient with paraplegia of healed disease be evaluated?

The patient should be evaluated:

1. **Clinically** evaluated for signs of recrudescence/reactivation of disease. Symptoms and signs of active disease should be searched. The patients with recrudescence generally have a recent onset neural deficit which is gradually progressive with clinical signs of active disease (history of pain and local spinal tenderness).

2. **Hematologically** by complete blood picture with ESR (low Hb with raised ESR, as seen in active disease).

3. **X-ray:** Besides the radiological evidence of a healed disease, one may encounter dimineralization above or at the apex of kyphosis or distal to it. The reactivation may be above/below, in a healthy segment. Usual radiological signs of TB spine are observed. The degree of kyphotic deformity needs to be assessed and on recrudescence/reactivation, the deformity shows progression. One may observe non-union and non-incorporation of graft in previously operated cases.

4. *Other imaging:* MRI for signs of active disease and/or spinal cord signal changes (presence of syringohydromelia, myelomalacia, thinning of cord, arachnoiditis). PET scan may be useful for detecting persistence or reactivation of infection/inflammation.

4. Jain AK.Tuberculosis of the spine: a fresh look at an old disease. J Bone Joint Surg Br 2010 Jul;92(7):905–13.

55. Bilsel N, Aydingoz O, Hanci M, Erdoğİan F. Late onset Pott's paraplegia. Spinal Cord 2000; 38, 669–674.

56. Hsu LCS, Cheng CL, Leong JCY. Pott's paraplegia of late onset. The cause of compression and results after anterior decompression. J Bone Joint Surg [Br] 1988;70-B :534–8.

29. Jain AK, Kumar J. Tuberculosis of spine: neurological deficit. Eur Spine J 2013; 22 (Suppl 4):S624–S633.

27. Jain AK. Treatment of tuberculosis of the spine with neurologic complications. Clin Orthop Relat Res 2002 May;(398):75 84.

3. Cheung WY, Keith DK Luk. Clinical and radiological outcomes after conservative treatment of TB spondylitis: is the 15 years' follow-up in the MRC study long enough? Eur Spine J 2013; 22 (Suppl 4):S594–S602.

Ref 55: *"Hodgson et al described two basic groups in preoperative evaluation of the lesion. Group A: paraplegia with active disease, which included two subtypes: (1) External pressure on the cord; (2) penetration of the dura by infection; Group B: paraplegia of healed disease, which included two subtypes: (1) Transection of the cord by a bony ridge; (2) constriction of the cord by granulation and fibrous tissue. The distraction of the spinal cord in the kyphotic area may cause ischemia and spinal tract atrophy and gliosis can be the outcome. Both the effects of this distraction and the direct compression to the spinal cord may be the cause of the paraplegia."*

Ref 29: *"Paraplegia with healed disease may occur when the initial lesion has healed with a residual severe deformity 10 to 20 years before. It is produced by stretching the spinal cord over an internal anterior bony projection, producing gliosis. MRI shows severe atrophy of the cord and/or syringohydromyelia, or constricting scarring of and around the dura. Reactivation of the disease is found in 30 to 40% of cases on exploration. Symptomatic severe stenosis of the lumbar canal and ossification of the ligamentum flavum adjacent to severe kyphosis may produce an incomplete neurological deficit."*

Q. 29. What are the indications for surgery in late onset paraplegia (paraplegia with healed disease)?

Indications for surgical intervention in healed post tubercular kyphosis include:

1. Degree of kyphotic deformity >60°
2. Progression of kyphosis
3. Non-union and non-incorporation of graft in operated cases
4. Suspicion of reactivation of disease
5. Development of neural deficit (late onset paraplegia).

55. Bilsel N, Aydingoz O, Hanci M, Erdoğan F. Late onset Pott's paraplegia. Spinal Cord 2000; 38:669–674.

56. Hsu LCS, Cheng CL, Leong JCY. Potts paraplegia of late onset. The cause of compression and results after anterior decompression. J Bone Joint Surg [Br] 1988;70-B:534–8.

29. Jain AK, Kumar J. Tuberculosis of spine: neurological deficit. Eur Spine J 2013; 22 (Suppl 4):S624–S633.

27. Jain AK. Treatment of tuberculosis of the spine with neurologic complications. Clin Orthop Relat Res 2002 May;(398):75–84.

3. Cheung WY, Keith DK Luk. Clinical and radiological outcomes after conservative treatment of TB spondylitis: is the 15 years' follow-up in the MRC study long enough? Eur Spine J 2013; 22 (Suppl 4): S594–S602.

Ref 55: *"The most common symptoms in the middle-aged patients with kyphosis are slowly progressing weakness and numbness of the lower extremities together with urinary incontinence and unsteady spastic gait. Luk reported that tuberculosis under control by chemotherapy could still recur many years later. Once the signs of neurological dysfunction appear, the treatment must be decompression and even if the adequate decompression can be achieved, the results are not guaranteed."*

2. *"Non-union and instability at the kyphus may also contribute to the late-onset paraplegia. When there is non-union at the kyphus, it opens and closes with movements, resulting in dynamic damage to spinal cord and neurological deficits. Because of the post-TB kyphosis that commonly occurs at the thoracolumbar junction, the compensatory hyperlordosis at the adjacent levels may also lead to accelerated facet joint degeneration, spinal canal stenosis and neurological deficit."*

Q. 30. How should we prognosticate late onset paraplegia?

The patients developing late onset paraplegia in a healed TB spine are likely to show poor or no neural recovery. The surgical treatment is still suggested to prevent further progression of neural deficit at later follow-up. While those developing late onset paraplegia following recrudescence of disease are likely to show some neural recovery after treatment.

Factors (reported for paraplegia with active disease) favoring a better outcome include:

1. Young age
2. Lower dorsal/lumbar level of lesion
3. Good nutritional status
4. Preserved cord volume and morphology on MRI imaging
5. Duration and progression of late onset paraplegia: Long-standing paraplegia or a very gradual onset of paraplegia has a poor chances of recovery.
6. Drug sensitivity test (in case of reactivation of disease) should be performed to rule out drug resistance. The patients having

reactivation with drug resistant organism are likely to show poor neural recovery.

7. The condition of spinal cord on MRI: The spinal cord with mild to moderate cord atrophy with edema may show some neural improvement while the spinal cord showing myelomalacia/syringomyelia are bad prognostic indicator.

---

27. Jain AK. Treatment of tuberculosis of the spine with neurologic complications. Clin Orthop Relat Res 2002 May;(398):75–84.

28. Jain AK, Jena A, Tuli SM. Correlation of clinical course with magnetic resonance imaging in tuberculous myelopathy. Neurology India, 2000; 48(2):132–139.

29. Jain AK, Kumar J. Tuberculosis of spine: neurological deficit. Eur Spine J 2013; 22 (Suppl 4):S624–S633.

5. Zhang Z. Late onset Pott's paraplegia in patients with upper thoracic sharp kyphosis. Int Orthop (SICOT) (2012) 36:381–385.

Ref 27: *"Numerous factors have been identified that determine the neural recovery in patients with Pott's paraplegia. Younger age and good nutritional status are associated with better neural recovery. The cervicodorsal junction and upper dorsal spine affection show poor neural recovery because the spinal canal is narrow. The patients with paraplegia with active disease have a better chance of neural recovery as compared with patients with paraplegia with healed disease. Patients with severe kyphosis have poor neural recovery. Patients with neurologic complications of gradual onset and shorter duration have better neurologic recovery than patients with neurologic complications of a longer duration and rapid onset. Rapidly progressive paraplegia signifies a mechanical insult because of pressure from disk or sequestrae, pathologic subluxation or dislocation, or vascular catastrophe, and shows the worst prognosis. In long-standing compression, some permanent changes in the cord may be responsible for nonrecovery or poor recovery. Patients with severe paraplegia (Stage IV paraplegia) have poor neural recovery. Patients with typical anterior vertebral body disease have a better neural recovery as compared with patients with grossly unstable panvertebral lesions.*

Ref 28: *Jain et al. studied MRI observations in 43 patients with tuberculosis of the spine with neurologic complications sequentially and correlated them with the clinical behavior of the disease. Extradural compression attributable to fluid on MRI scans resolves well with treatment and patients have a good neural recovery in comparison with extradural compression of mixed or granulomatous (dry) nature showing constriction of the cord. Patients with preserved cord volume with edema or myelitis of the cord on MRI scans have a good neural recovery. Myelomalacia of the spinal cord was found to be a poor prognostic* *sign of neural recovery. The magnitude of thinning of the spinal cord did not always correlate with severity of neural deficit; however, thinning of the cord in association with myelomalacia, syrinx, or both carries a bad prognosis. The patient is likely to have better neural recovery if, on surgical decompression, pus and granulation tissue are drained (wet lesion) in comparison with thick inspissated pus, caseous tissue, fibrous tissue, bony sequestrae or bony salient and disk (dry lesion). Evoked potential studies are helpful in objectively documenting the respective sensory and motor deficit in patients with Pott's paraplegia. The motor evoked potential is more frequently abnormal as compared with sensory evoked potential and correlates with respective clinical improvement."*

"Several factors influence the neurological recovery rate in late onset Pott's paraplegics, such as the patient's general condition; age; the condition of the spinal cord; the level, duration and severity of paraplegia; the time of onset before the initiation of treatment; type of treatment; and the patient's drug sensitivity."

Q. 31. How should we treat late onset paraplegia?

The mainstay of treatment of late onset paraplegia with kyphosis in TB spine is anterior decompression of the spinal cord and stable fusion of the spinal column. Internal kyphectomy is indicated for a patient of late onset paraplegia with healed disease while anterior debridement and decompression with or without post-instrumentation is indicated in late onset paraplegia secondary to recrudescence of disease. The surgical correction of kyphotic deformity can be contemplated, if the neural deficit is minimal and deformity is not grotesque especially in children and young adults where the proximal and distal compensatory curvatures are still flexible and can be reversed with the segmental instrumentation.

However, in severe healed kyphotic deformity with moderate to severe neural deficit, only internal kyphectomy should be performed to provide more space (also described as anterior transposition of cord) to the kinked spinal cord.

3. Cheung WY, Keith DK Luk. Clinical and radiological outcomes after conservative treatment of TB spondylitis: is the 15 years' follow-up in the MRC study long enough? Eur Spine J 2013; 22 (Suppl 4):S594–S602.

52. Wong YW, Leong JC, Luk KD. Direct internal kyphectomy for severe angular tuberculous kyphosis. Clin Orthop Relat Res 2007 Jul;460:124–9.

29. Jain AK, Kumar J. Tuberculosis of spine: neurological deficit. Eur Spine J 2013; 22 (Suppl 4):S624–S633.

57. Jain AK, Dhammi IK, Jain S, Mishra P. Kyphosis in spinal tuberculosis – Prevention and correction. Indian J Orthop 2010 Apr-Jun; 44(2):127–136.

58. Rajasekaran S, Vijay K, Shetty AP. Single-stage closing-opening wedge osteotomy of spine to correct severe post-tubercular kyphotic deformities of the spine: a 3-year follow-up of 17 patients. Eur Spine J 2010 Apr;19(4):583–92.

Ref 52: *"For severe kyphosis with paraplegia of healed disease presenting at late adulthood, salvage of slowly progressive neurology is the main goal of treatment. Correction of the rigid and severe spinal deformity is no longer a priority. The decompression of the internal gibbus and stabilize the kyphosis with strut bone grafting via the costotransversectomy approach for this group of patients is still a preferred treatment."*

Ref 58: *"More recently, Rajasekaran et al. described a single-stage closing–opening wedge osteotomy to correct severe kyphosis as a result of TB infection...*
...Thus, the best indication for this procedure would be for children or young adults where the compensatory curves are still flexible and can be reversed with the segmental instrumentation."

Q. 32. Should ATT be given in paraplegia with healed disease (late onset paraplegia) after surgical decompression?

ATT should be given in all cases of TB spine with healed disease when surgical intervention is performed. In cases with documented healed disease, ATT should be given for 6–9 months post-surgery. In cases where there is clinical and/or histopatho-logical demonstration of recrudescence, a full course of ATT should be prescribed and drugs may be adjusted according to drug sensitivity pattern, if available. The duration of ATT is to be decided based on the clinical imaging criteria of bone healing.

55. Bilsel N, Aydingoz O, Hanci M, Erdoğlan F. Late onset Pott's paraplegia. Spinal Cord 2000; 38,669–674.

56. Hsu LCS, Cheng CL, Leong JCY. Pott's paraplegia of late onset. The cause of compression and results after anterior decompression. J Bone Joint Surg [Br] 1988;70-B:534–8.

58. Rajasekaran S, Vijay K, Shetty AP. Single-stage closing-opening wedge osteotomy of spine to correct severe post-tubercular kyphotic deformities of the spine: a 3-year follow-up of 17 patients. Eur Spine J 2010 Apr;19(4):583–92.

1. *"Although no indication of active disease in any patient existed preoperatively, infectious fluid was observed within small cavities during the operation of each patient. All patients received antituberculosis drug therapy postoperatively for a period of 9 ± 12 months although Koch bacillus could not be grown in the specimens taken. Isoniazid, rifampicin, pyrazinamid and streptomycin were used in all patients."*

2. *"Patients with healed disease received antituberculous drugs for two to three months as prophylaxis against recurrence."*

3. *"None of the patients had evidence of active tuberculosis. However, to prevent the recurrence of the disease, patients were prescribed full course of antituberculous drugs (ATDs) for a minimum period of 9 months.*

ATYPICAL PRESENTATION OF TB SPINE

Q. 33. What is the definition of atypical presentations of TB spine?

The cases of TB spine which do not have typical clinico-radiological localization/presentation of lesion are clubbed together as atypical presentations of TB spine. This term was described in the pre-MRI era when the diagnosis was based on clinicoradiological grounds. With the introduction of MRI, few of the atypical presentations are diagnosed clearly. They are still relevant because the suspicion for possible underlying tuberculosis is made on clinicoradiological ground and patients are subjected for MRI.

The atypical lesions/presentations are:

1. *Intraspinal extramedullary tuberculous granulomas*: These patients present with compressive radiculopathy/myelopathy with or without clinical localization. The plain X-ray may not show any evidence of disease. MRI shows an extradural granulomas compressing the dural sleeve (spinal cord or cauda equina).

2. *Intramedullary tuberculoma*: These patients present with compressive myelopathy with no finding on X-rays. On MRI, it may show an intramedullary lesion which on T2WI shows intramedullary lesion which has hypointense lesion in periphery with central hyperintensity and peripheral edema. On T1WI with gadolinium enhancement, intense peripheral enhancement is seen.

3. *Single vertebral disease*: Typically TB spine is a paradiscal disease, where two or more contiguous vertebral bodies are affected. Rarely it may show single vertebral involvement. Hence, it is described as atypical presentation of TB spine. The differential diagnosis in such cases may be Calves disease, lymphoma, giant cell tumor and hemangioma. The MRI is diagnostic.

4. *Large paravertebral abscess with little or no demonstrable bony focus*: Rarely TB spine may show large prevertebral abscess and X-rays fail to show any VB affection. However, MRI in such cases may show a small disease focus in a verterbral body.

5. Isolated epidural abscess with no demonstrable bony focus.

6. *Isolated involvement of neural arch and appendages*: The tubercular focus may be affecting only laminae/spinous process/pedicle, while vertebral body is unaffected.

7. *Sclerotic lesions and intervertebral bony bridging*: Classicaly the tubercular lesion shows dimineralization on plain X-ray, rarely the vertebral body may be sclerotic with lateral osteophytes on the vertebral body.

8. *Multifocal (skipped) lesion*: The spine has tubercular affection at two locations with normal intermediate segment.

9. Rarely, a herniated intervertebral disk and a failed back syndrome may be secondary to tubercular affection of the vertebral bodies.

4. Jain AK. Tuberculosis of the spine: a fresh look at an old disease. J Bone Joint Surg Br 2010 Jul;92(7):905–13.

59. Jain AK, Sethi A, Sethi R, Kumar S. Atypical presentation of spinal tuberculosis. Indian J Orthop 1997;31(3):164–170.

60. Kumar S, Jain AK, Dhammi IK, Aggarwal AN. Treatment of intraspinal tuberculoma. Clin Orthop Relat Res 2007 Jul;460:62–6.

61. Kumar KA. Clinical study and classification of posterior spinal tuberculosis. Int Orthop 1985;9(3):147-52.

62. Yuan K, Zhong ZM, Zhang Q, Xu SC, Chen JT. Evaluation of an enzyme-linked immunospot assay for the immunodiagnosis of atypical spinal tuberculosis (atypical clinical presentation/atypical radiographic presentation) in China. Braz J Infect Dis 2013 Sep-Oct;17(5):529–37.

63. Arora S, Sabat D, Maini L, Sural S, Kumar V, Gautam VK, Gupta A, Dhal A. Isolated involvement of the posterior elements in spinal tuberculosis: a review of twenty-four cases. J Bone Joint Surg Am 2012 Oct 17;94(20):e151.

64. Pande KC, Pande SK, Babhulkar SS. An atypical presentation of tuberculosis of the spine. Spinal Cord 1996; 34, 716–719.

65. Ahmadi J, Bajaj A, Destian S, Segall HD, Zee CS. Spinal tuberculosis: atypical observations at MR imaging. Radiology 1993 Nov; 189(2):489–93.

Q. 34. How do we investigate them?

The other features of atypical spinal TB include the following aspects:

1. Worm-eaten destruction of vertebral end plate
2. Destruction of centricity of the vertebral body or concentric collapse of vertebral body
3. Tuberculous abscess with no identifiable osseous lesion
4. Contiguous or skipped vertebral body destruction
5. Lytic lesion in pedicle/spinous process.

The X-ray picture might be unremarkable in many cases. Hence MRI and/or CT scan are essential to localize the disease and make a presumptive diagnosis.

The diagnosis can be confirmed with a CT-guided/open biopsy and/or aspiration of pus where accessible. Samples should be sent for PCR, BACTEC/culture and histopathology. Surgical decompression is indicated.

62. Yuan K, Zhong ZM, Zhang Q, Xu SC, Chen JT. Evaluation of an enzyme-linked immuno spot assay for the immuno diagnosis of atypical spinal tuberculosis (atypical clinical presentation/atypical radiographic presentation) in China. Braz J Infect Dis 2013 Sep-Oct;17(5):529–37.

63. Arora S, Sabat D, Maini L, Sural S, Kumar V, Gautam VK, Gupta A, Dhal A. Isolated involvement of the posterior elements in spinal tuberculosis: a review of twenty-four cases. J Bone Joint Surg Am 2012 Oct 17;94(20):e151.

4. Jain AK. Tuberculosis of the spine: a fresh look at an old disease. J Bone Joint Surg Br 2010 Jul;92(7):905–13.

59. Jain AK, Sethi A, Sethi R, Kumar S. Atypical presentation of spinal tuberculosis. Indian J Orthop 1997;31(3):164–170.

Q. 35. How do we treat when isolated lesions are diagnosed?

Antitubercular chemotherapy remains the cornerstone of treatment in all diagnosed cases. In addition to ATT, additional steps required in specific situations include:

1. *Spinous process disease*: Aspiration of cold abscess, if present. However, in the presence of neural deficit, the excision of spinous process and hemilaminectomy/laminectomy is indicated.

2. *Disease of laminae*: When disease of laminae is associated with neural deficit, surgical decompression by laminectomy is to be performed. The disease of laminae without neural deficit is to be treated by ATT alone.

3. *Disease of facet joint*: Isolated facet diseases are to be treated by non-operative method (ATT and suitable braces). When both facet joints are diseased along with vertebral body disease, then posterior instrumented stabilization is indicated.

4. *Extradural granuloma*: Laminectomy and removal of extra-dural granuloma is indicated. The granuloma is exposed to whole length and removed up to proximal and distal extent to visualize the spinal cord in the whole length. The sheet of granulation tissue present posterior to the dura is removed and no attempt is made to remove granuloma lying anterior to the spinal cord.

5. *Intradural granuloma*: The intramedullary granuloma resolves on ATT. The patients should be treated by ATT with close monitoring (at least once a week) of neural deficit. On deterioration of neural deficit, myelotomy may be indicated, however, it is seldom required and the intramedullary granuloma resolves on ATT. Expert consultation with a neurosurgeon is desirable.

59. Jain AK, Sethi A, Sethi R, Kumar S. Atypical presentation of spinal tuberculosis. Indian J Orthop 1997;31(3):164–170.
60. Kumar S, Jain AK, Dhammi IK, Aggarwal AN. Treatment of intraspinal tuberculoma. Clin Orthop Relat Res 2007 Jul;460:62–6.
61. Kumar K. A clinical study and classification of posterior spinal tuberculosis. Int Orthop 1985;9(3):147–52.
62. Yuan K, Zhong ZM, Zhang Q, Xu SC, Chen JT. Evaluation of an enzyme-linked immunospot assay for the immunodiagnosis of atypical spinal tuberculosis (atypical clinical presentation/atypical radiographic presentation) in China. Braz J Infect Dis 2013 Sep-Oct;17(5):529–37.
63. Arora S, Sabat D, Maini L, Sural S, Kumar V, Gautam VK, Gupta A, Dhal A. Isolated involvement of the posterior elements in spinal tuberculosis: a review of twenty-four cases. J Bone Joint Surg Am 2012 Oct 17;94(20):e151.
65. Pande KC, Pande SK, Babhulkar SS. An atypical presentation of tuberculosis of the spine. Spinal Cord (1996) 34, 716–719.

FAILURE OF CONSERVATIVE TREATMENT

Therapeutically Refractory Disease or Suspected (Presumptive) Drug Resistance

Q. 36. How to define a failure of conservative treatment (presumptive drug resistance)?

If a patient on conservative treatment does not show any improvement at 5–6 months of bed rest and ATT.

a. *Clinical*: Persistent or worsening of symptoms with localized tenderness, and/or increasing deformity.

b. *Hematological*: Persistently raised ESR or showing rising trend.

c. MRI shows deterioration of lesion at 5–6 months

d. Appearance of new lesion

e. Failure to show healing of ulcer/sinus

f. New cold abscess/lymph node appears

g. Would dehiscence in a postoperative case

Rule out paradoxical response:

a. In cases of suspected drug resistance, patient continues to remain stationary or worsens on treatment from the beginning.

b. Whereas in case of paradoxical response, patient initially improves and then shows deterioration.

Drug sensitivity shall show a sensitive and susceptible organism. Continuation of standard ATT is all that is required in case of paradoxical response.

---

65. Jain AK, Dhammi IK, Modi P, Kumar J, Sreenivasan R, Saini NS. Tuberculosis spine: Therapeutically refractory disease. Indian J Orthop 2012 Mar; 46(2):171–8.

3. Cheung WY, Keith DK Luk. Clinical and radiological outcomes after conservative treatment of TB spondylitis: is the 15 years' follow-up in the MRC study long enough? Eur Spine J (2013) 22 (Suppl 4):S594–S602.

Q. 37. How to investigate and treat when failure of conservative treatment (presumptive drug resistance) is documented?

How do we investigate a therapeutically non-responding TB spine?

What is the objective of surgery?

What investigation should be undertaken once the tissue procured?

CT-guided aspiration of pus/tissue biopsy should be performed. In cases where the aspirate/biopsy proves inconclusive, the lesion should be surgically debrided to reduce the disease load, procure tissue to subject it for investigations to ascertain the diagnosis and perform culture sensitivity for AFB.

Immunocompetence should be confirmed by testing for HIV, diabetes mellitus, liver/kidney disease. Complete and differential blood counts are indicated.

The diagnosis has to be ascertained by procuring tissue and samples to be sent for:

1. Histopathology, cytopathology to make histological diagnosis
2. Gram's stain
3. AFB staining
4. Culture and drug sensitivity testing (conventional LJ medium/BACTEC) for *Mycobacterium* (rule out fungal/brucellar infections)
5. *Molecular tests*: GeneXpert/Line probe assay/CB-NAAT for rapid drug sensitivity testing where available.

9. Bhojraj S, Nene A. Lumbar and lumbosacral tuberculous spondylodiscitis in adults: Redefining the indications for surgery. J Bone Joint Surg [Br] 2002;84-B:530–4.

65. Jain AK, Dhammi IK, Modi P, Kumar J, Sreenivasan R, Saini NS. Tuberculosis spine: Therapeutically refractory disease. Indian J Orthop 2012 Mar;46(2):171–8.

3. Cheung WY, Keith DK Luk. Clinical and radiological outcomes after conservative treatment of TB spondylitis: is the 15 years' follow-up in the MRC study long enough? Eur Spine J (2013) 22 (Suppl 4):S594–S602.

Ref 65: *"The disease may be drug-resistant, however, and therefore a poor response to standard chemotherapy at the end of 6 to 12 weeks does not imply that surgery is indicated. Our protocol in patients with clinical or radiological progression of disease despite receiving antituberculous treatment, was to start* *second-line drugs empirically, in consultation with a chest physician and to attempt a CT-guided needle biopsy in order to obtain tissue for culture. We had eight such patients who required second-line treatment before they showed a satisfactory response."*

"Though the majority of the patients respond well to anti-TB treatment, paradoxical response occurs in about 15% of cases. It usually develops 2 weeks to a few months after starting the anti-TB treatment. It is defined as clinical or radiological worsening of pre-existing tuberculous lesions or the development of new lesions not attributable to the normal course of disease, in a patient who initially improved with anti-TB drugs. It is a diagnosis by exclusion, which can only be made after excluding secondary bacterial infection, non-compliance to drug treatment and development of drug resistance. Up to 10% of patients with central nervous system TB report paradoxical response and this number may be as high as 30% in HIV-infected patients. The paradoxical response is a component of immune reconstitution inflammatory syndrome or immune restoration syndrome, which results from an exuberant inflammatory response toward incubating opportunistic pathogens."

Patients demonstrating a paradoxical response are more likely to have lower baseline lymphocyte counts, followed by a surge. This surge may be profound in HIV-infected patients recently started on HAART. Pregnancy may also be a risk factor for the paradoxical response.

Q. 38. Role of GeneXpert/Line probe assay in cases with failure of conservative treatment?

"The rapid TB test, known as GeneXpert MTB/RIF, is a fully automated diagnostic molecular test. It has the potential to revolutionize and transform TB care and control.

The test:
- Simultaneously ascertain the diagnosis of TB and rifampicin drug resistance.
- Provides accurate results in less than two hours so that patients can be offered proper treatment on the same day
- Has minimal biosafety requirements and training needs, and can be housed in non-conventional laboratories.

The articles on these test for osteoarticular TB are not available in literature (studies are required). However, the recommendations are avilable for pulmonary TB and neural and lymph node tuberculosis. The evidence is to be generated for bone and joint tuberculosis.

---

66. WHO October 2014: Tuberculosis diagnostics: Xpert MTB/RIF Test
    http://www.who.int/tb/publications/Xpert_factsheet.pdf

67. Held M, Laubscher M, Zar HJ, Dunn RN GeneXpert polymerase chain reaction for spinal tuberculosis an accurate and rapid diagnostic test. Bone Joint J 2014;96-B:1366–9.

*Index TB guidelines: Guidelines for extrapulmonary tuberculosis-2016. MOHFW, Govt of India.

Ref 65: *For diagnosis of pulmonary TB and rifampicin resistance*

- *Strong recommendation:*
  - *Xpert MTB/RIF should be used as the initial diagnostic test in adults and children presumed to have MDR-TB or HIV-associated TB*
- *Conditional recommendations (recognising major resource implications):*
  - *Xpert MTB/RIF may be used as the initial diagnostic test in adults and children presumed to have TB.*
  - *Xpert MTB/RIF may be used as a follow-up test to microscopy in adults presumed to have TB but not at risk of MDR-TB or HIV-associated TB, especially in further testing of smear-negative specimens*

For diagnosis of extrapulmonary TB and rifampicin resistance:

Strong recommendation: Xpert MTB/RIF should be used as the initial diagnostic test in testing cerebrospinal fluid specimens from patients presumed to have TB meningitis.

Conditional recommendation: Xpert MTB/RIF may be used as a replacement test for usual practice (including conventional microscopy, culture, and/or histopathology) for testing of specific non-respiratory specimens (lymph nodes and other tissues) from patients presumed to have extrapulmonary TB.

Ref 67: *"One of the disadvantages of PCR testing is that, in contrast to TB culture, PCR testing will give a positive result even if the pathogens are not viable. In these patients, active TB has to be confirmed clinically and by means of various imaging modalities. Another concern about the GeneXpert method is that it tests drug resistance only for rifampicin, therefore, a monoresistance for isoniazid can only be detected with other PCR testing methods, such as GenoType MTBDR plus or GenoType Mycobacterium CM lineprobe assays (Hain Lifescience, Nehren, Germany). In our series, we discovered one patient with isoniazid monoresistance. According to current treatment guidelines, isoniazid monoresistance does not alter the conventional TB regime for patients without isoniazid monoresistance. In conclusion, the GeneXpert test is more sensitive and gives faster access to results than the gold standard. Consequently, we recommend its use as the initial test in the diagnosis of patients with TB of the spine."*

Q. 39. While waiting for culture report in a case of suspected drug resistance is it justified to treat the patient as presumptive drug resistance by a second line ATT. While waiting for culture report what drug treatment should be started?

While waiting for culture report, these cases should be treated as presumptive drug resistance. Nowadays with the advent of BACTEC culture and PCR based tests like GeneXpert and Line Probe Assay, one can know about the presence of drug resistance very soon. Rifampicin by GeneXpert and rifampicin and isoniazid by Line Probe Assay in a few hours to a few days. These patients should be started on inj. amikacin/kanamycin, ethionamide, cycloserine, levofloxacin and pyrazinamide. Once the culture reports are available, then the drug treatment has to be tailored according to culture report.

Q. 40. If culture is sterile then what treatment is to be initiated?

In the presence of sterile tubercular culture report and histopathology report suggestive of tuberculosis, the patient should be treated by second-line drugs (presumptive drug resistance) as per the standard protocol of drug resistance.

Q. 41. What drugs should be started routinely in 2nd line therapy?

Based on WHO guidelines for the treatment of drug resistance and on findings of this study, the following guidelines can be considered while formulating the second-line regimens in indicated cases:

Table 6.2. Dosage and weight band recommendations for second-line drugs—ATT

S. no.	Drugs	Patient wt. (16–25 kg)	Patient wt. (26–45 kg)	Patient wt. (45–70 kg)	Patient wt. (>70 kg)
1.	Rifampicin	300 mg	450 mg	600 mg	600 mg
2.	Isoniazid	200 mg	200 mg	300 mg	450 mg
3.	Kanamycin	500 mg	500 mg	750 mg	1000 mg
4.	Levofloxacin	250 mg	500 mg	750 mg	1000 mg
5.	Ethionamide	375 mg	500 mg	750 mg	1000 mg
6.	Ethambutol	400 mg	800 mg	1200 mg	1600 mg
7.	Pyrazinamide	500 mg	1250 mg	1500 mg	2000 mg

(Contd...)

Table 6.2. Dosage and weight band recommendations for second-line drugs—ATT (*Contd...*)

S. no.	Drugs	Patient wt. (16–25 kg)	Patient wt. (26–45 kg)	Patient wt. (45–70 kg)	Patient wt. (>70 kg)
8.	Cycloserine	250 mg	500 mg	750 mg	1000 mg
9.	Na-PAS (80% bioavailability)	5 g	10 g	12 g	16 g
10.	Pyridoxine	50 mg	100 mg	100 mg	100 mg
11.	Moxifloxacin	200 mg	400 mg	400 mg	400 mg
12.	Capreomycin	500 mg	750 mg	1000 mg	1000 mg
13.	Amikacin	500 mg	500 mg	750 mg	1000 mg
14.	High dose INH	400 mg	600 mg	900 mg	900 mg
15.	Clofazimine	100 mg	200 mg	200 mg	200 mg
16.	Linezolid	300 mg	600 mg	600 mg	600 mg
17.	Amoxy-clav (for child 80 mg/kg in two doses)	875/125 mg BD	875/125 BD	875/125 2 morn+ 1 even	875/125 2 morn+ 1 even
18.	Clarithromycin	250 mg BD	500 mg BD	500 mg BD	750 mg BD

(*Reference*: Technical and Operational guidelines for TB control in India 2016, MOH&FW, Govt of India)

* The dosages have to be adjusted as per weight of the patient, if obese.

- *Individualized treatment is the best for drug-resistant tuberculosis spine patients, but in situations where culture sensitivity facilities are not available or when there is progression of disease inspite of the standard antitubercular treatment and in situations of repeated negative culture, an objectively designed empiric second-line regimen can be considered.*

- *Regimen should include at least four new drugs which have not been taken by the patient in the past. It is not recommended to add a single drug to the failing regimen: "Addison syndrome". Selection of drugs should be based on their hierarchical order from groups 1–5, bactericidal activity and adverse effect profile. Total duration of treatment should not be less than 18–24 months.*

- *No two drugs of the same pharmacological group or sharing the same drug adverse effect should be clubbed together in the regimen.*

- *Among the group-1 drugs, only pyrazinamide can be included in the regimen as it was found to be effective in more than 50% MDR strains. This level of resistance, however, makes it undependable. Pharmacologically pyrazinamide has an advantage when used in the initial part of the treatment as it acts well in closed cavities and acidic environments.*

- *According to WHO, any second-line regimen should have at least 6 months of initial injectable kanamycin or amikacin or capreomycin. Injectable kanamycin or amikacin can be added, as favorable susceptible patterns were found in most of our cases (resistance in 5.5% each). Pharmacologically also they are bactericidal against tuberculosis bacilli. Aminoglycosides have mainly ototoxic and nephrotoxic adverse effects which should be carefully monitored.*

- *Among the group-3 (fluoroquinolones), moxifloxacin can be added. In this study, resistance to moxifloxacin was 15.5% as compared to ofloxacin (38.8%). In vitro studies have shown decreasing efficacy from moxifloxacin = gatifloxacin [levofloxacin] ofloxacin against M. tuberculosis. Fluoroquinolones are bactericidal against tuberculosis bacilli and are also well tolerated; with adverse effect profile including mainly gastrointestinal disturbances. Thus, can be safely included in the regimen.*

- *From group-4, PAS being resistant in less than 9%, and cycloserine can be included. Ethionamide had more resistance (34.4%) than PAS in our study group. Overall ethionamide is less-toxic than PAS, but with enteric coated PAS, gastrointestinal side effects can be avoided. Giving PAS along with ethionamide should be avoided as their adverse effects are counterproductive.*

- *An important and useful adjunct can be clofazamine due to favorable susceptibility and toxicity profile.*

- *To adjudge clinical recovery, all drug-resistant tuberculosis patients can be serially monitored with three monthly complete blood count (CBC), erythrocyte sedimentation rate (ESR), C-reactive protein (CRP) and MRI along with drug-toxicity effects so as to modify drug combinations suitably.*

  In conclusion, our study highlights the growing threat posed by the development of widespread resistance to antituberculous drugs in the management of tuberculosis spine.

Complications arise due to delays in diagnosis, obtaining samples and by inappropriate administration of second-line drugs. Based on our findings, we recommend:

- *Having a high index of suspicion for the presence of drug resistance. Routine biopsy, culture and drug sensitivity testing of all patients even in the patients proposed for conservative management.*
- *Use of drug susceptibility patterns wherever available to guide selection of appropriate second-line drugs.*
- *In cases of non-availability of sensitivity despite the repeated attempts; use of data from large series like this, to plan best empirical chemotherapy protocol.*
- *Consideration to be made to relative drug toxicities, efficacy and compatibility when selecting second-line drugs.*

68. Mohan K1, Rawall S, Pawar UM, Sadani M, Nagad P, Nene A, Nene A. Drug resistance patterns in 111 cases of drug-resistant tuberculosis spine. Eur Spine J 2013 Jun;22 Suppl 4:647–52.

Q. 42. What is the duration for second-line treatment?

The duration of second-line treatment is generally two years and more as per guidelines for drug resistant pulmonary TB. However, no data exists for spinal tuberculosis. It is suggested to evaluate these patients by contrast MRI scan at 12, 18 months and 24 months of treatment to see the sequential changes as resolving tuberculosis lesion and in the end attainment of MRI-based healed status (fatty replacement of marrow as bright vertebral body in T1WI and absence of enhancement on contrast MRI). PET scan at 2 years may be helpful to ascertain absence of biological activity. Although no scinetific data exist on PET scan.

Q. 43. What is the role of vitamin D_3 as an adjunct to ATT?

Vitamin D supplementation during TB treatment remains controversial; a few studies have reported clinical improvement in pulmonary TB and 1 study reported no effect.

Given the controversy, it is recommended that daily recommended vitamin D allowance (400–600 IU) be provided to patients undergoing antitubercular therapy. Therapeutic dosage to be restricted to those with documented vitamin D deficiency.

69. Martineau AR, Honecker FU, Wilkinson RJ, Griffiths CJ. Vitamin D in the treatment of pulmonary tuberculosis. J Steroid Biochem Mol Biol 2007 Mar;103(3-5):793–8.

70. Salahuddin N, Ali F, Hasan Z, Rao N, Aqeel M, Mahmood F. Vitamin D accelerates clinical recovery from tuberculosis: results of the SUCCINCT Study [Supplementary Cholecalciferol in recovery from tuberculosis]. A randomized, placebo-controlled, clinical trial of vitamin D supplementation in patients with pulmonary tuberculosis. BMC Infect Dis 2013 Jan 19;13:22.

71. Wejse C, Gomes VF, Rabna P, Gustafson P, Aaby P, Lisse IM, et al. Vitamin D as supplementary treatment for tuberculosis: a double-blind, randomized, placebo-controlled trial. Am J Respir Crit Care Med 2009;179:843–50.

72. A Cochrane Review CD006086 Sinclair D, Abba K, Grobler L, Sudarsanam TD. Nutritional supplements for people being treated for active tuberculosis (2011) (Review), found that

73. WHO: Guideline: Nutritional care and support for patients with tuberculosis, 2013.

74. Sinclair D, Abba K, Grobler L, Sudarsanam TD. Nutritional supplements for people being treated for active tuberculosis (2011) (Review). Cochrane Database Syst Rev 2011 Nov 9;(11):CD006086.

75. WHO: Guideline: Nutritional care and support for patients with tuberculosis, 2013.

Q. 44. What is the role of steroids in spinal TB?

There is no role for steroids in the treatment of spinal TB. The steroid was not used ever by author in his clinical practice in spinal tuberculosis. It may be given as bolus when performing anterior transposition of the spinal cord in a case of paraplegia with healed disease where inadvertent cord handling has happened and patient has neural deterioration after surgical decompression.

Ref 76: *A Cochrane Review CD002244 Prasad K, Singh MB. Corticosteroids for managing tuberculous meningitis (Review) states:*
"Corticosteroids are commonly used in addition to antituberculous drugs for treating the condition. They help reduce swelling and congestion of the meninges, and thus decrease pressure inside the brain and the attendant risk of death or disabling residual neurological deficit among survivors. This review identified seven trials involving 1140 people that evaluated either dexamethasone or prednisolone given in addition to antituberculous drugs; only

one trial was of high quality. Overall, the trials showed that corticosteroids help reduce the risk of death or a risk of death or disabling residual neurological deficit. Only one trial evaluated the effects of corticosteroids in HIV-positive people, but the effects were unclear. Given the results of the review, all HIV-negative people with tuberculous meningitis should receive corticosteroids, but more trials are needed in HIV positive people."

1. The steroid use is advocated for intracranial tuberculoma/ involvement of meninges.

"No published controlled trials have examined whether patients with intra-cranial tuberculomas without meningitis or spinal cord tuberculosis benefit from adjunctive corticosteroids,although they are widely advocated. Anecdotally, they improve symptom and seizure control and reduce tuberculoma size and peri-lesional edema. Duration of therapy varies depending on response; it is common for symptoms to return once the dose is reduced...

There is insufficient evidence to recommend routine adjunctive cortico-steroids for all patients with tuberculomas without meningitis, or with spinal cord tuberculosis. However, they may be helpful in those patients whose symptoms are not controlled, or are worsening, on antituberculosis therapy, or who have acute spinal cord compression secondary to vertebral tuberculosis (B, II). Similar doses to those used for TBM should be given..."

Q. 45. What is the role of high protein diet in treating spinal TB?

Malnutrition can lead to secondary immunodeficiency that increases the host's susceptibility to infection. High protein diet is generally recommended by clinicians during the treatment of TB. It is thought to counteract the chronic wasting associated with the disease. However, there is no evidence to support the role of high protein diet in treating spinal TB.

77. Gupta KB, Gupta R, Atreja A, Verma M, Vishvkarma S. Tuberculosis and nutrition. Lung India/: Official Organ of Indian Chest Society. 2009;26(1):9–16.

78. Yang L, Liu Z. Analysis and therapeutic schedule of the postoperative recurrence of bone tuberculosis. J Orthop Surg Res 2013; 8: 47.

72. Sinclair D, Abba K, Grobler L, Sudarsanam TD. Nutritional supplements for people being treated for active tuberculosis (2011) (Review) Cochrane Database Syst Rev 2011 Nov 9;(11):CD006086.

73. WHO: Guideline: Nutritional care and support for patients with tuberculosis, 2013.

Ref 72: *A Cochrane Review CD006086 Sinclair D, Abba K, Grobler L, Sudarsanam TD. Nutritional supplements for people being treated for active Tuberculosis (2011) (Review), found that:*

"We currently don't know if providing free food to tuberculosis patients, as hot meals or ration parcels, reduces death or improves cure. Providing free food probably does improve weight gain during treatment, and may improve quality of life but further research is necessary.

We don't know if vitamins reduce death in HIV-negative people but they probably don't work in HIV-positive people with tuberculosis.

No studies have assessed whether vitamins improve tuberculosis cure. Vitamins probably don't improve weight gain, and no studies have assessed their effect on quality of life."

Ref 73: *WHO: Guideline: Nutritional care and support for patients with tuberculosis, 2013.*

"There is no evidence to recommend that nutritional management of severe acute malnutrition should be different for those with active TB than for those without active TB.

- *There is no evidence to recommend that nutritional management of severe acute malnutrition should be different in children with active TB than for those without active TB.*
- *Concerns about weight loss or failure to gain weight should trigger further clinical assessment (e.g. resistance to TB drugs, poor adherence, comorbid conditions) and nutrition assessment of the causes of undernutrition, in order to determine the most appropriate interventions.*

  WHO guideline: *Nutritional care and support for patients with tuberculosis 25.*
- *Closer nutritional monitoring and earlier initiation of nutrition support (before the first 2 months of TB treatment are completed) should be considered, if the nutritional indicator is approaching the cut-off value for a diagnosis of severe acute malnutrition.*
- *There is no evidence to recommend that nutritional management of moderate undernutrition should be different for children (less than 5 years of age) with active TB than for those without.*
- *Efforts should be made, within the sound principles of nutrition assessment, counselling and support, to ensure that TB patients are receiving the recommended intake of micronutrients, preferably through food or fortified foods. If that is not possible, micronutrient supplementation at 1 × the recommended nutrient intake is warranted."*

HIP

Q. 1. How common is tuberculosis of hip joint?

Tuberculosis of the hip constitutes approximately 15–20% of all cases of osteoarticular tuberculosis.

---

1. Tuli SM. Tuberculosis of the Skeletal System (Bones, Joints, Spine and Bursal sheaths) 4th ed. New Delhi: Jaypee Brothers Medical Publishers Pvt. Ltd.; 2010.
2. Babhulkar S, Pande S. Tuberculosis of the hip. Clin Orthop Relat Res. 2002 May; (398):93–9.
3. Martini M. Ed. Tuberculosis of the Bone and Joint. Springer-Verlag, Heidelberg; 1988: 87–96.

Q. 2. What is the common age of presentation?

Disease usually starts during first three decades, but no age is immune.

---

4. Saraf SK, Tuli SM. Tuberculosis of hip: A current concept review. Indian J Orthop 2015 Jan-Feb; 49(1): 1–9.
1. Tuli SM. Tuberculosis of the Skeletal System (Bones, Joints, Spine and Bursal sheaths) 4th ed. New Delhi: Jaypee Brothers Medical Publishers Pvt. Ltd.; 2010.

Q. 3. What are the clinical features (history and examination) to diagnose tuberculosis of hip?

The turberculosis of hip may progress from synovitis to early arthritis, advanced arthritis with or without subluxation/dislocation.

TB hip in synovitis stage: Patient presents with
- Pain, limp, deformity and fullness around the hip.
- Insidious in onset and are progressive in nature when without treatment.
- Child may wake up during night.
- Constitutional features like loss of weight and appetite with evening rise of temperature may be present in some cases.

On examination:
- The gait is antalgic
- Apparent lenghtening of the affected limb

- Tenderness in the scarpa's triangle
- Attitude and presence of flexion, abduction and external rotation deformity of the hip with restriction of range of movements at hip.

Stage of early arthritis: With progressive destruction of the joint, the local symptoms (as mentioned above) become more prominent. There is history of night cries. On examination,

- Presence of fullness around hip with tenderness in Scarpa's triangle.
- Presence of attitude of flexion, adduction and internal rotation with apparent limb shortening. On examination, the flexion, adduction and internal rotation deformity is demonstrated.
- Muscles are in spasm and wasting is also evident. The restriction of range of movement is about 50% of the normal range with painful spasm.

Stage of advanced arthritis:

- The destruction of joint leads to characteristic flexion, adduction and internal rotation deformity.
- The hip movements are painful and grossly restricted with shortening of the limb.
- Pathological dislocation/subluxation may occur as a result of gross destruction of the femoral head or superior acetabular margin (wandering acetabulum), adding further shortening and deformity.

Note. The attitude of the limb and deformity does not always correspond with the stage of arthritis, particularly when patients have been treated with traction.

1. Tuli SM. Tuberculosis of the Skeletal System (Bones, Joints, Spine and Bursal sheaths) 4th ed. New Delhi: Jaypee Brothers Medical Publishers Pvt. Ltd.; 2010.
4. Saraf SK, Tuli SM. Tuberculosis of hip: A current concept review. Indian J Orthop 2015 Jan-Feb; 49(1):1–9.
5. Sankaran B. Tuberculosis of bones and joints. Indian J Tuberculosis 1993; 40:109–19.

Q. 4. Which is the most commonly accepted clinical classification of TB hip?

The classification which is most commonly accepted is described by Tuli SM. The tuberculosis of hip is classified as (1) synovitis, (2) early arthritis, (3) advanced arthritis, (4) advanced arthritis with complications.

1. In synovitis stage, the patient develops flexion, abduction and external rotation deformity with apparant lengthening. the X-rays show regional osteopenia with haziness of articular margins.

2. In early arthritis, the patient develops flexion, adduction and internal rotation deformity with apparant shortening. The X-rays show rarefaction, osteopenia, bony erosion in femoral head , acetabulum and both with no or slight reduction in joint space.

3. In advanced arthritis, the patient develops flexion, adduction and internal rotation deformity with true shortening. The X-rays show besides all the above described features the articular surfaces are destroyed and joint space is grossly reduced.

4. In advanced arthritis with subluxations/dislocations, the patient develops flexion, adduction and internal rotation deformity with gross shortening. The X-rays show gross reduction/destruction of joint spaces with or without wandering acetabulum.

1. Tuli SM. Tuberculosis of the Skeletal System (Bones, Joints, Spine and Bursal sheaths) 4th ed. New Delhi: Jaypee Brothers Medical Publishers Pvt. Ltd.; 2010.

Q. 5. How to ascertain diagnosis of TB hip in various stages of the disease?

TB synovitis: The differential diagnoses in this stage are conditions which cause synovial inflammation like traumatic synovitis, transient synovitits, early stage of Perthes disease, low grade pyogenic infection, juxta-articular disease, early stage of slipped capital femoral epiphyses and avascular necrosis of the femoral head.

- Plain radiograph may be non-contributory in most of these cases or may show regional osteopenia.
- Ultrasonography may show joint effusion. The anterior synovial recess may be increased with or without thickening of anterior joint capsule. Ultrasound-guided aspiration may be useful to procure fluid for cytological evidence of diagnosis.
- MRI may show synovial effusion and bone edema. In this stage of disease, aspiration cytology or open biopsy is indicated to ascertain diagnosis.

Early arthritis:
- X-rays show regional osteopenia, indistinct joint margins and slight diminution of the joint space. These findings are generally diagnostic.
- MRI may show bone edema and joint effusion and minimal bone destruction.
- Open biopsy is indicated to make a diagnosis.

Advance arthritis: The X-ray in advanced stage of the disease is characteristic of diagnosis with severe localized osteopenia, gross destruction of head of femur and acetabulam. Surgical intervention (joint debridement excisional arthroplasty will allow to procure tissue to ascertain bacteriological/histological/molecular diagnosis).

Q. 6. What is the management of tuberculosis of hip in the stage of synovitis?

In the endemic regions for TB, like India, a clinical diagnosis supported by radiographs is adequate for starting of treatment which may not be the case in stage of synovitis. In early synovitis stage, clinicoradiological diagnosis is difficult hence further imaging to ascertain diagnosis is imperative. However, to establish the diagnosis, the patient is subjected to further examination like USG examination of hip joint; synovial effusion from the joint can be aspirated under USG guidance and is subjected to examination of its physical properties, culture, AFB smear examination and molecular diagnosis. MRI is useful to know the extent of involvement. In most of the patients, the above investigations can give a clue about the diagnosis. In some cases, the presence of concomitant pulmonary TB lesion could be enough reason to start ATT.

Aspiration/needle biopsy should be performed to establish microbiological/histopathological/molecular diagnosis. If the tissue/fluid yield is inadequate then open biopsy in indicated.

The patient should be started on ATT, analgesics and skin traction or skeletal traction. Since these limbs have abduction deformity, the traction should be applied to both the lower limbs. The traction in the 'well leg' should be more than the affected limb.

In a typical case, the pain starts subsiding 4 weeks after treatment and at that time, the active assisted exercises of the hip is added. The prognosis after ATT, traction/rest and mobilization exercises is very good in this stage and the surgical interventions usually are not required. The expected outcome in a well-treated case is attainment of almost near normal function.

6. Tuli SM. General principles of osteoarticular tuberculosis. Clin Orthop Relat Res 2002;398:11–19.

7. Shanmugasundaram TK. Tuberculosis of spine. Ind J Tuberculosis 1982;29:213–21.

Q. 7. What is the management of tuberculosis of hip in stage of early arthritis?

Traction (skin or skeletal on the affected limb), ATT, and analgesics supplementation is necessary till muscle spasm is relieved. Patient is advised to mobilize the joint without bearing weight over the involved limb. Range of motion exercises are started whenever patient is able to co-operate. Tissue confirmation of diagnosis is necessary, if there is failure to respond on chemotherapy. Synovectomy and joint debridement are performed with the objective to reduce the disease load and ascertain diagnosis. Palpable abscesses and large joint effusions are aspirated/drained. The expected outcome is a painless, mobile hip with 50–70% range of motion.

4. Saraf SK, Tuli SM. Tuberculosis of hip: A current concept review. Indian J Orthop 2015 Jan-Feb; 49(1):1–9.

Q. 8. What is the management of tuberculosis of hip in stage of advance arthritis?

In this stage of disease, the diagnosis can be made confidently on clinicoradiological grounds. Traction, ATT followed by arthrolysis of joint with joint debridement is indicated. Traction is applied to the affected side to correct the flexion and adduction deformity. The granulation tissue, sequestra and fibrous tissues are excised carefully without compromising with the vascularity of remaining part of upper end of the femur. After surgery, the skeletal traction is applied, and movements of the hip are allowed under supervision as soon as patient is able to participate in physiotherapy. The expected outcome depends on the radiological type of disease and the age of the patient. The children usually show good outcome.

4. Saraf SK, Tuli SM. Tuberculosis of hip: A current concept review. Indian J Orthop 2015 Jan-Feb; 49(1):1–9.

6. Tuli SM. General principles of osteoarticular tuberculosis. Clin Orthop Relat Res 2002;398:119.

8. Babhulkar S, Pande S. Tuberculosis of the hip. Clin Orthop Relat Res 2002;398:939.

Q. 9. What is the management of tuberculosis of hip in advanced arthritis with subluxation/dislocation?

Gross destruction of joint along with deformities and shortening requires operative intervention in the form of either excisional arthroplasty or arthrodesis. In excisional arthroplasty, the joint is debrided and the destroyed femoral head and neck is excised. The limb is maintained in traction and the range of motion exercises are permitted while on traction to achieve painless mobile joint. Such joints are usually unstable with gross shortening of the limb.

1. Tuli SM. Tuberculosis of the Skeletal System (Bones, Joints, Spine and Bursal sheaths) 4th ed. New Delhi: Jaypee Brothers Medical Publishers Pvt. Ltd.; 2010.

4. Saraf SK, Tuli SM. Tuberculosis of hip: A current concept review. Indian J Orthop 2015 Jan-Feb; 49(1):1–9.

8. Tuli SM, Mukherjee SK. Excision arthroplasty for tuberculous and pyogenic arthritis of the hip. J Bone Joint Surg Br 1981 Feb; 63-B(1):29–32.

10. Kim YY, Ahn BH, Bae DK, Ko CU, Lee JD, Kwak BM, et al. Arthroplasty using the Charnley prosthesis in old tuberculosis of the hip. Clinical experience with 810 year follow up evaluation. Clin Orthop Relat Res 1986; 211:116–21.

11. Jupiter JB, Karchmer AW, Lowell JD, Harris WH. Total hip arthroplasty in the treatment of adult hips with current or quiescent sepsis. J Bone Joint Surg Am 1981; 63:194–200.

Q. 10. What is the role of joint debridement in TB hip?

It is expected that patient will start showing significant relief in pain and spasm within 6–8 weeks on non-operative treatment. When patient does not respond to chemotherapy, then synovectomy and joint debridement are indicated.

The joint debridement is generally indicated in synovitis and early arthritis stage of the disease. In joint debridement, all of the synovial tissue, loose bodies, loose articular cartilage are removed and curettage of juxta-articular lesions is performed. The tissue obtained is sent for AFB smear, and culture, molecular diagnosis, histopathological evaluation to ascertain diagnosis [CB-NAAT (GeneXpert) and Line Probe Assay (LPA)]. Postoperatively, the limb is mobilized on traction (active and active assisted) and ATT. After 6 weeks, the patient may be mobilized with orthosis. Generally, patients attain good outcome.

4. Saraf SK, Tuli SM. Tuberculosis of hip: A current concept review. Indian J Orthop 2015 Jan-Feb; 49(1):1–9.

Q. 11. What is the management of stiff hip joint with fixed deformities after the disease has achieved healed status?

There are multiple options:

a. *Corrective osteotomy*: Patients presenting with sound ankylosis of short fibrous nature or bony ankylosis in unacceptable, deformed, non-functioning position require upper femoral corrective osteotomy. It corrects the alignment and believed to increase the local vascularity, therefore, can convert the painful fibrous union to painless bony union.

b. *Excision arthroplasty/girdlestone arthroplasty:* This procedure is generally performed in patients after completion of
growth. The joint is debrided and destroyed femoral head
and neck are excised. Excision arthroplasty provides a
mobile, painless hip joint with control of infection and
correction of deformity. The procedure is useful for those
patients who desire to do ground level activities.

Its other advantage is that it can be performed in the diseased
joints and hence reduces the disease load and help in effective
control of the disease. However, some degree of shortening
and instability is unavoidable. Delayed degenerative changes
in ipsilateral knee, contralateral hip and lumbosacral spine
also are the problems associated with excision arthroplasty.

c. *Arthrodesis:* Surgical fusion of the hip in the functional position relieves the pain and corrects the deformity, however,
it is at the cost of complete loss of movements. Its acceptance
in the society where squatting and sitting cross legged is
essential in day-to-day activity is very low.

1. Tuli SM. Tuberculosis of the Skeletal System (Bones, Joints, Spine
   and Bursal sheaths) 4th ed. New Delhi: Jaypee Brothers Medical
   Publishers Pvt. Ltd.; 2010.

4. Saraf SK, Tuli SM. Tuberculosis of hip: A current concept review.
   Indian J Orthop 2015 Jan-Feb; 49(1):1–9.

8. Tuli SM, Mukherjee SK. Excision arthroplasty for tuberculous
   and pyogenic arthritis of the hip. J Bone Joint Surg Br 1981 Feb; 63-
   B(1):29–32.

Q. 12. What are the stabilizing procedures in unstable hip?

After excision arthroplasty, the patient achieves mobile,
painless, unstable hip joint. To reduce instability, tectoplasty
or Milch pelvic support osteotomy can be done.

Tectoplasty is a procedure where a shelf is created above
the acetabulam to prevent upward movement of proximal
femur on vertical loading of hip.

The pelvic support osteotomy is performed at the level of
lesser trochanter. The proximal fragment abuts against the
lateral wall of the pelvis and angle at osteotomy site points
medially to provide a support of upper femur on the pelvis.
The disadvantages are:

a. It further shortens already shortened limb.
b. When performed in children, the angulation corrects spontaneously and proximal femur is no longer able to provide pelvic support. Hence resurgery is required after a few years.
c. After angulation osteotomy conversion to THR is difficult due to altered proximal femoral anatomy.

---

4. Saraf SK, Tuli SM. Tuberculosis of hip: A current concept review. Indian J Orthop 2015 Jan-Feb; 49(1):1–9.

12. Saito S, Takaoka K, Ono K. Tectoplasty for painful dislocation or subluxation of the hip. Long-term evaluation of a new acetabuloplasty. J Bone Joint Surg Br 1986;68:55–60.

13. Milch H. The pelvic support osteotomy. J Bone Joint Surg Am 1941; 23:581–595.

Q. 13. How safe is to use metal (total hip replacement) in the presence of active TB infection?

Metal implants have been used in patients with spinal tuberculosis and have been reported to have good results with no reactivation. In vitro study comparing the adherence and biofilm properties of *Mycobacterium tuberculosis* and *Staphylococcus epidermidis* suggested that tubercular bacilli rarely adheres to a metal surface and has little or no biofilm formation. This may partly explain the reason why a cementless prosthesis did not increase the risk of tuberculosis reactivation.

---

14. Ha KY, Chung YG, Ryoo SJ. Adherence and biofilm formation of Staphylococcus epidermidis and Mycobacterium tuberculosis on various spinal implants. Spine 2005; 30:38–43.

15. Wang Y, Wang J, Xu Z, Li Y, Wang H. Total hip arthroplasty for active tuberculosis of the hip. Int Orthop 2010; 34:111–14.

16. Govender S. The outcome of allografts and anterior instrumentation in spinal tuberculosis. Clin Orthop Relat Res 2002; 398:606.

Q. 14. Can total hip replacement (THR) be done in active disease?

There are few recent articles which support the use of THR in active stage of disease. Preoperative chemotherapy should be started 1 to 4 weeks to as much as 3 months before any surgical intervention in the presence of active infection. Postoperative chemotherapy is essential to control residual foci of TB. Although the first-line drugs for ATT have been standardized, there still is no consensus regarding the duration.

Sidhu *et al.* performed cemented THR in 23 patients with active tuberculous arthritis of the hip. His patients had received at least 3 months of antitubercular therapy before surgery and treatment was continued for a total of 18 months. With a mean follow up of 4.7 years, no activation of the infection or implant loosening was recorded. Wang *et al.* recommend a combination of antituberculous drugs for at least 2 weeks prior to the operation and subsequently for at least 12 months after operation.

Author's view: The success of THR depends on:

a. Control of tuberculosis

b. Retention of the prosthesis in sound biomechanical alignment.

The control of active disease may not have any issue in presence of prosthetic implant. In active tuberculosis, joint is destroyed with regional osteopenia. The implant placed in diseased and structurally weak bone may not remain in sound biomechanical alignment and is likely to displace. Thus overall longevity of THR would suffer.

Hence, it is suggested that we should perform THR once the disease has healed (hip has attained healed status) and hip joint has attained structural strength.

---

17. Kim SJ, Postigo R, Koo S, Kim JH. Total hip replacement for patients with active tuberculosis of the hip: A systematic review and pooled analysis. Bone Joint J 2013;95B:578–82.

18. Neogi DS, Yadav CS, Ashok Kumar, Khan SA, Rastogi S. Total hip arthroplasty in patients with active tuberculosis of the hip with advanced arthritis. Clin Orthop Relat Res 2010 February; 468(2): 605–612.

19. Yoon TR, Rowe SM, Santosa SB, Jung ST, Seon JK. Immediate cementless total hip arthroplasty for the treatment of active tuberculosis. J Arthroplasty 2005; 20:923–926.

Q. 15. How long one should wait after healing of disease to perform THR? Should we start ATT when THR is performed in a hip with healed disease and what should be the duration of ATT?

THR in a patient with healed TB of the hip is now an accepted procedure. The patients with healed disease can undergo THR. The full course ATT should be given once THR is per- formed.

17. Kim SJ, Postigo R, Koo S, Kim JH. Total hip replacement for patients with active tuberculosis of the hip: A systematic review and pooled analysis. Bone Joint J 2013; 95B: 578–82.

20. Kim YH, Han DY, Park BM. Total hip arthroplasty for tuberculous coxarthrosis. J Bone Joint Surg Am 1987;69:718–27.

10. Kim YY, Ahn BH, Bae DK, Ko CU, Lee JD, Kwak BM, et al. Arthroplasty using the Charnley prosthesis in old tuberculosis of the hip. Clinical experience with 810 year follow up evaluation. Clin Orthop Relat Res 1986; 211: 116–21.

21. Sandhu HS, Kalhan BM, Dogra S. Management of tuberculosis of the hip joint. In: Shanmughasundaram TK, editor. Current Concepts in Bone and Joint Tuberculosis. 147, EVR Periyar Road, Madras, India: 1983.

18. Neogi DS, Yadav CS, Ashok Kumar, Khan SA, Rastogi S. Total hip arthroplasty in patients with active tuberculosis of the hip with advanced arthritis. Clin Orthop Relat Res 2010 February; 468(2): 605–612.

Q. 16. Which type of prosthesis is used—cemented/un- cemented/hybrid?

The presence of cemented or cementless implants seemingly has no influence on reactivation. In studies of THR in patients with quiescent TB, reactivation rates were similar for cemented and cementless THRs, which indicate thermal reaction from cement is irrelevant to reactivation. Neogi et al recommended uncemented prostheses for patients younger than 60 years, and in patients older than 60 years hybrid with cemented femoral component. Studies have shown that in patients with large aceta- bular defects, morcellized allograft can be used successfully.

22. Yoon TR, Rowe SM, Santosa SB, Jung ST, Seon JK. Immediate cementless total hip arthroplasty for the treatment of active tuberculosis. J Arthroplasty 2005; 20:923–926.

23. Eskola. Cementless total replacement for old tuberculosis of the hip. J Bone Joint Surg Br 1988;70:603–606.

18. Neogi DS, Yadav CS, Ashok Kumar, Khan SA, Rastogi S. Total hip arthroplasty in patients with active tuberculosis of the hip with advanced arthritis. Clin Orthop Relat Res 2010 February; 468(2): 605–612.

Q. 17. What are the results of long-term follow-up available of THR performed in active TB arthritis?

- Sidhu *et al.* performed cemented THR in 23 patients with active tuberculous arthritis of the hip. With a mean follow-up of 4.7 years, no activation of the infection or implant-loosening was recorded.

- Kim *et al.* performed a systematic review and evaluated the outcome of THR in patients with active TB of the hip in referenced articles published between 1950 and 2012. A total of 65 patients of histologically confirmed TB were reviewed with a mean follow-up was 53.2 months (24–108). Anti-tubercular treatment continued postoperatively between 6 and 15 months. Their analysis concluded that THR in patients with active TB of the hip is a safe procedure. The mean Harris hip score at averaged 4 years was 85.

- Yoon *et al.* reported advanced active tuberculous arthritis of the hip patients treated with cementless THR. Post-operatively, antituberculous medications were continued for 1-year. With average follow-up of 4.8 years, reactivation of the infection was not detected.

- Wang *et al.* reported no case of hip dislocation, loosening of implant or recrudescence after mean follow-up of 49 months.
  Hence, THR is a safe procedure in active tubercular arthritis as far as available limited literature is concerned.

24. Sidhu AS, Singh AP, Singh AP. Total hip replacement in active advanced tuberculous arthritis. J Bone Joint Surg Br 2009;91:1301–4.

17. Kim SJ, Postigo R, Koo S, Kim JH. Total hip replacement for patients with active tuberculosis of the hip: a systematic review and pooled analysis. Bone Joint J 2013 May; 95-B(5):578–82.

25. Yoon TR, Rowe SM, Santosa SB, Jung ST, Seon JK. Immediate cementless total hip arthroplasty for the treatment of active tuberculosis. J Arthroplasty 2005; 20: 923–926.

15. Wang Y, Wang J, Xu Z, Li Y, Wang H. Total hip arthroplasty for active tuberculosis of the hip. Int Orthop 2010 December; 34(8): 111–114.

Q. 18. When to stop ATT in TB hip after total hip replacement?

This question was answered in one of the few articles available on the subject. Preoperative multidrug chemotherapy containing at least two bactericidal drugs for 4 weeks in absence of draining sinus or any other active focus. This period of 4 weeks allows stabilization of the lesion, improvement in soft tissue contractures with traction, and better planning of the reconstructive procedure. Postoperatively, if the patient's general condition shows marked improvement and the ESR and CRP return to normal by the fifth month, then ATT was continue until 1 year; however, if the ESR and CRP took more than 5 months to return to normal, the authors continued ATT until 18 months.

18. Neogi DS, Yadav CS, Ashok Kumar, Khan SA, Rastogi S. Total hip arthroplasty in patients with active tuberculosis of the hip with advanced arthritis. Clin Orthop Relat Res 2010 February; 468(2):605–612.

Q. 19. What is the follow-up protocol for TB hip and what are the parameters of healing?

Tuberculosis hip patients should be followed up every 6 weeks for the initial 6 months. The observations should be made about:

- Constitutional features: Reduction of pain around hip, healing of sinuses, improved range of movements.
- Hematological: Erythrocyte sedimentation rate (ESR), C-reactive protein (CRP), and liver function tests (LFT).
- Radiographic outcome: It should be assessed by taking anteroposterior and lateral radiographs every 8 weeks. Radiograph should be compared with pretreatment X-rays to access for change in overall bone density, joint margins, any new and progressive radiolucent lines or cavities.
- In THR cases, implant subsidence, migration dislocation, etc. should be noted.
- MRI would show resolution of edema of soft tissues and bones and synovial fluid collection.

1. Tuli SM. Tuberculosis of the Skeletal System (Bones, Joints, Spine and Bursal sheaths) 4th ed. New Delhi: Jaypee Brothers Medical Publishers Pvt. Ltd.; 2010.

18. Neogi DS, Yadav CS, Ashok Kumar, Khan SA, Rastogi S. Total hip arthroplasty in patients with active tuberculosis of the hip with advanced arthritis. Clin Orthop Relat Res 2010 February; 468(2):605–612.

KNEE

Q. 1. What is the incidence of knee involvement in osteoarticular tuberculosis? What is the common age of presentation?

There is no exact data available. Incidence of TB knee is approximately 8–10% of all osteoarticular cases. It is the third most common osteoarticular site involved by tuberculosis after spine and hip. No direct data available. The incidence of EPTB is higher in children.

1. Hoffman EB, Allin J, Campbell JA, Leisegang FM. Tuberculosis of the knee. Clin Orthop Relat Res 2002 May;(398):100–106.

2. Watts HG, Lifeso RM. Tuberculosis of bones and joints. J Bone Joint Surg Am 1996 Feb;78(2):288–98.

3. Fraser Wares, Balasubramanian R, Mohan A, Sharma SK. Extrapulmonary tuberculosis: Management and control. In: Agarwal and Chauhan (Eds). Tuberculosis Control in India. Directorate General of Health Services/Ministry of Health and Family Welfare 2005 India. Elsevier India.

4. Mittal R, Trikha V, Rastogi S. Tuberculosis of patella. Knee 2006 Jan; 13(1):54–6.

5. Arora VK, Agarwal SP. Paediatric Tuberculosis: An experience from LRS institute of tuberculosis and respiratory diseases. In: Agarwal and Chauhan (Eds). Tuberculosis Control in India. Directorate General of Health Services/Ministry of Health and Family Welfare 2005 India. Elsevier India.

6. Murray RC. Tuberculosis of the knee. A follow-up investigation of old cases. Br Med J 1940 Jul 6;2(4148):10–2.

Q. 2. What are the clinical features to diagnose tuberculosis of knee (early disease *vs* advanced disease)?

The patients of tuberculosis of the knee reports with insidious onset pain, which is not associated with any specific cause (no history of significant trauma). Some may report with hip pain. The pain is gradually increasing and associated with limp. They gradually advance from minor flexion deformity to severe deformity, mild reduction of range of motion to gross restriction of range of motion depending upon the severity/stage of the disease.

In early disease, the patient presents with the history of:
1. Pain
2. Limp
3. Swelling (warm, red, swollen and tender joint)
4. Fever (low grade, evening rise of temperature)
5. Weight loss, anorexia

On examination, the knee joint is usually swollen with fluid in the joint, observed as patellar tap and obliteration of both medial and lateral parapatellar hollows along with supra-patellar fullness. The joint line is tender. The local temperature is raised and synovium is thickened giving a doughy feeling. The muscles show wasting and the range of motion is restricted only terminally in synovitis stage. Inguinal and external iliac lymphadenopathy may be palpated/observed.

In advanced disease, in addition to the above:
1. Further restriction of motion
2. Deformity [ranges from mild flexion deformity to grotesque triple deformity (flexion, posterior subluxation, external rotation and valgus)
3. Discharging sinuses (may or may not be there)

1. Hoffman EB, Allin J, Campbell JA, Leisegang FM. Tuberculosis of the knee. Clin Orthop Relat Res 2002 May;(398):100–106.
7. Kerri O, Martini M. Tuberculosis of the knee. Int Orthop 1985; 9:153–157.
8. Lee AS, Campbell JA, Hoffman EB. Tuberculosis of the knee in children. J Bone Joint Surg Br 1995 Mar;77(2):313–8.
9. Tuli SM. Tuberculosis of the skeletal system. 3rd ed. New Delhi, India: Jaypee Brothers Medical Publishers; 2004.

Q. 3. What are the radiological features of tuberculosis of knee joint in early and advanced stages?

The radiological features depend upon the stage of the disease.

1. *Synovitis stage*
   a. Regional osteoporosis (osteopenia)
   b. Increased soft tissue shadow (due to synovial hypertrophy, effusion)

2. *Early arthritis stage*: Besides all the above
  a. Loss of definition of articular surfaces
  b. Marginal erosions
  c. Diminution of joint space
  d. Destruction of joint space

3. *Advanced arthritis stage*
  a. Marked diminution of joint space
  b. Gross destruction and deformation of joint
  c. Osteolytic cavities in lower end femur and upper end of tibia
  d. Sequestra
  e. Triple deformity

9. Tuli SM. Tuberculosis of the skeletal system. 4th ed. New Delhi, India: Jaypee Brothers Medical Publishers; 2010.

10. Key LA. Tuberculosis of the knee-joint in adults. Br Med J 1940 Sep 28;2(4160):408–422.

11. Golding FC. Tuberculosis of the knee-joint: Section of Radiology. Proc R Soc Med 1941 Oct;34(12):823–34.

"X-ray changes in the early tuberculous knee-joint are as a rule inconclusive rather than definite. One or more of the following abnormalities are usually to be seen—(1) a general appearance of haziness; (2) increased width of the normal soft-tissue shadow-woolliness, distortion of shape, or actual obliteration' of the normal triangular shadow of the infrapatellar pouch seen in the lateral view; (3) osteoporosis; (4) diminished joint space, often only on one side; (5) lack of definition, or thinning of the cortical bone. After an average interval of four months from the onset of symptoms, an abscess cavity or cavities are usually present in bone; localized marginal erosion may also be seen. The later bone changes are obvious. In general, destructive bone changes are more advanced than appear from X-ray examination." All X-ray changes are listed below:

1. *Decalcification of the bone*
2. *Enlargement of joint capsule*
3. *Presence of abscess outside capsule*
4. *Enlargement of epiphyses and patella*
5. *Narrowing of joint space*
6. *Narrowing of cortex of shaft and widening of medulla*
7. *Presence of erosion of one-half of the condylar surface*

8. *Presence of erosion of both condylar surfaces*
9. *Presence of erosion of articular surface of patella*
10. *Coarse trabeculation of ends of bones*
11. *Posterior subluxation of tibia*
12. *Genu valgum*
13. *Genu varum*
14. *Hyperextension of the knee*
15. *Primary focus in patella*
16. *Presence of clearly defined single focus in epiphyses*
17. *Presence of clearly defined focus in region of metaphyses*
18. *Bone ankylosis as result of conservative treatment*
19. *Bone ankylosis as result of operative treatment*
20. *Recurrence after excision*
21. *Presence of periostitis*
22. *Presence of secondary infection (by sinus)*
23. *Evidence on film of this secondary infection*
24. *Sequestrum any of these changes in a case of TB knee of various stages.*

Q. 4. How can ultrasonography (USG) be useful in the diagnosis of TB knee?

Joint effusion and synovial proliferation are observed by ultrasonography of the tubercular knee. There are no pathognomonic features to differentiate TB from other causes of joint effusion. However, the effusion in the joint and synovial thickening can be appreciated on clinical examination alone and USG does not provide any additional information. Since knee is a superficial joint, USG is generally not required for guided aspiration.

9. Iagnocco A1, Coari G, Buzzi G, Guerrisi R, Valesini G. Magnetic resonance imaging of peripheral osteoarticular tuberculosis compared with sonography and standard radiographs. Rheumatol Int 2003 Jul;23(4):195–7.

10. De Backer AI, Mortelé KJ, Vanhoenacker FM, Parizel PM. Imaging of extraspinal musculoskeletal tuberculosis. Eur J Radiol 2006;57:119–30.

11. De Backer AI, Vanhoenacker FM, Sanghvi DA. Imaging features of extra axial musculoskeletal tuberculosis. Indian J Radiol Imaging 2009 Jul-Sep;19(3):176–86.

Q. 5. What are the specific MRI features in early knee disease/ advanced knee disease?

MRI features suggestive of TB of the knee joint are:

1. Joint effusion
2. Low signal foci in synovial fluid
3. Synovial thickening
4. Low to intermediate signal of the proliferating synovium on T2-weighted images
5. High signal of the proliferating synovium and post-contrast enhancement
6. Presence of marrow signal abnormalities suggesting bone edema, bone abscess
7. Soft tissue abscess with ulcerations
8. Sinus formation

Author's view: However, to diagnose TB of the knee, the MRI is seldom required and the diagnosis may be ascertained on aspiration cytology/core biopsy. In a very early disease (stage of synovitis) besides the changes in the synovium, the presence of concomitant bone edema/affection may be better appreciated on MRI.

10. De Backer AI, Mortelé KJ, Vanhoenacker FM, Parizel PM. Imaging of extraspinal musculoskeletal tuberculosis. Eur J Radiol 2006;57:119–30.

11. De Backer AI, Vanhoenacker FM, Sanghvi DA. Imaging features of extra axial musculoskeletal tuberculosis. Indian J Radiol Imaging 2009 Jul-Sep;19(3):176–86.

12. Sanghvi DA, Iyer VR, Deshmukh T, Hoskote SS. MRI features of tuberculosis of the knee. Skeletal Radiol 2009 Mar;38(3):267–73.

13. Choi JA, Koh SH, Hong SH, Koh YH, Choi JY, Kang HS. Rheumatoid arthritis and tuberculous arthritis: differentiating MRI features. Am J Roentgenol 2009 Nov;193(5):1347–53.

1. *"The findings in our study indicate that tuberculosis must be considered when hypointense synovial proliferation is seen on T2-weighted MR images of the knee joint. Other findings, such as joint fluid collection, post-contrast enhancement of synovium, presence of marrow signal abnormalities, and soft tissue abscess with ulcerations and sinus formation, support the diagnosis of TB."*

2. *"Uniform synovial thickening, large size of bone erosion, rim enhancement at site of bone erosion, and extra-articular cystic masses were more frequent and more numerous in tuberculous arthritis. MRI may be helpful in the differentiation between RA and tuberculous arthritis"*

Q. 6. How FNAC/biopsy are to be taken (aspiration/arthroscopic/open biopsy)?

Tissue for/culture/smear/molecular diagnostic tests like GeneXpert and histopathological examination can be taken by any of the following routes (percutaneous, arthroscopic, and open). Arthroscopic joint evaluation and synovial biopsy allow histopathological examination and microbiological tests to improve diagnostic accuracy. Arthroscopic technique offers the advantage of direct visualization of joint, early diagnosis and hence allows for subtotal excision of tubercular synovium, granulation tissue and pannus over cartilage.

Arthroscopic subtotal synovectomy is useful in synovitis stage of disease followed by early postoperative mobilization and ATT to preserve/regain the joint function.

14. Guo L, Yang L, Duan XJ, Chen GX, Zhang Y, Dai G. Arthroscopically assisted treatment of adolescent knee joint tuberculosis. Orthop Surg 2010 Feb;2(1):58–63.

15. Shen HL, Xia Y, Li P, Wang J, Han H. Arthroscopic operations in knee joint with early-stage tuberculosis. Arch Orthop Trauma Surg 2010 Mar;130(3):357–61.

16. Aggarwal VK, Nair D, Khanna G, Verma J, Sharma VK, Batra S. Use of amplified Mycobacterium tuberculosis direct test (Gen-probe Inc., San Diego, CA, USA) in the diagnosis of tubercular synovitis and early arthritis of knee joint. Indian J Orthop 2012;46:531–5.

17. Titov AG, Nakonechniy GD, Santavirta S, Serdobintzev MS, Mazurenko SI, Konttinen YT. Arthroscopic operations in joint tuberculosis. Knee 2004 Feb;11(1):57–62.

Q. 7. How do we classify the tuberculosis of the knee?

Ans. Tuberculosis of knee is classified clinically into various stages. The commonly used clinical classification is (Tuli based on Babhulkar and Pande 2002):

1. *Stage 1.* Synovitis
2. *Stage 2.* Early arthritis
3. *Stage 3.* Advanced arthritis
4. *Stage 4.* Advanced arthritis with triple deformity

Radiological classification by Kerri and Martini:

1. *Stage 1.* Normal: Osteopenia with soft-tissue swelling with or without epiphyseal hypertrophy

2. *Stage 2*. Osteomyelitic: Epiphyseal or metaphyseal cysts. Normal joint space
3. *Stage 3*. Arthritic: Narrow joint space without gross anatomical disorganization
4. *Stage 4*. Arthritic: Gross anatomical disorganization

Konig and Volkmann's Pathological Classification (1890)

1. *Tumor albus*: It is described as white swelling occurring in a tubercular bone and joint. This term may be given for white-skinned person. However, for dark-skinned person, the patient present as swelling around knee.
2. *Caries sicca*: Bone infection (tuberculosis) in a dry form with little or no exudate. Generally seen in shoulder.
3. *Tubercular hydrops*: It is described as excessive collection of fluid in the knee joint secondary to synovitis of the knee.
4. *Cold abscess knee*
5. *Frame knee*: It is desscribed as a stage where the following treatment by plastering the epiphysis around the knee are fused and patient develops marked shortening and stiffness (decreased range of motion).

The modern imaging has improved the diagnostic ability in early stage of disease hence severe form of disease generally do not occur.

9. Tuli SM. Tuberculosis of the skeletal system. 3rd ed. New Delhi, India: Jaypee Brothers Medical Publishers; 2004.
18. Pritchard FH. Recent Scandinavian Contributions on Tuberculosis of the Knee-Joint and Its Surgical Treatment. Ann Surg 1890 Sep;12(3):203–13.
19. Kerri O, Martini M. Tuberculosis of the knee. Int Orthop 1985; 9:153–157.

Q. 8. Can we start antitubercular treatment without histo-logical proof?

Generally, in synovitis stage, one requires tissue diagnosis before starting patient on ATT. The diagnosis may be obtained by aspiration cytology/open biospy/arthroscopic subtotal synovectomy. Delay of a few days in the treatment of limb lesion does not give rise to severe consequences as tuberculosis is a slowly progressive disease. In early and advance arthritis stages, generally clinicoradiological diagnosis is adequate to initiate ATT. Since knee being a superficial joint, generally tissue diagnosis is possible with minimally invasive methods and should always be attempted.

10. Key LA. Tuberculosis of the knee-joint in adults. Br Med J 1940 Sep 28;2(4160):408–422.

20. Jain AK, Jena SK, Singh MP, Dhammi IK, Ramachadran VG, Dev G. Evaluation of clinico-radiological, bacteriological, serological, molecular and histological diagnosis of osteoarticular tuberculosis. Indian J Orthop 2008 Apr;42(2):173–7.

Q. 9. What is the management of tuberculosis of the knee?

All cases need to be put on antitubercular therapy [2 HRZE + 10 HRE]. In addition, according to the stage of disease, ancillary treatment includes:

1. *Synovitis stage*:
   a. Rest to the limb.
   b. Traction (skeletal/skin) to prevent/correct flexion deformity.
   c. Gentle assisted knee bending exercises for 5 minutes every hour.

Intra-articular instillation of streptomycin and isoniazid once weekly was reported in old literature. However, no evidence is in favor of instillation of drugs. The ATT drugs are found in adequate concentration in the diseased tissue after oral intake.

If at 6 weeks, there is no improvement in signs/symptoms at all, synovectomy (open/arthroscopic) may be performed. The tissue should be submitted for histology, AFB smear, culture for TB, CB-NAAT(GeneXpert) and Line Probe Assay (LPA).

2. *Early arthritis stage*:
   a. Modified Russell's traction to prevent correct triple deformity. This type of traction corrects the subluxation of tibia and then flexion deformity of the knee. Once the deformity is corrected, the knee may be mobilized on ATT.
   b. Joint debridement (open/arthroscopic) may be indicated, if it does not show clinicoradiological improvement.

c. Corrective plaster cast/bracing in case joint is unstable after debridement.

3. *Advanced arthritis stage*:

a. In children, double traction is applied to correct knee deformity followed by corrective plaster for 6 months. Arthrodesis should be deferred till completion of skeletal growth.

b. In adults, with painful arthritic knee or fibrous ankyloses, joint debridement till healthy bleeding cancellous bone is visualized should be undertaken followed by compression arthrodesis by Charnley's clamp. The knee arthrodesis will provide a painless, stable joint.

4. *Healed tubercular knee with/without deformity*:

a. Corrective supracondylar femoral osteotomy to restore available range of motion into a functional range of motion arc.

b. Total knee replacement arthroplasty may also be performed.

1. Hoffman EB, Allin J, Campbell JA, Leisegang FM. Tuberculosis of the knee. Clin Orthop Relat Res 2002 May;(398):100–106.

6. Murray RC. Tuberculosis of the knee: A followup investigation of old cases. Br Med J 1940 Jul 6;2(4148):10–2.

8. Lee AS, Campbell JA, Hoffman EB. Tuberculosis of the knee in children. J Bone Joint Surg Br 1995 Mar;77(2):313–8.

9. Tuli SM. Tuberculosis of the skeletal system. 3rd ed. New Delhi, India: Jaypee Brothers Medical Publishers; 2004

10. Key LA. Tuberculosis of the knee-joint in adults. Br Med J 1940 Sep 28;2(4160):408–422.

17. Guo L, Yang L, Duan XJ, Chen GX, Zhang Y, Dai G. Arthroscopically assisted treatment of adolescent knee joint tuberculosis. Orthop Surg 2010 Feb; 2(1):58–63.

21. Ahern RT, Arden GP. Intra-articular streptomycin in tuberculosis of the knee. Br Med J 1952 Mar 1;1(4756):466–8.

22. Kant KS, Agarwal A, Suri T, Gupta N, Verma I, Shaharyar A. Tuberculosis of knee region in children: a series of eight cases. Trop Doct 2014 Jan;44(1):29–32.

Q. 10. What is the management of stiff knee joint with fixed deformity?

There are two options available:

1. Corrective osteotomy, if sound knee fusion is present.
2. Total knee arthroplasty.

---

9. Tuli SM. Tuberculosis of the skeletal system. 3rd ed. New Delhi, India: Jaypee Brothers Medical Publishers; 2004.

Q. 11. What are the indications of corrective osteotomy in healed disease?

In cases where the disease has healed with painless range of motion (minimum of 20°), a corrective osteotomy is indicated when:

1. There is varus or valgus deformity. Osteotomy is done to correct biomechanical alignment.
2. To put residual range of motion in functional arc, a supra-condylar femoral osteotomy may be performed.

---

9. Tuli SM. Tuberculosis of the skeletal system. 3rd ed. New Delhi, India: Jaypee Brothers Medical Publishers; 2004.

Q. 12. What is role of total knee replacement (TKR) in tuberculosis of knee? Can TKA be done in active disease? How long one should wait after healing of disease to perform TKA? Should we start ATT when TKA is done in healed disease and what is the suggested duration of ATT?

Ans. Data is limited in number and follow-up to recommend TKA in active disease. Since the knee joint is a superficial joint with inflamed soft tissue in tuberculosis, hence TKR should not be performed in active disease. It may be performed after 2–3 years of healing, under ATT cover. As a general rule, all cases of healed tuberculosis when planned for any impant surgery like TKA, it must be under cover of a full course of ATT. Large scale studies are required to generate a recommendation.

---

23. Gale DW, Harding ML. Total knee arthroplasty in the presence of active tuberculosis. J Bone Joint Surg Br 1991 Nov;73(6):1006–7.

24. TekinKoruk S, Sipahioðlu S, Caliir C. Periprosthetic tuberculosis of the knee joint treated with antituberculosis drugs: a case report. Acta Orthop Traumatol Turc 2013;47(6):440–3.

26. Marmor M, Parnes N, Dekel S. Tuberculosis infection complicating total knee arthroplasty: report of 3 cases and review of the literature. J Arthroplasty 2004 Apr;19(3):397–400.

27. Wray CC, Roy S. Arthroplasty in tuberculosis of the knee. Two cases of missed diagnosis. Acta Orthop Scand 1987 Jun;58(3):296–8.

28. Habaxi KK, Wang L, Miao XG, Alimasi WQ, Zhao XB, Su JG, Yuan H. Total knee arthroplasty treatment of active tuberculosis of the knee: a review of 10 cases.Eur Rev Med Pharmacol Sci 2014; 18(23):3587–92.

29. Oztürkmen Y, Uzümcügil O, Karamehmetoðlu M, Leblebici C, Caniklioðlu M. Total knee arthroplasty for the management of joint destruction in tuberculous arthritis. Knee Surg Sports Traumatol Arthrosc 2014 May;22(5):1076–83.

30. Kim YH. Total knee arthroplasty for tuberculous arthritis. J Bone Joint Surg Am 1988 Oct;70(9):1322–30.

31. Eskola A, Santavirta S, Konttinen YT, Tallroth K, Lindholm ST. Arthroplasty for old tuberculosis of the knee. J Bone Joint Surg Br 1988 Nov;70(5):767–9.

PubMed search "total knee arthroplasty in active tuberculosis" yielded 11 results. Of the 7 relevant results pertaining to TKR in active disease, one was a case report with 10-year follow-up, three were case reports were the diagnosis was missed and there were 2 case series with (n = 10, 12, knees) TKR done in active disease and one case series (n = 22) where it was done after subsidence of signs of infection. Gale et al[23] reported a 10-year follow-up of a patient with active pulmonary and knee tuberculosis with active rheumatoid arthritis who remained disease-free at follow-up.

Habaxi et al[27] operated on 10 patients with active disease after instituting 2–4 weeks of ATT. At 14-month follow-up, none of their patients had aseptic loosening, although there was 1/10 case with recurrence at 3 months post-op and had to undergo revision arthroplasty. ATT was continued for 1–1.5 years postoperatively. Oztürkmen et al[28] operated on 12 patients with active disease in a two-stage procedure. First stage involved joint debridement and placement of an antibiotic cement spacer for 6 months along with ATT; this was followed by cemented TKR in the second stage. ATT was continued for 1 year postoperatively. At mean 6-year follow-up 10/12 knees showed no loosening, 2/12 showed only 1 mm radiolucency. There were no cases with recurrence of infection. Marmor et al[25] had to revise TKA in 2/3 patients where the diagnosis had initially been missed. Kim[29] used uncemented TKA in 18 knees and cemented in 4 after a disease-free interval ranging from 3 months to 5 years. There was no component loosening. However, one patient had to undergo implant removal and arthrodesis due to recurrent active infection.

Eskola et al[30] reviewed 6 patients treated by TKA 35 years after primary infection and found that at 6.3 years mean follow-up 5/6 patients were disease free. One patient had recurrence of the disease 18 months after the surgery and was successfully treated with ATT for one year.

Q. 13. When to stop ATT?

Ans. No specific end point mentioned in literature. Most studies have treated patients with ATT for up to 18 months. However, in view of data available from spinal tuberculosis, the joint should be evaluated by contrast MRI at 9, 12 and 18 months following ATT in order to monitor and ensure MRI based healing of the lesion (no contrast enhancement, fatty replacement of bone marrow in the lesion).

ANKLE

Q. 1. What are the clinical symptoms/presentations of tuberculosis of ankle, in synovitis stage/advanced arthritis?

TB of the ankle and foot can affect any age. It is more common in children and young adults. It comprises of less than 5% of total osteoarticular tuberculosis. The disease can present as acute/chronic arthritis, bursitis, tenosynovitis, synovitis or osteitis. The disease may start in synovium or from bone (distal end of tibia, malleolus, talus or calcaneum).

In **early stage** of disease (synovitis or early arthritis), the patient presents:
1. Pain
2. Weight loss and anorexia
3. Limp (antalgic gait)
4. Swelling (warm, red, swollen tender joint)
5. Synovial thickening (doughy/boggy on palpation)
6. Fever (low grade, evening rise of temperature, night sweats)
7. Regional lymphadenopathy
8. Restricted range of motion of ankle

While in **advanced disease**, we observe (in addition to the above):
1. Wasting of calf muscles
2. Joint effusion
3. Deformity (ranges from mild plantar flexion deformity to grotesque pathological anterior subluxation/dislocation of ankle)
4. Discharging sinuses

---

1. Shams F, Asnis D, Lombardi C, Segal-Maurer S. A report of two cases of tuberculous arthritis of the ankle. J Foot Ankle Surg 2009 Jul-Aug;48(4):452–6.
2. Samuel S, Boopalan PR, Alexander M, Ismavel R, Varghese VD, Mathai T. Tuberculosis of and around the ankle. J Foot Ankle Surg 2011 Jul-Aug;50(4):466–72.

3. Korim M, Patel R, Allen P, Mangwani J. Foot and ankle tuberculosis: case series and literature review. Foot (Edinb) 2014 Dec;24(4):176–9.

4. Dhillon MS, Tuli SM. Osteoarticular tuberculosis of the foot and ankle. Foot Ankle Int 2001 Aug;22(8):679–86.

5. Tuli SM. Tuberculosis of the ankle and foot. In: Tuli SM, ed. Tuberculosis of the skeletal system. 3rd ed. New Delhi, India: Jaypee Brothers Medical Publishers (P) Ltd.; 2004:127–34.

6. Gursu S, Yildirim T, Ucpinar H, Sofu H, Camurcu Y, Sahin V, Sahin N. Long-term follow-up results of foot and ankle tuberculosis in Turkey. J Foot Ankle Surg 2014 Sep-Oct;53(5):557–61.

7. Chen SH, Wang T, Lee CH. Tuberculous ankle versus pyogenic septic ankle arthritis: a retrospective comparison. Jpn J Infect Dis. 2011; 64(2):139–42.

8. Agarwal A, Qureshi NA, Khan SA, Kumar P, Samaiya S. Tuberculosis of the foot and ankle in children. J Orthop Surg (Hong Kong) 2011 Aug;19(2):213–7.

9. Inoue S, Matsumoto S, Iwamatsu Y, Satomura M. Ankle tuberculosis: a report of four cases in a Japanese hospital. J Orthop Sci 2004; 9(4):392–8.

10. Dhillon MS, Nagi ON. Tuberculosis of the foot and ankle. Clin Orthop Relat Res 2002;398:107–13.

11. Nayak B, Dash RR, Mohapatra KC, Panda G. Ankle and foot tuberculosis: a diagnostic dilemma. J Family Med Prim Care 2014 Apr;3(2):129–31.

Q. 2. What are the findings on plain X-rays in early and advanced TB ankle?

Radiographic (roentgenographic) features are usually noted 2 to 4 months after disease onset and only a joint effusion may be apparent in the very early stage.

1. *Synovitis stage*:
   a. Regional osteopenia (osteoporosis)
   b. Increased soft tissue shadow (due to synovial hypertrophy, effusion)

2. *Early arthritis stage*:
   a. Loss of definition of articular surfaces
   b. Marginal erosions
   c. Diminution of joint space

d. Destruction of joint space (eccentric)

e. Sinus

3. *Advanced arthritis stage*:

a. Marked diminution of joint space

b. Gross destruction and deformation of joint

c. Osteolytic cavities

d. Sequestra

e. Anterior dislocation of ankle joint.

f. Sclerosis, and fibrous ankylosis

12. Choi WJ, Han SH, Joo JH, Kim BS, Lee JW. Diagnostic dilemma of tuberculosis in the foot and ankle. Foot Ankle Int 2008; 29:711–5.

13. De Backer AI, Mortelé KJ, Vanhoenacker FM, Parizel PM. Imaging of extraspinal musculoskeletal tuberculosis. Eur J Radiol 2006;57:119–30.

14. De Backer AI, Vanhoenacker FM, Sanghvi DA. Imaging features of extraaxial musculoskeletal tuberculosis. Indian J Radiol Imaging 2009 Jul-Sep;19(3):176–86.

15. Dhillon MS, Aggarwal S, Prabhakar S, Bachhal V. Tuberculosis of the foot: an osteolytic variety. Indian J Orthop 2012;46:206–11.

4. Dhillon MS, Tuli SM. Osteoarticular tuberculosis of the foot and ankle. Foot Ankle Int 2001 Aug;22(8):679–86.

10. Dhillon MS, Nagi ON. Tuberculosis of the foot and ankle. Clin Orthop Relat Res 2002;398:107–13.

5. Tuli SM. Tuberculosis of the ankle and foot. In: Tuli SM, ed. Tuberculosis of the skeletal system. 3rd ed. New Delhi, India: Jaypee Brothers Medical Publishers (P) Ltd.; 2004:127–34.

16. Ruggieri M, Pavone V, Polizzi A, Smilari P, Di Fede GF, Sorge G, et al. Tuberculosis of the ankle in childhood: clinical, roentgengraphic and computed tomography findings. Clin Pediatr (Phila) 1997;36:529–34.

Q. 3. What is the role of ultrasonography in TB ankle? How efficient is ultrasound for US guided FNAC for TB synovitis?

There are **no pathognomonic findings** on USG as such. It may also be helpful during aspiration of these effusions for microbiological and cytological/histological examination and molecular diagnosis. It may show:

1. Cold abscesses and joint effusions

2. Collections in bursae

3. Synovial hypertrophy

13. De Backer AI, Mortelé KJ, Vanhoenacker FM, Parizel PM. Imaging of extraspinal musculoskeletal tuberculosis. Eur J Radiol 2006;57: 119–30.

14. De Backer AI, Vanhoenacker FM, Sanghvi DA. Imaging features of extraaxial musculoskeletal tuberculosis. Indian J Radiol Imaging 2009 Jul-Sep;19(3):176–86.

Q. 4. What are CT scan findings in TB ankle? Is contrast CT better for diagnosis of TB ankle?

CT scan findings are **non-specific** for ankle tuberculosis. Findings include:

1. Erosions and lytic areas of destruction in the involved bone (geographical extent of lesion can be delineated)
2. Cavitation
3. Narrowing of joint
4. Sequestra
5. Soft tissue extension can be delineated

CT scan has been used for CT-guided biopsy from lesions. The use of contrast has not been mentioned but uniform enhancement of abscess wall has been reported as in other foci of osteoarticular TB.

10. Dhillon MS, Nagi ON. Tuberculosis of the foot and ankle. Clin Orthop Relat Res 2002;398:107–13.

4. Dhillon MS, Tuli SM. Osteoarticular tuberculosis of the foot and ankle. Foot Ankle Int 2001 Aug;22(8):679–86.

13. De Backer AI, Mortelé KJ, Vanhoenacker FM, Parizel PM. Imaging of extraspinal musculoskeletal tuberculosis. Eur J Radiol 2006;57: 119–30.

14. De Backer AI, Vanhoenacker FM, Sanghvi DA. Imaging features of extraaxial musculoskeletal tuberculosis. Indian J Radiol Imaging 2009 Jul-Sep;19(3):176–86.

3. Korim M, Patel R, Allen P, Mangwani J. Foot and ankle tuberculosis: case series and literature review. Foot (Edinb) 2014 Dec;24(4): 176–9.

1. "CT scan is useful to delineate the bony anatomy and delineate cortical breaks or collapse of the articular surface. It is useful to plan reconstructive procedures (Korim et al)."

2. *"CT scan is particularly useful for evaluating the degree of bone destruction, sequestrum formation (although rare), and surrounding soft tissue extension (Vanhoenacker et al.)."*

3. *"CT scans help in defining the geographic extent of the lesion and can clearly show the sequestration and cortical breaks. They also outline the extent of the bone destruction and are helpful in facilitating biopsy. Plain radiographs, CT scans, and MRI done during the follow-up of these patients who are receiving multidrug therapy sometimes may show advancing of the lesion, even after 3 to 4 months of treatment. This is because the imaging appearances lag behind the biologic process of repair. Even after complete clinical and radiologic healing, there may be residual cavities observed on serial CT scans or on radiographs."*

4. *"During the destructive phase of the disease, we have found that the use of CT scans helps in defining the geographic extent of the lesion and can clearly show any sequestration. It also outlines the extent of the bone destruction and is very helpful in facilitating biopsy We have also done. The serial CT scans in a few cases in an attempt to demonstrate the effects of medical therapy. Although it is not as informative as MRI in showing the bone edema and marrow changes. We were able to see that there was complete resorption of sequestrae in some cases."* It is important to note that even after complete clinical and radiological healing, there may be residual cavities noted on serial CT scans. These are of little consequence regarding the durability of healing and chances of recrudescence. These are filled with fibrous or fibro-osseous tissue and do not warrant surgical intervention. Radiographs, CT scans and MRI done during the follow up of these patients on multi-drug therapy may show *"advancing"* of a lesion even after three to four months of treatment."

Q. 5. What are MRI findings of TB ankle? Is contrast MRI better for diagnosis of TB ankle?

Nonspecific features suggestive of TB ankle include:

1. Bony regions showing hypointense (low) signal on T1-weighted images and hyperintense (high) signal on T2-weighted images suggestive of marrow edema.
2. Regions of necrosis seen as intermediate signal intensity on T2-weighted images.
3. Thickening of synovium
4. Tenosynovitis
5. Soft tissue abscesses
6. Intraosseous abscess and cavitation
7. Joint effusion

8. Contrast enhancement (gadolinium) of hypertrophic synovium and abscesses.

Zacharia *et al*[17] reported that a combination of low–intermediate signal intensity areas on T1WI, somewhat higher signal intensity areas on T2WI (due to caseous necrosis), and prominent soft-tissue changes in the form of cold abscesses with peripheral rim enhancement, and tenosynovitis might provide a clue to the diagnosis of tubercular arthritis of ankle.

Prakash *et al*[18] reported that a combination of intraosseous abscess, soft tissue abscess and tenosynovitis as suggestive of tubercular arthritis of ankle in a patient with a long history of symptoms.

17. Zacharia TT, Shah JR, Patkar D, Kale H, Sindhwani V. MRI in ankle tuberculosis: Review of 14 cases. Australas Radiol 2003 Mar;47(1): 11–6.

3. Korim M, Patel R, Allen P, Mangwani J. Foot and ankle tuberculosis: case series and literature review. Foot (Edinb) 2014 Dec;24(4):176–9.

18. Prakash M, Gupta P, Sen RK, Sharma A, Khandelwal N. Magnetic resonance imaging evaluation of tubercular arthritis of the ankle and foot. Acta Radiol 2014 Oct 20.

4. Dhillon MS, Tuli SM. Osteoarticular tuberculosis of the foot and ankle. Foot Ankle Int 2001 Aug; 22(8):679–86.

13. De Backer AI, Mortelé KJ, Vanhoenacker FM, Parizel PM. Imaging of extraspinal musculoskeletal tuberculosis. Eur J Radiol 2006; 57:119–30.

14. De Backer AI, Vanhoenacker FM, Sanghvi DA. Imaging features of extraaxial musculoskeletal tuberculosis. Indian J Radiol Imaging 2009 Jul-Sep;19(3):176–86.

1. *"Our study revealed various morphological patterns of ankle joint involvement. The earliest findings were ankle and subtalar joint effusions that were hypointense on T1WI and hyperintense on T2WI. Hypointense foci on T2WI within the effusion were suggestive of calcified loose bodies and provide a reliable clue to the diagnosis. Further sequela of the disease was in the form of bone marrow signal alterations of varying grades. The altered signal intensities were in the form of fat replacement on T1WI and bone marrow edema on T2WI."*
"Tenosynovitis was a common finding in ankle tuberculosis with the anterior tendon group involved in six cases, medial in nine cases, lateral in six cases and posterior in 12 cases. The serous form (Stage I) was the most common compared

to the serofibrinous (Stage II) and fungoid forms (Stage III). Abnormal soft-tissue collections, representing granulation tissue or abscess, were detected in 10 cases."

2. "Magnetic resonance evaluated soft-tissue changes in the form of cellulitis, granulation tissue and abscess formation tenosynovitis and neurovascular involvement. Low–intermediate SI areas on T1WI, somewhat higher SI areas on T2WI (due to caseous necrosis), and prominent soft-tissue changes in the form of cold abscesses with peripheral rim enhancement mighty provide a clue to the diagnosis."

"MRI demonstration of cortical fractures, early cavitations, and soft tissue fluid collection has the potential to suggest the diagnosis at the predestructive stage of the disease. Sequential MRIs done after adequate medical therapy show return to normal architecture of the bone, with normal signal intensity."

"Cross-sectional imaging is more reliable at picking up early disease. MRI is good at looking at soft tissue architecture and collections (Korim et al)."

3. "In a study of MRI in 17 patients, Prakash et al emphasized that diagnosis of TB of foot and ankle is not based on radiology alone, instead clinicoradiological diagnosis is important. In the MRI, the average number of bones involved were 2.5 (1–8), more than two-thirds had bone marrow alterations, and erosion (58%) and intraosseous abscess were noted 47% cases. Synovial thickening was noted in all patients which involved multiple joints in all cases. Nearly 50% cases had tenosynovitis, medial group in all cases, and rarer in anterior group of tendons. Joint effusion was seen in 11/17 cases, most commonly at subtalar joint."

"Soft tissue involvement with diffuse gadolinium enhancement was seen in all cases. The multiplicity of findings of intraosseous abscess, soft tissue abscess and tenosynovitis favor the diagnosis of tubercular arthritis."

Q. 6. What is the role of FNAC from the draining enlarged / matted lymph nodes (popliteal/inguinal) to establish the diagnosis of new case of tuberculosis of ankle.

Enlarged lymph nodes have been reported by many studies. However, no study has documented FNAC from draining lymph nodes as a mode to establish the diagnosis.

The histological/cytological evidence (from the draining lymph nodes) of tuberculosis is adequate to treat the patient as a case of tuberculosis. It can be taken as supportive evidence only. One should always look for palpable lymph nodes in popleteal/inguinal region.

Q. 7. How to establish the diagnosis of ankle tuberculosis in synovitis stage and in arthritis stage?

Ans. The diagnosis is established on the following criteria:

1. Clinical and hematological parameters (raised ESR, relative lymphocytosis and monocytosis)

2. Radiological evidence (as above)

3. Imaging evidence (as above)

4. *Needle/CT* guided/USG guided/open biopsy

5. *Microbiological*: Smear for AFB/culture/BACTEC

6. *Molecular*: GeneXpert/Line Probe Assay.

In early disease in the stage of synovitis, when clinico-radiological evidence is nonspecific, a tissue biopsy is a must to establish a diagnosis. In a region where facilities are lacking in, a patient coming from an endemic region with classical clinico-radiological evidence of advanced arthritis can be presumptively diagnosed on the same and ATT may be instituted. However, wherever possible tissue should be procured by needle biopsy/aspiration and sent for histopathological, microbiological and molecular tests for confirmation partaculary in synovitis or early arthritis stage.

4. Dhillon MS, Tuli SM. Osteoarticular tuberculosis of the foot and ankle. Foot Ankle Int 2001 Aug;22(8):679–86.

10. Dhillon MS, Nagi ON. Tuberculosis of the foot and ankle. Clin Orthop Relat Res 2002;398:107–13.

6. Gursu S, Yildirim T, Ucpinar H, Sofu H, Camurcu Y, Sahin V, Sahin N. Long-term follow-up results of foot and ankle tuberculosis in Turkey. J Foot Ankle Surg 2014 Sep-Oct;53(5):557–61.

7. Chen SH, Wang T, Lee CH. Tuberculous ankle versus pyogenic septic ankle arthritis: a retrospective comparison. Jpn J Infect Dis 2011;64(2):139–42.

8. Agarwal A, Qureshi NA, Khan SA, Kumar P, Samaiya S. Tuberculosis of the foot and ankle in children. J Orthop Surg (Hong Kong) 2011 Aug;19(2):213–7.

9. Inoue S, Matsumoto S, Iwamatsu Y, Satomura M. Ankle tuberculosis: a report of four cases in a Japanese hospital. J Orthop Sci 2004; 9(4):392–8.

1. "When the diagnosis was unconfirmed by biopsy, but clinical and radiological features were highly suggestive of tuberculosis, a therapeutic trial of antitubercular therapy (ATT for 30 to 45 days) was instituted. Resolution of clinical features was considered diagnostic."

2. "We also advocate tissue diagnosis when the disease is not endemic; in our country, most subacute/chronic infections with an insidious course and typical clinical features are treated as tubercular until proven otherwise."

3. "Fine needle aspiration cytology (for those with an abscess), a trocar bone biopsy (for those with osseous lesions), an open biopsy to collect synovial and bone specimens (for those with joint involvement), and an edge biopsy of sinuses (for those with sinuses) were performed. The specimens were subjected to acid-fast staining (Ziehl-Neelsen) and histopathological examination. Diagnosis was based on a smear positive for acid-fast bacilli (n = 2), histopathology (n = 15), or clinicoradiological findings (n = 4)."

Q. 8. In a suspected case of TB ankle, can ATT be started on clinicoradiological (X-ray/MRI) basis alone in an endemic area?

In early disease (in the stage of synovitis), when clinicoradiological evidence is nonspecific, a tissue biopsy is mandatory to establish a diagnosis. In a region where facilities are lacking or in, a patient coming from an endemic region with classical clinicoradiological evidence of advanced arthritis, can be diagnosed on the same and ATT may be instituted. However, wherever possible tissue should be procured by needle biopsy/aspiration and sent for histopathological, microbiological and molecular tests for confirmation.

4. Dhillon MS, Tuli SM. Osteoarticular tuberculosis of the foot and ankle. Foot Ankle Int 2001 Aug;22(8):679–86.

10. Dhillon MS, Nagi ON. Tuberculosis of the foot and ankle. Clin Orthop Relat Res 2002;398:107–13.

6. Gursu S, Yildirim T, Ucpinar H, Sofu H, Camurcu Y, Sahin V, Sahin N. Long-term follow-up results of foot and ankle tuberculosis in Turkey. J Foot Ankle Surg 2014 Sep-Oct;53(5):557–61.

7. Chen SH, Wang T, Lee CH. Tuberculous ankle versus pyogenic septic ankle arthritis: a retrospective comparison. Jpn J Infect Dis 2011;64(2):139–42.

8. Agarwal A, Qureshi NA, Khan SA, Kumar P, Samaiya S. Tuberculosis of the foot and ankle in children. J Orthop Surg (Hong Kong) 2011 Aug;19(2):213–7.

9. Inoue S, Matsumoto S, Iwamatsu Y, Satomura M. Ankle tuberculosis: a report of four cases in a Japanese hospital. J Orthop Sci 2004;9(4):392–8.

19. Gavaskar AS, Chowdary N. Tibiotalocalcaneal arthrodesis using a supracondylar femoral nail for advanced tuberculous arthritis of the ankle. J Orthop Surg (Hong Kong) 2009 Dec;17(3):321–4.

18. Prakash M, Gupta P, Sen RK, Sharma A, Khandelwal N. Magnetic resonance imaging evaluation of tubercular arthritis of the ankle and foot. Acta Radiol 2014 Oct 20.

Q. 9. What are the indications of a biopsy in suspected TB of the ankle?

Indications for tissue diagnosis are:

1. To establish a diagnosis in the synovitis stage.

2. To establish a definitive diagnosis when clinicoradiological picture is ambiguous especially when a patient is from a non-endemic region.

3. To establish a diagnosis when ATT given for 30 to 45 days shows no improvement in signs/symptoms.

4. The lesions sitting astride the physis. In such cases, chondro-blastoma in differential diagnosis.

5. To obtain tissue for culture and drug sensitivity testing when the response to ATT is suboptimal.

20. Jain AK, Jena SK, Singh MP, Dhammi IK, Ramachadran VG, Dev G. Evaluation of clinico-radiological, bacteriological, serological, molecular and histological diagnosis of osteoarticular tuberculosis. Indian J Orthop 2008 Apr; 42(2):173–7.

15. Dhillon MS, Aggarwal S, Prabhakar S, Bachhal V. Tuberculosis of the foot: An osteolytic variety. Indian J Orthop 2012;46:206–11.

21. Dhillon MS, Sharma S, Gill SS, Nagi ON. Tuberculosis of bones and joints of the foot: an analysis of 22 cases. Foot Ankle 1993 Nov-Dec;14(9):505–13.

6. Gursu S, Yildirim T, Ucpinar H, Sofu H, Camurcu Y, Sahin V, Sahin N. Long-term follow-up results of foot and ankle tuberculosis in Turkey. J Foot Ankle Surg 2014 Sep-Oct;53(5):557–61.

7. Chen SH, Wang T, Lee CH. Tuberculous ankle versus pyogenic septic ankle arthritis: a retrospective comparison. Jpn J Infect Dis 2011; 64(2):139–42.

8. Agarwal A, Qureshi NA, Khan SA, Kumar P, Samaiya S. Tuberculosis of the foot and ankle in children. J Orthop Surg (Hong Kong) 2011 Aug;19(2):213–7.

1. *"The diagnosis of osteoarticular tuberculosis in endemic areas is clinico-radiological. It is justified to treat the patients clinicoradiologically in classical lesions of the bone. The clinical and radiological response can be observed in 8–12 weeks. However, there are certain cases with doubtful diagnosis, where tissue is required to ascertain diagnosis.*

2. *In the bone of the appendicular skeleton, tissue may be procured by fine needle aspiration cytology (FNAC) or core biopsy. Delay of a few days in the treatment of the limb lesion does not give rise to severe consequences, as tuberculosis is a slowly progressive disease."*

3. *"In many cases, the suspicion of bone tumor was entertained by the treating physician and the biopsy was done keeping that in mind; the true nature of the lesion was revealed only after tissue biopsy showed features suggestive of tuberculosis. Some form of tissue sampling was mandatory for all suspicious osteolytic lesions of the foot even in endemic regions as it could establish the diagnosis with relative certainty. This became doubly important when the radiographic presentation of the disease was that of a destructive lesion limited to the bone, and when the disease-affected population groups were routinely not affected by the disease."*

4. *"When the diagnosis was unconfirmed by biopsy, but clinical and radiological features were highly suggestive of tuberculosis, a therapeutic trial of antitubercular therapy (ATT for 30 to 45 days) was instituted. Resolution of clinical features was considered diagnostic."*

"We also advocate tissue diagnosis when the disease is not endemic; in our country, most subacute/chronic infections with an insidious course and typical clinical features are treated as tubercular until proven otherwise."

Q. 10. What is the preferred mode of biopsy in suspected case of TB ankle (open, USG guided, image intensifier guided or CT guided)?

Tissue for AFB smear/culture/smear/GeneXpert and histopathological examination can be taken by any of the following routes (percutaneous, USG guided, arthroscopic, and open). A percutaneous needle biopsy/FNAC is a simple OPD procedure and is recommended for most of the cases.

Any mode of biopsy can be used to obtain tissue depending upon the facilities, skills of treating surgeon and type of lesion. If the disease is superficial or the abscess or lesion is clinically palpable, the percutaneous techniques can be used. When the lesion is not clinically appreciable or is deeply located, then biopsy using guidance of ultrasonography or CT can be used. Ultrasound is more suitable for soft tissue collections and superficial bony lesions. CT comes with disadvantage of exposure to ionizing radiation. If no guidance facilities are available or surgeon is not confident or inadequate samples have been obtained repeatedly by percuatneous methods, an open biopsy should be considered.

Ulcer edge biopsy and sinus tract curettage may be confirmatory and is also advised in applicable cases. However, the possibility of bacterial contamination/colonization/ secondary infection of sinus tract by local skin flora and *Staph. aureus* should be kept in mind while sending the curetted material for microbiological/molecular investigations.

Arthroscopic technique offers the advantage of direct visualization of joint and hence allows for excision of tubercular synovium, granulation tissue and pannus over cartilage, but should be done only by experienced surgeons.

8. Agarwal A, Qureshi NA, Khan SA, Kumar P, Samaiya S. Tuberculosis of the foot and ankle in children. J Orthop Surg (Hong Kong) 2011 Aug;19(2):213–7.

11. Nayak B, Dash RR, Mohapatra KC, Panda G. Ankle and foot tuberculosis: a diagnostic dilemma. J Family Med Prim Care 2014 Apr;3(2):129–31.

22. Agarwal A, Kant KS, Suri T, Gupta N, Verma I, Shaharyar A. Tuberculosis of the calcaneus in children. J Orthop Surg (Hong Kong) 2015 Apr;23(1):84–9.

19. Gavaskar AS, Chowdary N. Tibiotalocalcaneal arthrodesis using a supracondylar femoral nail for advanced tuberculous arthritis of the ankle. J Orthop Surg (Hong Kong) 2009 Dec;17(3):321–4.

18. Prakash M, Gupta P, Sen RK, Sharma A, Khandelwal N. Magnetic resonance imaging evaluation of tubercular arthritis of the ankle and foot. Acta Radiol 2014 Oct 20.

Q. 11. How do we classify the severity of disease?

Korim *et al.* (2014) discuss the four stages proposed by Martini and Ouahes and refined by Chen *et al.*

Stage 1. Infection of synovial lining with little bony erosion or localized osteoporosis.

Stage 2. Marked erosions or areas of frank TB osteomyelitis but the joint space is maintained.

Stage 3. More synovial and bony involvement with a loss of joint space.

Stage 4. Involvement of more than 1 peritalar joint surface or concomitant pyogenic arthritis with substantial disorganization of osseous architecture.

---

23. Chen SH, Lee CH, Wong T, Feng HS. Long-term retrospective analysis of surgical treatment for irretrievable tuberculosis of the ankle. Foot Ankle Int 2013 Mar;34(3):372–9.
 3. Korim M, Patel R, Allen P, Mangwani J. Foot and ankle tuberculosis: case series and literature review. Foot (Edinb) 2014 Dec;24(4):176–9.
24. Martini M, BenkeddacheY, MedjaniY, Gottesman H. Tuberculosis of the upper limb joints. Int Orthop 1986;10:17–23.

Q. 12. What is the stage-wise treatment for TB foot? What is the role of immobilization (Plaster/AFO) in early part of treatment?

Just like other joints, nonoperative treatment with ATT (2 HRZE/10 HRE) for at least 12 months (may be 18 months), rest to the joint in functional position (using plaster of Paris cast for 4–6 weeks) and gentle nonweight-bearing mobilization (ankle foot orthosis) thereafter, as tolerated, should be instituted as treatment in all cases. A majority of patients heal with good functional outcome. Surgery is rarely indicated in early stage of disease.

---

 8. Agarwal A, Qureshi NA, Khan SA, Kumar P, Samaiya S. Tuberculosis of the foot and ankle in children. J Orthop Surg (Hong Kong) 2011 Aug;19(2):213–7.
 5. Tuli SM. Tuberculosis of the ankle and foot. In: Tuli SM, ed. Tuberculosis of the skeletal system. 3rd ed. New Delhi, India: Jaypee Brothers Medical Publishers (P) Ltd.; 2004:127–34.
 4. Dhillon MS, Tuli SM. Osteoarticular tuberculosis of the foot and ankle. Foot Ankle Int 2001 Aug;22(8):679–86.
10. Dhillon MS, Nagi ON. Tuberculosis of the foot and ankle. Clin Orthop Relat Res 2002;398:107–13.
25. Watts HG, Lifeso RM. Current concepts review: tuberculosis of bone and joints. J Bone Joint Surg [Am] 1996;78-A:288–98.

Q. 13. How do you monitor treatment response?

Patients are to be followed up weekly for first 6 weeks, and every 3 months thereafter for at least 2 years. During visit at 6th week and on subsequent visits thereafter, routine ESR, hemogram, liver and kidney profile and X-ray to monitor progress should be done.

A declining trend in ESR towards normal values by 12 months, remineralization of osteopenic bony lesion, restoration of trabeculae on X-ray healing of sinuses, absence of bony tenderness and resumption of function (passive range of subtalar movement, ankle movement, forefoot movement) denotes good treatment response.

8. Agarwal A, Qureshi NA, Khan SA, Kumar P, Samaiya S. Tuberculosis of the foot and ankle in children. J Orthop Surg (Hong Kong) 2011 Aug;19(2):213–7.

5. Tuli SM. Tuberculosis of the ankle and foot. In: Tuli SM, ed. Tuberculosis of the skeletal system. 3rd ed. New Delhi, India: Jaypee Brothers Medical Publishers (P) Ltd.; 2004:127–34.

4. Dhillon MS, Tuli SM. Osteoarticular tuberculosis of the foot and ankle. Foot Ankle Int 2001 Aug;22(8):679–86.

10. Dhillon MS, Nagi ON. Tuberculosis of the foot and ankle. Clin Orthop Relat Res 2002;398:107–13.

Q. 14. Define end point of treatment (ATT) of ankle TB.

Cardinal signs of healed disease include:
1. Healing of sinuses
2. Disappearance of local/systemic symptoms
3. Normalization of ESR on repeated examinations
4. Radiological evidence (lags behind clinical signs). The radio-logical evidence of healing include: Remineralization of the osteopenic bones, obliteration of bone cavities, restoration of trabeculae. MRI should not be done within 6 months of ATT and is useful to assess healing of the lesion at 12 and 18 months.

Contrast MRI at 12 and 18 months showing resolution of bone edema, fatty replacement of bone marrow and no enhancement by gadolinium contrast is indicative of healing of the lesion.

Various studies have advocated continuing ATT up to 18 months.

4. Dhillon MS, Tuli SM. Osteoarticular tuberculosis of the foot and ankle. Foot Ankle Int 2001 Aug;22(8):679–86.

10. Dhillon MS, Nagi ON. Tuberculosis of the foot and ankle. Clin Orthop Relat Res 2002;398:107–13.

6. Gursu S, Yildirim T, Ucpinar H, Sofu H, Camurcu Y, Sahin V, Sahin N. Long-term follow-up results of foot and ankle tuberculosis in Turkey. J Foot Ankle Surg 2014 Sep-Oct;53(5):557–61.

Q. 15. What are the indications of surgery in TB ankle?

Osteoarticular TB is a medical disease. At best surgical intervention is an adjunct to systemic antitubercular treatment. In a majority of cases, ATT for 12 to 18 months and rest to the ankle is all that is needed to achieve complete resolution of disease.

Indications for surgery include:
1. Impending collapse of bone producing ankle deformity
2. Drainage of large abscess
3. Joint debridement (arthroscopic/open)
4. To obtain tissue for diagnosis when nonoperative treatment based on clinicoradiological diagnosis fails to show adequate clinical response.
5. To obtain tissue for drug sensitivity testing when drug resistance is suspected and the response to ATT is suboptimal
6. Correction of deformity in healed tubercular foot.
7. Arthrodesis (open/arthroscopy assisted) using internal fixation (intramedullary nail, Steinmann pin, bridge plating), external fixation (ring fixator, Charnley clamps) or strut bone grafts (fibula/iliac crest) in cases of:
   a. Advanced painful arthritis of the ankle with gross destruction and deformity.
   b. Healed tuberculous ankle with painful fibrous ankylosis.

4. Dhillon MS, Tuli SM. Osteoarticular tuberculosis of the foot and ankle. Foot Ankle Int 2001 Aug;22(8):679–86.

10. Dhillon MS, Nagi ON. Tuberculosis of the foot and ankle. Clin Orthop Relat Res 2002;398:107–13.

6. Gursu S, Yildirim T, Ucpinar H, Sofu H, Camurcu Y, Sahin V, Sahin N. Long-term follow-up results of foot and ankle tuberculosis in Turkey. J Foot Ankle Surg 2014 Sep-Oct;53(5):557–61.

26. Tang KL, Li QH, Chen GX, Guo L, Dai G, Yang L. Arthroscopically assisted ankle fusion in patients with end-stage tuberculosis. Arthroscopy 2007;23:919–22.

5. Tuli SM. Tuberculosis of the ankle and foot. In: Tuli SM, ed. Tuberculosis of the skeletal system. 3rd ed. New Delhi, India: Jaypee Brothers Medical Publishers (P) Ltd.; 2004:127–34.

19. Gavaskar AS, Chowdary N. Tibiotalocalcaneal arthrodesis using a supracondylar femoral nail for advanced tuberculous arthritis of the ankle. J Orthop Surg (Hong Kong) 2009 Dec;17(3):321–4.

27. Jain M, Singh R. Ankle arthrodesis in tubercular arthritis using anterior bridge plating: a report of 2 cases. Foot (Edinb) 2014 Jun;24(2):81–5.

1. *"Since articular cartilage destruction in osteoarticular TB begins peripherally as tubercular granulation, tissue does not form proteolytic enzymes within the joint, and the central areas of articular cartilage in most joints are preserved for relatively long periods of time. This forms the basis for a good functional recovery even without surgery."*

2. *"Surgical intervention is at best an adjunct to the systemic antitubercular medical therapy. No surgical resection is a substitute for a prolonged course of appropriate chemotherapy. The role of surgery is usually limited to biopsy when the diagnosis is uncertain or debridement in the non-responsive cases, or resection with or without arthrodesis for deformity or for painful joints. Sequestrae do not need to be routinely removed, as they are resorbed with ATT alone. Residual osseous cavities are filled with fibrous or fibro-osseous tissue and need no operative intervention. We have observed such patients for 10 to 15 years with maintenance of healed status."*

3. *"Some surgical procedures such as sinus tract excision may hasten healing, and curettage of juxta-articular cavities that threaten to invade an adjacent joint may improve the overall prognosis by minimizing chances of joint involvement."*

Q. 16. What is the role of arthrodesis in TB ankle?

The TB of the ankle responds favorably to ATT and arthrodesis is seldom indicated as such.

Arthrodesis of the ankle (with/without talectomy) is indicated only in cases of:
1. Crippling deformity of ankle joint.
2. Painful fibrous ankylosis in healed TB.

3. Whenever ankle joint is subjected to open surgical debridement.

It can also be done in active disease. ATT needs to be restarted (full course) when surgical intervention is planned for healed disease. Post-surgery foot is to be kept in plaster for 3–6 months initially without weight bearing followed by and protected weight bearing later on till radiological evidence of fusion is seen

---

10. Dhillon MS, Nagi ON. Tuberculosis of the foot and ankle. Clin Orthop Relat Res 2002;398:107–13.

28. Martini M, Adjrad A, Daoud A. Tuberculous osteoarthritis of the foot and ankle joint. Int Orthop 1984;8(3):203–9. French [abstract]

5. Tuli SM. Tuberculosis of the ankle and foot. In: Tuli SM, ed. Tuberculosis of the skeletal system. 3rd ed. New Delhi, India: Jaypee Brothers Medical Publishers (P) Ltd.; 2004:127–34.

19. Gavaskar AS, Chowdary N. Tibiotalocalcaneal arthrodesis using a supracondylar femoral nail for advanced tuberculous arthritis of the ankle. J Orthop Surg (Hong Kong) 2009 Dec;17(3):321–4.

26. Tang KL, Li QH, Chen GX, Guo L, Dai G, Yang L. Arthroscopically assisted ankle fusion in patients with end-stage tuberculosis. Arthroscopy 2007;23:919–22.

27. Jain M, Singh R. Ankle arthrodesis in tubercular arthritis using anterior bridge plating: a report of 2 cases. Foot (Edinb) 2014 Jun;24(2):81–5.

1. *"In some cases where the joint is significantly destroyed and remains painful, arthrodesis (triple arthrodesis in the hindfoot, Lisfranc joint arthrodesis or ankle arthrodesis) may give a stable and pain-free joint. Whenever arthrodesis is done, plaster casts may need to be worn for long periods of time (3–6 months) until obvious fusion is seen on radiographs."*

"The authors have reviewed 26 cases of tuberculosis of the foot and 32 of the ankle, which they have treated personally. All the patients were adults and most presented with advanced destruction of bone and joints. Bacterial and histological confirmation of the diagnosis was obtained in 56 patients. All were treated by chemotherapy; the drugs and regime varied over the years. All responded well to this treatment, but one relapsed after 24 months. Orthopedic problems were usually managed by immobilization in plaster casts, but 6 patients required arthrodesis, 5 of the ankle and one triple fusion. The functional results of the standard treatment were generally good. Arthrodesis is seldom needed and should be performed only for permanent pain or crippling deformity."

"If surgical treatment be indicated in a joint involvement, the operation should be combined with deliberate arthrodesis."

Ref 19: *"Seven patients of advanced TB arthritis with severe pain on walking, with gross destruction of the articular cartilage of the tibiotalar joint with severe periarticular rarefaction on radiographs underwent tibiocalcaneal arthrodesis under spinal anaesthesia under a tourniquet by anterolateral approach. The articulating surfaces were debrided and shaped for maximum contact and the synovium was removed piecemeal circumferentially from the ankle and subtalar joint (Gavaskar and Chowdary)."*

Ref 26: *"Arthroscopic assisted arthrodesis enables visualization of joint surfaces, decreases blood loss and morbidity, preserves the mortice and thus enables early functional recovery. Arthroscopic assisted debridement and ankle arthrodesis using a retrograde nail attained good fusion and cosmesis (Tang et al.)".*

Q. 17. If ankle arthrodesis is done for arthritic pain after healed TB, is ATT required again?

As a general rule, if any surgical intervention is performed on any bone/joint after achieving healed status, one should start ATT and give it for 3–6 months.

Q. 18. What is the prognosis after ATT in TB ankle?

There is favorable response to ATT. The disease heals with good functional outcome, if treatment is started in synovitis or early arthritis stage on ATT and protected weight bearing till healing. The functional outcome is poor in cases which present in or progress to advanced arthritis and a fusion procedure is advocated to obtain a painless joint.

10. Dhillon MS, Nagi ON. Tuberculosis of the foot and ankle. Clin Orthop Relat Res 2002;398:107–13.

28. Martini M, Adjrad A, Daoud A. Tuberculous osteoarthritis of the foot and ankle joint. Int Orthop 1984;8(3):203–9. French [abstract]

5. Tuli SM. Tuberculosis of the ankle and foot. In: Tuli SM, ed. Tuberculosis of the skeletal system. 3rd ed. New Delhi, India: Jaypee Brothers Medical Publishers (P) Ltd.; 2004:127–34.

19. Gavaskar AS, Chowdary N. Tibiotalocalcaneal arthrodesis using a supracondylar femoral nail for advanced tuberculous arthritis of the ankle. J Orthop Surg (Hong Kong) 2009 Dec;17(3):321–4.

26. Tang KL, Li QH, Chen GX, Guo L, Dai G, Yang L. Arthroscopically assisted ankle fusion in patients with end-stage tuberculosis. Arthroscopy 2007;23:919–22.

27. Jain M, Singh R. Ankle arthrodesis in tubercular arthritis using anterior bridge plating: a report of 2 cases. Foot (Edinb). 2014 Jun;24(2):81–5.

1. *"Multidrug chemotherapy remains the mainstay of treatment, followed by active mobilization to achieve good functional results. Healing and restoration of function is excellent in patients with early-stage lesions. In patients with advanced-stage lesions, the prognosis is poorer and associated with residual bone changes and restriction of movements."*

Ref 19: *"Early mobilization and multidrug chemotherapy can achieve good results in early stages of tubercular arthritis (Gavaskar and Chowdary). While cases of advanced arthritis requiring ankle arthrodesis achieved fusion in 13 weeks and returned to their preoperative level of independence without any relapse, major complication or hardware failure (Gavaskar and Chowdary)".*

FOOT

Q. 1. What are the clinical presentations of tuberculosis of foot in early and advanced disease?

It can affect any age. However, it is more common in children and young adults. Calcaneum and talus are the most commonly involved bones whereas any bone in the foot as well as multiple bones can be involved at the same time. Differential diagnosis of calcaneal tuberculosis includes pyogenic or fungal infections, benign bone tumors or malignancies (e.g. Ewing's sarcoma).

The tubercular sinus can also be infected and this may lead to misdiagnosis. In **early disease,** they may present with:

1. Pain
2. Swelling (warm, red, tender)
3. Limp ("Heel-up" if calcaneus is primary site)

Rarely,

4. Fever (low grade, evening rise of temperature)
5. Regional lymphadenopathy
6. Weight loss, anorexia

In **advanced disease**, in addition to the above:

1. Synovial thickening (doughy/boggy on palpation)
2. Joint effusion
3. Deformity (depending on collapse of tarsal involved)
4. Discharging sinuses
5. Cold abscess.

Four different types of pathological presentations are described (Dhillon and Tuli 2001 based on Jellis 1988):

1. *Periarticular granuloma*—most common, progresses to involve joint, if left untreated.
2. *Central granuloma*—encountered in metatarsals of children.
3. *Primary isolated synovitis*—hematogenous origin.
4. Tubercular tenosynovitis and bursitis.

"Tubercular bacilli reach the joint space via the bloodstream. Skeletal tuberculosis of the foot is basically of four types:"

1. A periarticular granuloma of bone may form due to localization of the bacilli in the epiphyseal region; this may ultimately spread to the neighboring joint by direct erosion or through subsynovial vessels, and is the most common presentation of the disease.

2. A central granuloma of the bone is uncommon and is more frequently seen in children. This is due to endarteritis of the nutrient artery and may show a cavity with or without a sequestrum.

3. Primary hematogenous synovitis in isolation is rarely seen in the foot, although it is theoretically possible.

4. Tenosynovitis and bursitis are late sequelae of established infection and usually occur by spread from neighboring involved structures; however, isolated tubercular tenosynovitis as a primary manifestation of the disease also observed."

The foot bones are smaller in size and all joints are interconnected. As a result even if one bone and/or joint is primarily involved but eventually all joints and bones of midfoot are involved by the disease.

1. Tuli SM. Tuberculosis of the ankle and foot. In: Tuli SM, ed. Tuberculosis of the skeletal system. 3rd ed. New Delhi, India: Jaypee Brothers Medical Publishers (P) Ltd.; 2004:127–34.

2. Agarwal A, Kant KS, Suri T, Gupta N, Verma I, Shaharyar A. Tuberculosis of the calcaneus in children. J Orthop Surg (Hong Kong) 2015 Apr;23(1):84–9.

3. Jellis J. In: Helal B, Wilson D (eds). The Foot, London, Churchill Livingstone, 1988, pp 614–623.

4. Dhillon MS, Tuli SM. Osteoarticular tuberculosis of the foot and ankle. Foot Ankle Int 2001 Aug;22(8):679–86.

5. Dhillon MS, Aggarwal S, Prabhakar S, Bachhal V. Tuberculosis of the foot: An osteolytic variety. Indian J Orthop 2012;46:206–11.

6. Gursu S, Yildirim T, Ucpinar H, Sofu H, Camurcu Y, Sahin V, Sahin N. Long-term follow-up results of foot and ankle tuberculosis in Turkey. J Foot Ankle Surg 2014 Sep-Oct;53(5):557–61.

7. Mittal R, Gupta V, Rastogi S. Tuberculosis of the foot. J Bone Joint Surg 1999;81:997–1000.

8. Dhillon MS, Nagi ON. Tuberculosis of the foot and ankle. Clin Orthop Relat Res 2002;398:107–13.

9. Dhillon MS, Singh P, Sharma R, Gill SS, Nagi ON. Tuberculous osteomyelitis of the cuboid: a report of four cases. J Foot Ankle Surg 2000 Sep-Oct;39(5):329–35.

10. Dhillon MS, Sharma S, Gill SS, Nagi ON. Tuberculosis of bones and joints of the foot: an analysis of 22 cases. Foot Ankle 1993 Nov-Dec;14(9):505–13.

Q. 2. What are the findings on plain X-ray in early and advanced TB foot?

X-ray of the foot during the early phase can be unremarkable. We may see:

1. Localized osteoporosis
2. Increased soft tissue shadow
3. Fuzzy articular margins
4. Marginal erosions
5. Joint space may be normal or slightly narrow.

In advanced disease

1. Gross diminution of joint space
2. Irregular destruction of joint space
3. Cystic tuberculous cavities (with/without feathery "coke" like sequestrae) in large foot bone such as calcaneum. In this lesion, a well-defined lytic area is observed with loss of trabecular shadows. The cavity may contain a feathery sequestrum.
4. Pathological collapse of bone
5. Loss of articular cartilage leading to appearance of a coalesced mass of bones. This lesion is observed in all the tarsal bones except in talus and calcaneum (**rheumatoid appearance**)
6. Subperiosteal scalloping
7. Symmetrically scalloped "**kissing lesions**" of the two adjacent bones.

8. Ballooning of cortex, spindle-shaped expansion with successive layer of periosteal new bone **(spina ventosa)**. It is seen in short long bones such as metatarsal especially in children.
9. Sinuses.

1. Tuli SM. Tuberculosis of the ankle and foot. In: Tuli SM, ed. Tuberculosis of the skeletal system. 3rd ed. New Delhi, India: Jaypee Brothers Medical Publishers (P) Ltd.; 2004:127–34.

7. Mittal R, Gupta V, Rastogi S. Tuberculosis of the foot. J Bone Joint Surg 1999;81:997–1000.

4. Dhillon MS, Tuli SM. Osteoarticular tuberculosis of the foot and ankle. Foot Ankle Int 2001 Aug;22(8):679–86.

8. Dhillon MS, Nagi ON. Tuberculosis of the foot and ankle. Clin Orthop Relat Res 2002,398:107–13.

9. Dhillon MS, Singh P, Sharma R, Gill SS, Nagi ON. Tuberculous osteomyelitis of the cuboid: a report of four cases. J Foot Ankle Surg 2000 Sep-Oct;39(5):329–35.

10. Dhillon MS, Sharma S, Gill SS, Nagi ON. Tuberculosis of bones and joints of the foot: an analysis of 22 cases. Foot Ankle 1993 Nov-Dec;14(9):505–13.

Q. 3. What is the role of FNAC from the draining enlarged/matted lymph nodes (popliteal/inguinal) to establish the diagnosis of new case of tuberculosis of foot?

Enlarged lymph nodes have been reported by many studies. Although no article has reported outcome of FNAC in a series of such cases. It is advisable to undertake FNAC from enlarged lymph node.

Q. 4. Is there a role of ultrasonography and USG-guided FNAC in TB foot to detect cold abscess or synovial thickening for US-guided FNAC?

There are no pathognomonic findings on USG as such. There is no mention of use of ultrasound in tubercular foot in literature. However, it may show:

1. Cold abscesses and collections.
2. Synovial hypertrophy/tenosynovitis.

These are superficially palpable lesions hence most of the time one can aspirate or take a core biopsy without USG guide, whenever clinical localization is not possible, USG-guided aspiration/FNAC may be performed.

11. De Backer AI, Mortelé KJ, Vanhoenacker FM, Parizel PM. Imaging of extraspinal musculoskeletal tuberculosis. Eur J Radiol 2006;57:119–30.

12. De Backer AI, Vanhoenacker FM, Sanghvi DA. Imaging features of extraaxial musculoskeletal tuberculosis. Indian J Radiol Imaging 2009 Jul-Sep;19(3):176–86.

Q. 5. What are CT scan findings in TB foot? Is contrast CT better for diagnosis of TB foot?

Ans. CT scan findings are **non-specific** for foot tuberculosis. Findings include:

1. Erosions and lytic areas of destruction in the involved bone (Geographical extent of lesion can be delineated.)
2. Cavitation
3. Narrowing of joint
4. Sequestra

CT scan has been used for CT-guided biopsy from lesions. The use of contrast has not been mentioned but uniform enhancement of abscess wall has been reported as in other foci of osteoarticular TB.

8. Dhillon MS, Nagi ON. Tuberculosis of the foot and ankle. Clin Orthop Relat Res 2002;398:107–13.

4. Dhillon MS, Tuli SM. Osteoarticular tuberculosis of the foot and ankle. Foot Ankle Int 2001 Aug;22(8):679–86.

11. De Backer AI, Mortelé KJ, Vanhoenacker FM, Parizel PM. Imaging of extraspinal musculoskeletal tuberculosis. Eur J Radiol 2006;57:119–30.

12. De Backer AI, Vanhoenacker FM, Sanghvi DA. Imaging features of extra-axial musculoskeletal tuberculosis. Indian J Radiol Imaging 2009 Jul-Sep;19(3):176–86.

1. *"CT scans help in defining the geographic extent of the lesion and can clearly show the sequestration and cortical breaks. They also outline the extent of the bone destruction and are helpful in facilitating biopsy. Plain radiographs, CT scans, and MRI done during the follow-up of these patients who are receiving multidrug therapy sometimes may show advancing of the lesion, even after 3 to 4 months of treatment. This is because the imaging appearances lag behind*

the biologic process of repair. Even after complete clinical and radiologic healing, there may be residual cavities observed on serial CT scans or on radiographs".

2. *"During the destructive phase of the disease, we have found that the use of CT scans helps in defining the geographic extent of the lesion and can clearly show any sequestration. It also outlines the extent of the bone destruction and is very helpful in facilitating biopsy. We have also done serial CT scans in a few cases in an attempt to demonstrate the effects of medical therapy. Although it is not as informative as MRI in showing the bone edema and marrow changes, we were able to see that there was complete resorption of sequestrae in some cases."* It is important to note that even after complete clinical and radiological healing; there may be residual cavities noted on serial CT scans. These are of little consequence regarding the durability of healing and chances of recrudescence. These are filled with fibrous or fibro-osseous tissue and do not warrant surgical intervention. Radiographs, CT scans and MRI done during the follow-up of these patients on multi-drug therapy may show "advancing" of a lesion even after three to four months of treatment."

Q. 6. What are MRI findings of TB foot? Is contrast MRI better for diagnosis of TB foot?

MRI is more sensitive than specific to diagnose tuberculosis of foot. Nonspecific features suggestive of TB foot include:

1. Low signal on T1-weighted images and high signal on T2-weighted images suggestive of marrow edema.
2. Regions of necrosis seen as intermediate signal intensity on T2-weighted images.
3. Thickening of synovium
4. Soft tissue abscesses
5. Intraosseous abscess and cavitation
6. Joint effusion
7. Contrast enhancement of hypertrophic synovium and abscesses

Prakash et al reported that a combination of intraosseous abscess, soft tissue abscess and tenosynovitis is suggestive of tubercular arthritis of foot.

---

13. Korim M, Patel R, Allen P, Mangwani J. Foot and ankle tuberculosis: case series and literature review. Foot (Edinb) 2014 Dec;24(4):176–9.

14. Prakash M, Gupta P, Sen RK, Sharma A, Khandelwal N. Magnetic resonance imaging evaluation of tubercular arthritis of the ankle and foot. Acta Radiol 2014 Oct 20.

4. Dhillon MS, Tuli SM. Osteoarticular tuberculosis of the foot and ankle. Foot Ankle Int 2001 Aug;22(8):679–86.

13. De Backer AI, Mortelé KJ, Vanhoenacker FM, Parizel PM. Imaging of extraspinal musculoskeletal tuberculosis. Eur J Radiol 2006;57: 119–30.

14. De Backer AI, Vanhoenacker FM, Sanghvi DA. Imaging features of extraaxial musculoskeletal tuberculosis. Indian J Radiol Imaging 2009 Jul-Sep;19(3):176–86.

Ref 13: *"Cross-sectional imaging is more reliable at picking up early disease. MRI is good at looking at soft tissue architecture and collections (Korim et al)."*

2. *"In a study of MRI in 17 patients, Prakash et al, emphasized that diagnosis of TB of foot and ankle is not based on radiology alone, instead clinico-radiological diagnosis is important. In the MRI, the average number of bones involved were 2.5 (1–8), more than two-thirds had bone marrow alterations, and erosion (58%) and intra-osseous abscess were noted in 47% cases. Synovial thickening was noted in all patients which involved multiple joints in all cases.Nearly 50% cases had tenosynovitis, medial group in all cases, and rarer in anterior group of tendons. Joint effusion was seen in 11/17 cases, most commonly at subtalar joint. Soft tissue involvement with diffuse gadolinium enhancement was seen in all cases. The multiplicity of findings of intraosseous, abscess, soft tissue abscess and tenosynovitis favor the diagnosis of tubercular arthritis."*

3. *"MRI demonstration of cortical fractures, early cavitations, and soft tissue fluid collection has the potential to suggest the diagnosis at the pre-destructive stage of the disease. Sequential MRIs done after adequate medical therapy show return to normal architecture of the bone, with normal signal intensity."*

Q. 7. What are the differential diagnosis of TB foot and how to establish the diagnosis?

Ans. The diffenrential diagnoses include low grade pyogenic infection, mycoses, sarcoidosis, brucellosis are established on the following criteria:

1. Clinical and hematological parameters (raised ESR, relative lymphocytosis and monocytosis)
2. Radiological evidence (as above)
3. Imaging evidence (as above)
4. *Needle/CT* guided/USG guided/open biopsy
5. *Microbiological*: Smear for AFB/culture/BACTEC
6. *Molecular*: PCR/GeneXpert

In a region where facilities are lacking, a patient coming from an endemic region with classical clinicoradiological evidence of the disease, the ATT may be instituted.

However, since the lesion is superficial, tissue should be procured by needle biopsy/aspiration/core biopsy and sent for histopathological, microbiological and molecular tests for confirmation.

1. Tuli SM. Tuberculosis of the ankle and foot. In: Tuli SM, ed. Tuberculosis of the skeletal system. 3rd ed. New Delhi, India: Jaypee Brothers Medical Publishers (P) Ltd.; 2004:127–34.

7. Mittal R, Gupta V, Rastogi S. Tuberculosis of the foot. J Bone Joint Surg 1999;81:997–1000.

4. Dhillon MS, Tuli SM. Osteoarticular tuberculosis of the foot and ankle. Foot Ankle Int 2001 Aug;22(8):679–86.

8. Dhillon MS, Nagi ON. Tuberculosis of the foot and ankle. Clin Orthop Relat Res 2002;398:107–13.

9. Dhillon MS, Singh P, Sharma R, Gill SS, Nagi ON. Tuberculous osteomyelitis of the cuboid: a report of four cases. J Foot Ankle Surg 2000 Sep-Oct;39(5):329–35.

10. Dhillon MS, Sharma S, Gill SS, Nagi ON. Tuberculosis of bones and joints of the foot: an analysis of 22 cases. Foot Ankle 1993 Nov-Dec;14(9):505–13.

1. *"All the patients with only a soft-tissue lesion had a biopsy for confirmation, but those with bone lesions did not undergo this, and their diagnosis was based on clinical and radiological features."*

2. *"When the diagnosis was unconfirmed by biopsy, but clinical and radiological features were highly suggestive of tuberculosis, a therapeutic trial of antitubercular therapy (ATT for 30 to 45 days was instituted.) Resolution of clinical features was considered diagnostic."*

3. *"Out of 24 cases of osteolytic variety reported by Dhillon et al (2012), investigations revealed elevated ESR in all patients (25–90 mm/1st hr; most cases between 35 and 50 mm/1st hr), and positive Mantoux test in 21. ELISA was positive in nine of the 16 patients; PCR was done only in seven cases encountered after the year 2000, and was positive in six of the seven aspirates. Twenty-three patients were diagnosed on the basis of histopathology (n = 23), ELISA (n = 9), PCR (n = 6) or culture (n = 2), while one patient did not reveal any positive finding in any of the mentioned tests and was given a therapeutic trial of antitubercular chemotherapy, to which he responded favorably within nine weeks. All cases were subjected to aspiration or needle biopsy, to obtain tissue*

diagnosis, except two instances, where operative treatment was undertaken, primarily due to the impending joint involvement and collapse of the bone. Open biopsy and curettage was generally reserved for cases returning with a negative result on aspiration or needle biopsy.

4. In spite of a high index of suspicion for tuberculous infection, bony involvement in isolation can lead to some confusion, and diagnostic delays are common. The possible contributing factors include lack of constitutional symptoms so often related to osteoarticular tuberculosis elsewhere, confusion of radiographic features with bone tumors, and a relatively normal picture on laboratory investigations (including, at times, histopathology). Diagnosis of osteoarticular tuberculosis is often based on more than one test. Being a pauci-bacillary infection, culture from the infected tissue is seldom positive and the other ancillary evidence of infection then becomes important. Despite persistent efforts, a single diagnostic test for osteoarticular tuberculosis with high sensitivity and specificity has remained elusive, and chemotherapy is often instituted on clinical suspicion in endemic areas. Nevertheless, a full battery of diagnostic tests must be exhausted before adopting such an approach, especially in cases presenting at atypical locations, with unusual presentation, as is the case with osteolytic lesions in the foot. Adopting this principle we were able to find evidence supporting tuberculosis of foot in 23 of 24 cases (Dhillon et al, 2012)."

"We also advocate tissue diagnosis when the disease is not endemic; in our country, most subacute/chronic infections with an insidious course and typical clinical features are treated as tubercular until proven otherwise."

Q. 8. What are the indications of a biopsy in suspected TB foot?

Indications for tissue diagnosis are:

1. To establish a definitive diagnosis when clinicoradiological picture is ambiguous especially when a patient is from a non-endemic region.
2. To establish a diagnosis when ATT for 6 to 8 weeks shows no improvement in signs/symptoms.
3. When the differential diagnosis includes a fungal infection or conditions listed above.
4. To obtain tissue for culture and drug sensitivity testing when the response to ATT is suboptimal.

---

15. Jain AK, Jena SK, Singh MP, Dhammi IK, Ramachadran VG, Dev G. Evaluation of clinicoradiological, bacteriological, serological, molecular and histological diagnosis of osteoarticular tuberculosis. Indian J Orthop 2008 Apr;42(2):173–7.

5. Dhillon MS, Aggarwal S, Prabhakar S, Bachhal V. Tuberculosis of the foot· An osteolytic variety. Indian J Orthop 2012;46:206–11

10. Dhillon MS, Sharma S, Gill SS, Nagi ON. Tuberculosis of bones and joints of the foot: an analysis of 22 cases. Foot Ankle 1993 Nov-Dec;14(9):505–13

Q. 9. What is the role of sinus tract curettage for diagnosis of TB foot?

Sinus tract curettage/edge biopsy is an useful adjunct in establishing a diagnosis. Material can be sent for histopathology, culture (LJ medium/BACTEC/fungal/brucella), smear for AFB, PCR and GeneXpert analyses.

However, the possibility of bacterial contamination/colonization/secondary infection of sinus tract by local skin flora and *Staph. aureus* should be kept in mind while sending the curetted material for microbiological/molecular investigations.

16. Nayak B, Dash RR, Mohapatra KC, Panda G. Ankle and foot tuberculosis: a diagnostic dilemma. J Family Med Prim Care 2014 Apr;3(2):129–31.

2. Agarwal A, Kant KS, Suri T, Gupta N, Verma I, Shaharyar A. Tuberculosis of the calcaneus in children. J Orthop Surg (Hong Kong) 2015 Apr;23(1):84–9.

Q. 10. What are the investigations to be performed from the pus discharge of a sinus tract?

The pus discharge should be submitted for Gram's staining and pyogenic pus culture. The tissue obtained after biopsy should be sent for histopathology, culture (LJ medium/BACTEC/fungal/brucella), smear for AFB, PCR and GeneXpert analyses.

17. Chen SH, Lee CH, Wong T, Feng HS. Long-term retrospective analysis of surgical treatment for irretrievable tuberculosis of the ankle. Foot Ankle Int 2013 Mar;34(3):372–9.

15. Jain AK, Jena SK, Singh MP, Dhammi IK, Ramachadran VG, Dev G. Evaluation of clinicoradiological, bacteriological, serological, molecular and histological diagnosis of osteoarticular tuberculosis. Indian J Orthop 2008 Apr;42(2):173–7.

Ref 17: *"The diagnostic accuracy rates were 28.5% with aspiration of synovial fluid, 66.7% in histological analysis, and 44.4% in bacteriological analysis."*

Ref 15: *"AFB staining (direct) and AFB culture sensitivity was positive in six of fifty (12%) cases. Aerobic/anaerobic culture sensitivity was negative in all cases. Histology was positive for TB in all the cases. The PCR was positive in 49 of fifty (98%) cases."*

Q. 11. How do we classify the severity of disease?

Korim *et al.*, 2014, discuss the four stages proposed by Martini and Ouahes and refined by Chen *et al.*

Stage 1. Infection of synovial lining with little bony erosion or localized osteoporosis.

Stage 2. Marked erosions or areas of frank TB osteomyelitis but the joint space is maintained.

Stage 3. More synovial and bony involvement with a loss of joint space.

Stage 4. Involvement of more than one peritalar joint surface or concomitant pyogenic arthritis with substantial disorganization of osseous architecture.

---

17. Chen SH, Lee CH, Wong T, Feng HS. Long-term retrospective analysis of surgical treatment for irretrievable tuberculosis of the ankle. Foot Ankle Int 2013 Mar;34(3):372–9.
18. Korim M, Patel R, Allen P, Mangwani J. Foot and ankle tuberculosis: case series and literature review. Foot (Edinb) 2014 Dec;24(4):176–9.
19. Martini M, BenkeddacheY, MedjaniY, Gottesman H. Tuberculosis of the upper limb joints. Int Orthop 1986;10:17–23.

Q. 12. What is the role of immobilization (plaster/AFO) in early part of treatment of TB foot?

It is similar to that of tuberculosis of ankle. Nonoperative treatment with ATT (2HRZE + 10HRE) for at least 12 months (may be extended up to 18 months on a case to case basis). The joints should be put to the rest in functional position (using plaster) and gentle non-weight-bearing mobilization (using AFO) as tolerated later on, should be instituted as treatment in all cases. A majority of patients heal with good functional outcome. Surgery is rarely indicated.

10. Dhillon MS, Sharma S, Gill SS, Nagi ON. Tuberculosis of bones and joints of the foot: an analysis of 22 cases. Foot Ankle 1993 Nov-Dec;14(9):505–13.

1. Tuli SM. Tuberculosis of the ankle and foot. In: Tuli SM, ed. Tuberculosis of the skeletal system. 3rd ed. New Delhi, India: Jaypee Brothers Medical Publishers (P) Ltd.; 2004:127–34.

7. Mittal R, Gupta V, Rastogi S. Tuberculosis of the foot. J Bone Joint Surg 1999;81:997–1000.

4. Dhillon MS, Tuli SM. Osteoarticular tuberculosis of the foot and ankle. Foot Ankle Int 2001 Aug;22(8):679–86.

8. Dhillon MS, Nagi ON. Tuberculosis of the foot and ankle. Clin Orthop Relat Res 2002;398:107–13.

9. Dhillon MS, Singh P, Sharma R, Gill SS, Nagi ON. Tuberculous osteomyelitis of the cuboid: a report of four cases. J Foot Ankle Surg 2000 Sep-Oct;39(5):329–35.

6. Gursu S, Yildirim T, Ucpinar H, Sofu H, Camurcu Y, Sahin V, Sahin N. Long-term follow-up results of foot and ankle tuberculosis in Turkey. J Foot Ankle Surg 2014 Sep-Oct;53(5):557.

20. Watts HG, Lifeso RM. Current concepts review: tuberculosis of bone and joints. J Bone Joint Surg [Am] 1996;78-A:288–98.

Q. 13. How should the treatment response be monitored?

Patients should be called for follow up weekly/fortnightly for first 6 weeks (to assess drug tolerance), and every 2 months thereafter for at least 1 year. Each visit at the 6th week and thereafter should include investigations, viz. routine ESR, hemogram, liver and kidney function tests and X-ray to monitor progress. The indicators for good response to treatment are: (1) A declining trend in ESR leading to normal values by 12 months. (2) Remineralization, restoration of trabeculae on X-ray. (3) Healing of sinuses, absence of bony tenderness and resumption of function (passive range of subtalar movement, ankle movement, forefoot movement).

2. Agarwal A, Kant KS, Suri T, Gupta N, Verma I, Shaharyar A. Tuberculosis of the calcaneus in children. J Orthop Surg (Hong Kong) 2015 Apr;23(1):84–9.

5. Dhillon MS, Aggarwal S, Prabhakar S, Bachhal V. Tuberculosis of the foot: An osteolytic variety. Indian J Orthop 2012;46:206–11.

7. Mittal R, Gupta V, Rastogi S. Tuberculosis of the foot. J Bone Joint Surg 1999;81:997–1000.

Q. 14. What is the end point of treatment (ATT) of ankle/foot tuberculosis?

Generally as in other bone and joint tuberculosis, the end point is not defined. Cardinal signs of healed disease include:

1. Healing of sinuses
2. Disappearance of local/systemic symptoms
3. Normalization of ESR on repeated examinations
4. *Radiological evidence:*

   a. Remineralization (reduction of localized osteoporosis/ osteopenia)

   b. Obliteration of cavities

   c. Restoration of trabeculae

Various studies have advocated continuing ATT up to 18 months.

---

10. Dhillon MS, Sharma S, Gill SS, Nagi ON. Tuberculosis of bones and joints of the foot: an analysis of 22 cases. Foot Ankle 1993 Nov-Dec;14(9):505–13.

1. Tuli SM. Tuberculosis of the ankle and foot. In: Tuli SM, ed. Tuberculosis of the skeletal system. 3rd ed. New Delhi, India: Jaypee Brothers Medical Publishers (P) Ltd.; 2004:127–34.

7. Mittal R, Gupta V, Rastogi S. Tuberculosis of the foot. J Bone Joint Surg 1999;81:997–1000.

4. Dhillon MS, Tuli SM. Osteoarticular tuberculosis of the foot and ankle. Foot Ankle Int 2001 Aug;22(8):679–86.

8. Dhillon MS, Nagi ON. Tuberculosis of the foot and ankle. Clin Orthop Relat Res 2002;398:107–13.

9. Dhillon MS, Singh P, Sharma R, Gill SS, Nagi ON. Tuberculous osteomyelitis of the cuboid: a report of four cases. J Foot Ankle Surg 2000 Sep-Oct;39(5):329–35.

6. Gursu S, Yildirim T, Ucpinar H, Sofu H, Camurcu Y, Sahin V, Sahin N. Long-term follow-up results of foot and ankle tuberculosis in Turkey. J Foot Ankle Surg 2014 Sep-Oct;53(5):557–61.

"The cardinal signs of healed disease were taken to be—(1) disappearance of local/systemic symptoms (including sinuses); (2) no elevation/change in repeated erythrocyte sedimentation rate; (3) radiological evidence of remineralization, obliteration of cavities, restoration of trabeculae, and decrease in osteoporosis."

"It is important to note that the radiologic features lag behind the actual healing process and Dhillon and Nagi (2002) recommended at least 6–7 months of multimodal therapy before repeating cross-sectional imaging to reduce the rate of false positives for disease progression.

The disease was considered to be healed when the local or systemic symptoms disappeared, along with radiological evidence of remineralization, obliteration of cavities, decrease in regional osteoporosis, and restoration of the trabeculae (Mittal et al, 1999)."

Q. 15. What are the indications of surgery in TB foot?

In a majority of cases, ATT and rest to the foot is all that is needed for complete resolution of disease. Indications for surgery include:

1. Juxta-articular lesion (impending joint involvement)
2. Expanding lesion—large isolated lesion in the calcaneum.
3. Impending collapse of bone
4. Drainage of large abscess
5. Joint debridement
6. To obtain tissue for diagnosis when ATT was started on clinicoradiological diagnosis and now the lesion is not responding to conservative treatment.
7. To obtain tissue for drug sensitivity testing when drug resistance is suspected and the response to ATT is sub-optimal.
8. Correction of deformity in healed tubercular foot.
9. Arthrodesis in a healed tubercular foot with painful fibrous ankylosis

4. Dhillon MS, Tuli SM. Osteoarticular tuberculosis of the foot and ankle. Foot Ankle Int 2001 Aug;22(8):679–86.
7. Mittal R, Gupta V, Rastogi S. Tuberculosis of the foot. J Bone Joint Surg 1999;81:997–1000.
5. Dhillon MS, Aggarwal S, Prabhakar S, Bachhal V. Tuberculosis of the foot: An osteolytic variety. Indian J Orthop 2012;46:206–11.
8. Dhillon MS, Nagi ON. Tuberculosis of the foot and ankle. Clin Orthop Relat Res 2002;398:107–13.
6. Gursu S, Yildirim T, Ucpinar H, Sofu H, Camurcu Y, Sahin V, Sahin N. Long-term follow-up results of foot and ankle tuberculosis in Turkey. J Foot Ankle Surg 2014 Sep-Oct;53(5):557–61.

Ref 7: *"Surgical intervention was reserved for patients with either a juxta-articular focus threatening to involve a joint or for an impending collapse of a midfoot bone with cystic destruction (Mittal et al, 1999)."*

2. *"Since articular cartilage destruction in osteoarticular TB begins peripherally as tubercular granulation, tissue does not form proteolytic enzymes within the joint, and the central areas of articular cartilage in most joints are preserved for relatively long periods of time. This forms the basis for a good functional recovery even without surgery."*

3. *"Surgical intervention is at best an adjunct to the systemic anti-tubercular medical therapy. No surgical resection is a substitute for a prolonged course of appropriate chemotherapy. The role of surgery is usually limited to biopsy when the diagnosis is uncertain or debridement in the non-responsive cases, or resection with or without arthrodesis for deformity or for painful joints. Sequestrae do not need to be routinely removed, as they are resorbed with ATT alone. Residual osseous cavities are filled with fibrous or fibro-osseous tissue and need no operative intervention. We have observed such patients for 10 to 15 years with maintenance of healed status."*

4. *"Some surgical procedures such as sinus tract excision may hasten healing, and curettage of juxta-articular cavities that threaten to invade an adjacent joint may improve the overall prognosis by minimizing chances of joint involvement."*

5. *"Certain surgical procedures may be unique to the foot, as in one of the current patients, with a large cystic cavity in the cuboid and nonhealing sinuses, a mini-distractor was used to prevent the bone from collapsing. The lateral column length was maintained after debridement of the cuboid by using an external fixator in distraction mode, because only a shell of bone was left."*

6. *"Operative intervention may be indicated for non-responsive cases, uncertain diagnosis, or to save a joint threatened by a juxta-articular focus."*

7. *"Dhillon et al, 2012, reported two cases out of 24 osteolytic variety requiring surgery. One patient with impending cuboid collapse had curettage and fixation with an external fixator in distraction mode, until there was some evidence of remineralization. One patient with involvement of the calcaneus close to the posterior facet of the subtalar joint underwent surgical debridement due to the imminent danger of joint involvement. The lesions healed without joint involvement."*

8. *"Curettage, debridement, sequestrectomy, bone grafting, fistulectomy, synoviectomy, arthrodesis, and resection are among the preferred surgical choices."*

Q. 16. What is the role of triple arthrodesis in hindfoot TB? Can triple arthrodesis be done in active stage of TB of hindfoot?

Ans. The disease responds favorably to ATT and arthrodesis is seldom indicated as such.

Arthrodesis of the hindfoot is indicated only in cases of:
1. Crippling deformity of foot
2. Painful fibrous ankylosis in healed TB
3. Whenever talocalcaneonavicular joints are subjected to surgical debridement.

It can be done in active disease. Post-surgery foot is to be kept in plaster for 3–6 months without weight bearing till radiological evidence of fusion is seen.

---

8. Dhillon MS, Nagi ON. Tuberculosis of the foot and ankle. Clin Orthop Relat Res 2002;398:107–13.

21. Martini M, Adjrad A, Daoud A. Tuberculous osteoarthritis of the foot and ankle joint. Int Orthop 1984;8(3):203-9. French [abstract]

1. Tuli SM. Tuberculosis of the ankle and foot. In: Tuli SM, ed. Tuberculosis of the skeletal system. 3rd ed. New Delhi, India: Jaypee Brothers Medical Publishers (P) Ltd.; 2004:127–34.

1. *"In some cases where the joint is significantly destroyed and remains painful, arthrodesis (triple arthrodesis in the hindfoot, Lisfranc joint arthrodesis or ankle arthrodesis) may give a stable and pain-free joint. Whenever arthrodesis is done, plaster casts may need to be worn for long periods of time (3–6 months) until obvious fusion is seen on radiographs."*

Ref 8: *"The authors have reviewed 26 cases of tuberculosis of the foot and 32 of the ankle, which they have treated personally. All the patients were adults and most presented with advanced destruction of bone and joints. Bacterial and histological confirmation of the diagnosis was obtained in 56 patients. All were treated by chemotherapy; the drugs and regime varied over the years. All responded well to this treatment, but one relapsed after 24 months. Orthopedic problems were usually managed by immobilization in plaster casts, but 6 patients required arthrodesis, 5 of the ankle and one triple fusion. The functional results of the standard treatment were generally good. Arthrodesis is seldom needed and should be performed only for permanent pain or crippling deformity."*

"If surgical treatment be indicated in a joint involvement, the operation should be combined with deliberate arthrodesis. If talocalcaneonavicular joints are involved, a standard triple arthrodesis is necessary."

Q. 17. What is the prognosis after ATT in TB foot?

Ans. Usually there is a favorable response after ATT. Generally the disease heals with some or no loss of motion but no/minimal pain depending on the stage of the disease.

1. Tuli SM. Tuberculosis of the ankle and foot. In: Tuli SM, ed. Tuberculosis of the skeletal system. 3rd ed. New Delhi, India: Jaypee Brothers Medical Publishers (P) Ltd.; 2004:127–34.

2. Agarwal A, Kant KS, Suri T, Gupta N, Verma I, Shaharyar A. Tuberculosis of the calcaneus in children. J Orthop Surg (Hong Kong) 2015 Apr;23(1):84–9.

3. Jellis J. In: Helal B, Wilson D, (eds). The Foot, London, Churchill Livingstone, 1988, pp 614–623.

4. Dhillon MS, Tuli SM. Osteoarticular tuberculosis of the foot and ankle. Foot Ankle Int 2001 Aug;22(8):679–86.

5. Dhillon MS, Aggarwal S, Prabhakar S, Bachhal V. Tuberculosis of the foot: An osteolytic variety. Indian J Orthop 2012;46:206–11.

6. Gursu S, Yildirim T, Ucpinar H, Sofu H, Camurcu Y, Sahin V, Sahin N. Long-term follow-up results of foot and ankle tuberculosis in Turkey. J Foot Ankle Surg 2014 Sep-Oct;53(5):557–61.

7. Mittal R, Gupta V, Rastogi S. Tuberculosis of the foot. J Bone Joint Surg 1999;81:997–1000.

8. Dhillon MS, Nagi ON. Tuberculosis of the foot and ankle. Clin Orthop Relat Res 2002;398:107–13.

9. Dhillon MS, Singh P, Sharma R, Gill SS, Nagi ON. Tuberculous osteomyelitis of the cuboid: a report of four cases. J Foot Ankle Surg 2000 Sep-Oct;39(5):329–35.

10. Dhillon MS, Sharma S, Gill SS, Nagi ON. Tuberculosis of bones and joints of the foot: an analysis of 22 cases. Foot Ankle 1993 Nov-Dec;14(9):505–13.

Ref 5: *Dhillon et al, 2012, reported serial resorption of sequestra on radiographs with chemotherapy alone. At an average follow up of 8.3 years (range 2–15 years), none of the patients had rest pain during walking on level ground, although six patients complained of occasional discomfort or mild pain when walking on uneven ground. No significant restriction of motion was seen in these cases with purely osteolytic lesions. None of the patients had shown signs of recurrence.*

Q. 18. How to establish diagnosis of calcaneal tuberculosis in a patient with multiple persistent chronic sinuses which shows 'no growth' on culture including negative fungal culture and curettage report is inconclusive/shows chronic inflammation. Should ATT be given in such cases in endemic countries?

Studies have recommended a formal open biopsy to be done to obtain adequate tissue for analyses in cases where curettings sent are inconclusive. ATT should be started only after ascertaining diagnosis in such cases. Tissue should be obtained by formal open biopsy and sent for histopathological/microbiological/molecular tests to ascertain diagnosis and know pattern of sensitivity of organism, if adequate amount of tissue is obtained from a representative area, the diagnosis should be established beyond doubt and treated appropriately.

Q. 19. If discharge from sinus tract in a new case of tuberculosis of tarsal bones persists after 6–9 months ATT, should the same ATT be continued or should it be changed. In either case, how long should ATT be continued?

The lesion should be debrided in such cases and tissue should be sent for histology (to ascertain the diagnosis), AFB smear, AFB culture, smear and culture for pyogenic organisms, Gene Xpert, Line Probe Assay and fungal cultures. If the histology is suggestive of infective etiology with no fungal infection, the patient should be treated as presumptive drug resistance using second-line ATT after getting the drug sensitivity test for the *Mycobacterium TB* and/or GeneXpert and Line Probe report. The ATT regimen should be modified as per drug sensitivity available.

10. Dhillon MS, Sharma S, Gill SS, Nagi ON. Tuberculosis of bones and joints of the foot: an analysis of 22 cases. Foot Ankle 1993 Nov-Dec;14(9):505–13.

1. Tuli SM. Tuberculosis of the ankle and foot. In: Tuli SM, ed. Tuberculosis of the skeletal system. 3rd ed. New Delhi, India: Jaypee Brothers Medical Publishers (P) Ltd.; 2004:127–34.

7. Mittal R, Gupta V, Rastogi S. Tuberculosis of the foot. J Bone Joint Surg 1999;81:997–1000.

4. Dhillon MS, Tuli SM. Osteoarticular tuberculosis of the foot and ankle. Foot Ankle Int 2001 Aug;22(8):679–86.

8. Dhillon MS, Nagi ON. Tuberculosis of the foot and ankle. Clin Orthop Relat Res 2002;398:107–13.

9. Dhillon MS, Singh P, Sharma R, Gill SS, Nagi ON. Tuberculous osteomyelitis of the cuboid: a report of four cases. J Foot Ankle Surg 2000 Sep-Oct;39(5):329–35.

6. Gursu S, Yildirim T, Ucpinar H, Sofu H, Camurcu Y, Sahin V, Sahin N. Long-term follow-up results of foot and ankle tuberculosis in Turkey. J Foot Ankle Surg 2014 Sep-Oct;53(5):557.

25. Watts HG, Lifeso RM. Current concepts review: tuberculosis of boneand joints. J Bone Joint Surg [Am] 1996;78-A:288–98.

SHOULDER

Q. 1. What is the common age of presentation of tuberculosis of shoulder?

Tuberculosis of the shoulder is rare and constitutes 1–2 % cases of osteoarticular tuberculosis. It is more common in adults (>20 years). However, isolated reports of childhood affection also present.

1. Tuli SM. Tuberculosis of the shoulder. In: Tuli SM, ed. Tuberculosis of the skeletal system. 3rd ed. New Delhi, India: Jaypee Brothers Medical Publishers (P) Ltd.; 2004:135–43.

2. Kapukaya A, Subasi M, Bukte Y, Gur A, Tuzuner T, Kilnc N. Tuberculosis of the shoulder joint. Joint Bone Spine 2006 Mar;73(2):177–81.

3. Tkach PS, Chabanenko SV, Filiuk VV, Bezdetnyi AV. Osteochondral alloplasty of the humeral head in tuberculous omarthritis. Probl Tuberk 1991;(6):37–41. Russian [abstract]

4. Yalçinkaya F, Tümer N, Akar N, Ekim M, Bildirici Y. Tuberculous osteomyelitis: an unusual case of tuberculous infection in a child undergoing continuous ambulatory peritoneal dialysis. Pediatr Nephrol 1995 Aug;9(4):485–6.

5. Haygood TM, Williamson SL. Radiographic findings of extremity tuberculosis in childhood: back to the future? Radiographics 1994 May;14(3):561–70.

6. Richter R, Nübling W, Schulz HJ, Köhler G. Tuberculosis of the shoulder joint. Z Orthop Ihre Grenzgeb 1986 Jan-Feb;124(1):36–45. German. [abstract]

Q. 2. Is there an association with immunocompromised status or coexisting pulmonary TB in tuberculosis of shoulder?

Yes, the occurrence of osteoarticular tuberculosis in general is correlated with the immunocompromised states like:

• Steroid intake
• Diabetes mellitus
• Chronic renal failure
• HIV/AIDS
• Hypoproteinemia
• Pulmonary tuberculosis/disseminated/multifocal tuber-culosis.

7. Michalowska-Mitczuk D, Blasiñska-Przerwa K. Tuberculosis of shoulder bone. Pneumonol Alergol Pol. 2011;79(6):437–41. Polish.

8. Bansal S, Jindal S, Biswas R. Non-healing arm wound with a discharging sinus in an elderly patient with diabetes.BMJ Case Rep 2010 Sep 8;2010

4. Yalçinkaya F, Tümer N, Akar N, Ekim M, Bildirici Y. Tuberculous osteomyelitis: an unusual case of tuberculous infection in a child undergoing continuous ambulatory peritoneal dialysis. Pediatr Nephrol 1995 Aug;9(4):485–6.

9. Nakao S, Takeda A, Matsumoto H, Sasaki N, Sato K, Fujita Y, Yamazaki Y, Tobise K. A case of pulmonary tuberculosis complicated with multiple bone and joint tuberculosis. Kekkaku 2000 Jun;75(6):429–34. Japanese [abstract]

10. Salliot C, Allanore Y, Lebrun A, Guerini H, Champion K, Anract P, Kahan A. Disseminated extrapulmonary tuberculosis revealed by humeral osteomyelitis with chronic unremarkable pain. Joint Bone Spine 2005 May;72(3):263–6.

11. Tuli SM. Tuberculosis of the shoulder. In: Tuli SM, ed. Tuberculosis of the skeletal system. 3rd ed. New Delhi, India: Jaypee Brothers Medical Publishers (P) Ltd.; 2004:135–43.

Q. 3. What are the clinical symptoms/presentation of tuberculosis of shoulder (early/advanced) stage of disease?

In early disease, the presentation in the synovitis stage is very uncommon in tuberculosis of shoulder (PHOTO). They may present with:

1. Pain
2. Restricted range of motion (limitation of external rotation and abduction
3. Wasting of muscles (deltoid and supraspinatus primarily)

Rarely,

4. Fever (low grade, evening rise of temperature)
5. Regional lymphadenopathy
6. Weight loss, anorexia
7. Swelling (warm, red, swollen tender joint)

In advanced disease, the symptoms may be of long standing and in addition to the above,

1. Marked destruction of humeral head and glenoid and gross wasting of shoulder muscles are found. Rarely the deformity

(fibrous ankylosis with humeral head pulled up against glenoid and limb fixed in adduction and internal rotation) may develop

Rarely,

2. Swelling (warm, red, swollen tender joint)

3. Discharging sinuses around shoulder, arm and scapula

4. Cold abscess

Generally, the tuberculosis of shoulder presents in the advanced stage.

1. Tuli SM. Tuberculosis of the shoulder. In: Tuli SM, ed. Tuberculosis of the skeletal system. 3rd ed. New Delhi, India: Jaypee Brothers Medical Publishers (P) Ltd.; 2004:135–43.

2. Kapukaya A, Subasi M, Bukte Y, Gur A, Tuzuner T, Kilnc N. Tuberculosis of the shoulder joint. Joint Bone Spine 2006 Mar;73(2):177–81.

12. Li JQ, Tang KL, Xu HT, Li QY, Zhang SX. Glenohumeral joint tuberculosis that mimics frozen shoulder: a retrospective analysis. J Shoulder Elbow Surg 2012 Sep;21(9):1207–12.

13. Ba-Fall K, Niang A, Ndiaye AR, Lefebvre N, Chevalier B, Debonne JM, Mbaye PS, Margery J. Shoulder pain revealing tuberculosis of the humerus. Rev Pneumol Clin 2009 Feb;65(1):13-5. [abstract]

10. Salliot C, Allanore Y, Lebrun A, Guerini H, Champion K, Anract P, Kahan A. Disseminated extrapulmonary tuberculosis revealed by humeral osteomyelitis with chronic unremarkable pain. Joint Bone Spine 2005 May;72(3):263–6.

14. Monach PA, Daily JP, Rodriguez-Herrera G, Solomon DH. Tuberculous osteomyelitis presenting as shoulder pain. J Rheumatol 2003 Apr;30(4):851–6.

15. Kizildag B, Sener A, Komurcu E, Karatag O, Kosar S. Glenohumeral joint tuberculosis with multiple cold abscesses: an uncommon cause of shoulder pain. BMJ Case Rep 2013 Aug 23;2013.

16. Husen YA, Nadeem N, Aslam F, Shah MA. Tuberculosis of the scapula. J Pak Med Assoc 2006 Jul;56(7):336–8.

17. Kim RS, Lee JY, Jung SR, Lee KY. Tuberculoussubdeltoid bursitis with rice bodies. Yonsei Med J 2002 Aug;43(4):539–42.

18. Alkalay I, Kaufman T, Suprun H. Tuberculosis of the subdeltoid bursa. A case report. Isr J Med Sci 1980 Dec;16(12):853–5.

8. Bansal S, Jindal S, Biswas R. Non-healing arm wound with a discharging sinus in an elderly patient with diabetes. BMJ Case Rep 2010 Sep 8;2010.

9. Miller KD, Moore ME. Tuberculous arthritis of the shoulder: delayed diagnosis aided by arthrography. Clin Rheumatol 1983 Mar;2(1):61–4.

Q. 4. What is caries sicca?

Tuberculosis of the shoulder can have two types of manifestation. Dry form (caries sicca); and the exudative form. In caries sicca, as mentioned above, the lesion is dry. The bony destruction and exudates formation is less. The shoulder undergoes fibrous ankylosis; hence a gross restriction of motion is observed. However, rarely they may present with swelling, cold abscess and sinus formation in the deltoid region, along the biceps tendon or in the supraspinous fossa.

1. Tuli SM. Tuberculosis of the shoulder. In: Tuli SM, ed. Tuberculosis of the skeletal system. 3rd ed. New Delhi, India: Jaypee Brothers Medical Publishers (P) Ltd.; 2004:135–43.

11. Li JQ, Tang KL, Xu HT, Li QY, Zhang SX. Glenohumeral joint tuberculosis that mimics frozen shoulder: a retrospective analysis. J Shoulder Elbow Surg 2012 Sep;21(9):1207–12.

19. Lakhkar DL, Yadav M, Soni A, Kumar M. Unusual presentation of shoulder joint tuberculosis: A case report. Ind J Radiol Imag 2006 16:1:23–26.

20. Mangwani J, Gupta AK, Yadav CS, Rao KS. Unusual presentation of shoulder joint tuberculosis: A case report. J Orthop Surg (Hong Kong) 2001 Jun;9(1):57–60.

21. Nagaraj C, Singh S, Singh B, Trikha V, Rastogi S. Tuberculosis of the shoulder joint with impingement syndrome as initial presentation. J Microbiol Immunol Infect 2008 Jun;41(3):275–8.

Q. 5. What are the findings on plain radiography in early and advanced disease in TB of shoulder?

The shoulder must be subjected to anteroposterior and axillary views. X-ray of the shoulder joint during the early phase can be unremarkable.

However, the following findings may be present:

1. Localized osteoporosis (osteopenia)
2. Cloudy appearance of glenoid and humeral head

3. Fuzzy articular margins
4. Marginal erosions
5. Joint space may be normal or slightly reduced

In advanced disease,
1. Gross diminution of joint space
2. Irregular destruction of joint space
3. Cystic tuberculous cavities in proximal humerus
4. Pathological subluxation or dislocation of joint
- *Stage 1.* Localized osteoporosis, but no bony lesion
- *Stage 2.* One or more erosions or cavities in the bone and mild joint space narrowing
- *Stage 3.* Involvement of the entire joint without gross destruction including marked joint space narrowing
- *Stage 4.* Gross destruction

"The appearance of periarticular osteoporosis, marginal erosions and absent or mild joint space narrowing is most indicative of this disease. In rheumatoid arthritis, osteoporosis and marginal erosions are accompanied by early and significant loss of articular space."

1. Tuli SM. Tuberculosis of the shoulder. In: Tuli SM, ed. Tuberculosis of the skeletal system. 3rd ed. New Delhi, India: Jaypee Brothers Medical Publishers (P) Ltd.; 2004:135–43.
19. Lakhkar DL, Yadav M, Soni A, Kumar M. Unusual presentation of shoulder joint tuberculosis: A case report. Ind J Radiol Imag 2006 16:1:23–26.
22. Ostrowska M, Gietka J, Nesteruk T, Piliszek A, Walecki J. Shoulder joint tuberculosis. Pol J Radiol 2012; 77(4):55–59.
23. Martini M, BenkeddacheY, MedjaniY, Gottesman H. Tuberculosis ofthe upper limb joints. Int Orthop 1986;10:17–23.

Q. 6. What are the ultrasonographic (USG) findings of TB of shoulder?

No pathognomonic findings are described on USG. However, non-specific findings include:
1. Joint effusion
2. Collections in bursae

3. Cystic masses with hyperechoic contents resembling rice bodies
4. Rarely, proliferating synovium, rotator cuff tears.

The advantage of sonography is its capability to perform real-time cross-sectional imaging. It can be performed in any orientation. The tear of the rotator cuff can also be imaged.

19. Lakhkar DL, Yadav M, Soni A, Kumar M. Unusual presentation of shoulder joint tuberculosis: A case report. Ind J Radiol Imag 2006 16:1:23–26.

20. Pookarnjanamorakot C, Sirikulchayanonta V. Tuberculous bursitis of the subacromial bursa. J Shoulder Elbow Surg 2004 Jan-Feb;13(1):105–7.

Q. 7. What are CT scan findings in TB shoulder? Is contrast CT better?

The CT scan (plain and contrast enhanced) can demonstrate bone destruction better than MRI and soft tissue abscess can also be aprreciated. CT scan findings are **non-specific** for shoulder tuberculosis.

1. Erosions and lytic areas of destruction in humeral head, glenoid and scapula
2. Narrowing of glenohumeral joint
3. Soft tissue collection in between muscles (deltoid and subscapularis) which enhances on contrast CT.
4. Calcific foci in soft tissue around the joint are better appreciated.

19. Lakhkar DL, Yadav M, Soni A, Kumar M. Unusual presentation of shoulder joint tuberculosis: A case report. Ind J Radiol Imag 2006 16:1:23–26.

2. Kapukaya A, Subasi M, Bukte Y, Gur A, Tuzuner T, Kilnc N. Tuberculosis of the shoulder joint. Joint Bone Spine 2006 Mar;73(2):177–81.

Q. 8. What are MRI findings of TB shoulder?

In general, MRI can show non-specific findings and no pathognomonic features or constellation of features suggestive of tuberculosis are described in literature. Still MRI is useful in demonstrating the lesion before it can be appreciated on plain X-rays.

Nonspecific features suggestive of TB shoulder include:

1. Low signal on T1-weighted images and high signal on T2-weighted images suggestive of marrow edema

2. Regions of necrosis seen as intermediate signal intensity on T2-weighted images

3. Thickening of synovium, if present

4. Soft tissue abscesses, if present

5. Joint effusion, if present

6. Contrast enhancement of hypertrophic synovium and abscesses, if present. The other advantages of MRI are:

   - It demonstrates the lesion before evident on plain X-ray
   - Helpful in evaluating the extent of the lesion
   - It can show effusion, periarticular osteoporosis, bone lysis, sclerosis, periosteitis and thickened synovium. These findings are observed in tubercular and pyogenic osteomyelitis.

---

2. Kapukaya A, Subasi M, Bukte Y, Gur A, Tuzuner T, Kilnc N. Tuberculosis of the shoulder join.t Joint Bone Spine 2006 Mar;73(2):177–81.

19. Lakhkar DL, Yadav M, Soni A, Kumar M. Unusual presentation of shoulder joint tuberculosis: A case report. Ind J Radiol Imag 2006 16:1:23–26.

22. Ostrowska M, Gietka J, Nesteruk T, Piliszek A, Walecki J. Shoulder joint tuberculosis. Pol J Radiol 2012; 77(4):55–59.

14. Kizildag B, Sener A, Komurcu E, Karatag O, Kosar S. Glenohumeral joint tuberculosis with multiple cold abscesses: an uncommon cause of shoulder pain. BMJ Case Rep 2013 Aug 23;2013.

"Although non-specific, MRI is helpful in the differential diagnosis and for evaluating the extent of the lesions, and demonstrates lesions before they are evident on plain radiography. MRI usually shows a large effusion, periarticular osteoporosis, bone lysis, sclerosis, periostitis, and gross thickening of the synovial membrane. These MRI findings are seen in tuberculous osteomyelitis and chronic pyogenic osteomyelitis, and it is often difficult to differentiate the two conditions. In general, MRI has proved to be extremely sensitive in the early detection of osteomyelitis, because of the exquisite contrast it provides between the diseased areas and normal marrow. Infected areas are seen as regions of low signal intensity on T1-weighted images and as regions of high signal."

Q. 9. Can ATT be started on clinicoradiological basis alone in an endemic area? What are the triggers for diagnosis/ further workup in a case of TB shoulder?

The diagnosis of a rare disorder like shoulder tuberculosis that commonly presents in advanced stage should be based on clinicoradiological as well as histopathological/microbiological confirmation. Although in endemic regions, the clinical features, radiological/MRI appearance, and elevated ESR may be sufficient to diagnose tuberculosis.

The disease should be differentiated from neuropathic shoulder/rheumatoid arthritis/adhesive capsulitis/frozen shoulder syndrome which have similar presentations. It is not uncommon to diagnose a case of adhesive capsulitis ('frozen shoulder') with co-existent pulmonary tuberculosis as caries sicca. A biopsy is mandatory whenever any doubt exists.

2. Kapukaya A, Subasi M, Bukte Y, Gur A, Tuzuner T, Kilnc N. Tuberculosis of the shoulder joint. Joint Bone Spine 2006 Mar;73(2):177–81.

1. Tuli SM. Tuberculosis of the shoulder. In: Tuli SM, ed. Tuberculosis of the skeletal system. 3rd ed. New Delhi, India: Jaypee Brothers Medical Publishers (P) Ltd.; 2004:135–43.

Q. 10. What is the preferred mode of biopsy in suspected case of TB shoulder—open, USG-guided, image intensifier guided, CT-guided?

Tissue for PCR based molecular diagnosis/tubercular culture/ AFB smear/GeneXpert and histopathological examination can be taken by any of the following routes (percutaneous, USG-guided, CT-guided, arthroscopic, and open). The choice depends on location of lesion and its accessibility by any of the methods. In early disease, arthroscopic technique offers the advantage of direct visualization of joint and hence allows for excision of tubercular synovium, granulation tissue, rice bodies and pannus over cartilage. However, in advanced disease where arthroscopy is not feasible, an open debridement and biopsy is indicated.

17. Kim RS, Lee JY, Jung SR, Lee KY. Tuberculous subdeltoid bursitis with rice bodies. Yonsei Med J 2002 Aug;43(4):539–42.

2 Kapukaya A, Subasi M, Bukte Y, Gur A, Tuzuner T, Kilnc N. Tuberculosis of the shoulder joint. Joint Bone Spine 2006 Mar;73(2):177–81.

11. Li JQ, Tang KL, Xu HT, Li QY, Zhang SX. Glenohumeral joint tuberculosis that mimics frozen shoulder: a retrospective analysis. J Shoulder Elbow Surg 2012 Sep;21(9):1207–12.

Q. 11. How are the patients of tuberculosis of shoulder treated after the diagnosis?

Nonoperative treatment with ATT (2 HRZE/10 HRE) for at least 12 months, rest to the joint in functional position (using spica or brace or sling) and gentle mobilization as tolerated should be instituted as treatment in all cases. The ATT duration may be increased for 6 months more if the lesion has not attained healed status. A majority of patients heal with good functional outcome. Surgery is rarely indicated. Generally fibrous ankylosis is the goal. It is a non-weight-bearing joint; hence remains relatively pain free once healed.

Shoulder immobilization for 3 months in the form of spica (70° abduction, 30° forward flexion and internal rotation) was traditionally used to allow ankylosis of the glenohumeral joint in functional position. Active assisted movements were encouraged thereafter to achieve a functional shoulder via compensatory scapulothoracic movements.

There are no recent studies in literature wherein prolonged immobilization with spica is advocated. Gentle mobilization, and rest to the shoulder are now prescribed. Use of braces and shoulder slings to allow rest to the joint and allow gentle mobilization has been mentioned in some reports.

1. Tuli SM. Tuberculosis of the shoulder. In: Tuli SM, ed. Tuberculosis of the skeletal system. 3rd ed. New Delhi, India: Jaypee Brothers Medical Publishers (P) Ltd.; 2004:135–43.

2. Kapukaya A, Subasi M, Bukte Y, Gur A, Tuzuner T, Kilnc N. Tuberculosis of the shoulder joint. Joint Bone Spine 2006 Mar;73(2):177–81.

11. Li JQ, Tang KL, Xu HT, Li QY, Zhang SX. Glenohumeral joint tuberculosis that mimics frozen shoulder: a retrospective analysis. J Shoulder Elbow Surg 2012 Sep;21(9):1207–12.

25. Longo UG, Marinozzi A, Cazzato L, Rabitti C, Maffulli N, Denaro V. Tuberculosis of the shoulder. J Shoulder Elbow Surg 2011 Jun;20(4):e19–21.

21. Nagaraj C, Singh S, Singh B, Trikha V, Rastogi S. Tuberculosis of the shoulder joint with impingement syndrome as initial presentation. J Microbiol Immunol Infect 2008 Jun;41(3):275–8.

14. Kizildag B, Sener A, Komurcu E, Karatag O, Kosar S. Glenohumeral joint tuberculosis with multiple cold abscesses: an uncommon cause of shoulder pain. BMJ Case Rep 2013 Aug 23;2013.

20. Mangwani J, Gupta AK, Yadav CS, Rao KS. Unusual presentation of shoulder joint tuberculosis: A case report. J Orthop Surg (Hong Kong) 2001 Jun;9(1):57–60.

Q. 12. How the treatment response to be monitored?

The response to treatment is generally favorable. Patients are to be followed up weekly for 6 weeks, and every 3 months thereafter for at least 1 year or till the healed status is achieved. At each visit at the 6th week and thereafter should include a routine ESR, hemogram, liver and kidney profile and X-ray of the shoulder are to be performed to monitor progress.

A declining trend of ESR towards normal values by 12 months; remineralization, restoration of trabeculae on X-ray, healing of sinuses, absence of bony tenderness and resumption of function are indicators of good response to the treatment and signs of healing.

2. Kapukaya A, Subasi M, Bukte Y, Gur A, Tuzuner T, Kilnc N. Tuberculosis of the shoulder joint. Joint Bone Spine 2006 Mar;73(2):177–81.

1. Tuli SM. Tuberculosis of the shoulder. In: Tuli SM, ed. Tuberculosis of the skeletal system. 3rd ed. New Delhi, India: Jaypee Brothers Medical Publishers (P) Ltd.; 2004:135–43.

Q. 13. What are the indications of surgery in TB shoulder?

Non-operative management is usually the preferred treatment. The surgery is rarely indicated. The indications for surgery are:

1. *To establish diagnosis in early stage of diease or when cilinicoradiological diagnosis is doubtful*: Arthroscopic/CT guided/USG guided/formal arthrotomy can be done.
2. Drainage of abscess, if large.

3. Excision of sinuses, if present and unresponsive to ATT.

4. Joint debridement (open/arthroscopic) to remove loose bodies, rice bodies, granulation tissue and pannus to facilitate healing in cases not responding adequately to ATT.

5. Arthrodesis of a painful fibrous ankylosis.

6. Replacement arthroplasty in healed disease.

2. Kapukaya A, Subasi M, Bukte Y, Gur A, Tuzuner T, Kilnc N. Tuberculosis of the shoulder joint. Joint Bone Spine 2006 Mar;73(2):177–81.

1. Tuli SM. Tuberculosis of the shoulder. In: Tuli SM, ed. Tuberculosis of the skeletal system. 3rd ed. New Delhi, India: Jaypee Brothers Medical Publishers (P) Ltd.; 2004:135–43.

8. Bansal S, Jindal S, Biswas R. Non-healing arm wound with a discharging sinus in an elderly patient with diabetes. BMJ Case Rep 2010 Sep 8;2010.

17. Kim RS, Lee JY, Jung SR, Lee KY. Tuberculous subdeltoid bursitis with rice bodies. Yonsei Med J 2002 Aug;43(4):539–42.

26. Ogawa K, Nakamichi N. Advanced shoulder joint tuberculosis treated with débridement and closed continuous irrigation and suction: a report of 2 cases.Am J Orthop (Belle Mead NJ) 2010 Feb;39(2):E15-8.

1. *"Severe destructive tubercular lesions may not have as bad an outcome as anticipated. Good functional results are produced in the shoulder with conservative management and rehabilitation, despite the extent of joint destruction.*

2. *Better results have been reported with conservative management than with arthrodesis or excision. In our series, arthrodesis was performed in only one patient, and, according to the patients, this patient was less satisfied with the outcome than were those who were managed conservatively.*

Therefore, arthrodesis could be a treatment of last resort in the management of patients with shoulder tuberculosis. The pathology in tuberculosis lends itself to debridement of infected tissue because the shoulder is a non-weight-bearing joint and can accept more joint irregularity."

Q. 14. What is the role of resection arthroplasty in TB shoulder?

There is no role for resection arthroplasty mentioned in recent literature. Even previous studies have reported better results with nonoperative management than with excision arthroplasty.

2. Kapukaya A, Subasi M, Bukte Y, Gur A, Tuzuner T, Kilnc N. Tuberculosis of the shoulder joint. Joint Bone Spine 2006 Mar;73(2):177–81.

23. Martini M, BenkeddacheY, MedjaniY, Gottesman H. Tuberculosis of the upper limb joints. Int Orthop 1986;10:17–23.

Q. 15. What is the role of arthrodesis in TB shoulder?

Severe destructive tubercular lesions may not have as bad an outcome as anticipated. Good functional results are produced in the shoulder with conservative management and rehabilitation, despite the extent of joint destruction. Better results have been reported with conservative management than with arthrodesis or excision.

Arthrodesis is to be used as the treatment of last resort in cases where conservative management or surgical debridement heals with a painful fibrous ankylosis where replacement arthroplasty is not an option.

Both extra-articular and intra-articular techniques are described. Intra-articular method allows for joint debridement and internal fixation with screws/pins concomitantly and has been used ever since the advent of antitubercular drugs. In the present scenario, arthrodesis is rarely performed.

2. Kapukaya A, Subasi M, Bukte Y, Gur A, Tuzuner T, Kilnc N. Tuberculosis of the shoulder joint. Joint Bone Spine 2006 Mar;73(2):177–81.

27. González-Díaz R, Rodríguez-Merchán EC, Gilbert MS. The role of shoulder fusion in the era of arthroplasty. Int Orthop 1997;21(3):204–9.

1. Tuli SM. Tuberculosis of the shoulder. In: Tuli SM, ed. Tuberculosis of the skeletal system. 3rd ed. New Delhi, India: Jaypee Brothers Medical Publishers (P) Ltd.; 2004:135–43.

Q. 16. What is the role of replacement arthroplasty in TB shoulder?

There is only one report in recent literature mentioning the use of replacement arthroplasty for TB shoulder. Large scale studies are needed to generate a recommendation. There is no report of replacement arthroplasty for healed tuberculosis with painful fibrous ankylosis of shoulder.

PubMed search for "shoulder arthroplasty tuberculosis" yielded 13 results. Only one pertained to replacement arthroplasty in active shoulder TB. The other two were isolated case reports where there was post-surgical infection with tuberculosis in patients who had undergone shoulder arthroplasty for various reasons.

Luenam et al performed single stage cementless hemi-arthroplasty in 2 patients after joint debridement in active disease. Patients were put on ATT for 12 months. At 5-year follow-up, neither of the patients had recurrence of the disease or implant loosening.

Hattrup et al reported a case of *Mycobacterium* infection in a 78-year-old patient who had undergone replacement arthroplasty for avascular necrosis of humeral head. Patient was treated with removal of prosthesis and repeated debridements and put on ATT. Oncosurgical proximal humeral megaprosthesis was used to salvage her upper limb.

Lederman *et al.* reported a case of *Mycobacterium tuberculosis* infection of the shoulder that occurred 37 years after a shoulder hemiarthroplasty. Patient was on anticancer drugs for gastro-intestinal stromal tumor and succumbed to cancer 18 months after removal of prosthesis.

28. Luenam S, Kosiyatrakul A. Immediate cementless hemiarthroplasty for severe destructive glenohumeral tuberculous arthritis. Case Rep Orthop 2013 (2013). Id 426102, 7.

29. Hattrup SJ, Bhagia UT. Shoulder arthroplasty complicated by *Mycobacterium tuberculosis* infection: a case report. J Shoulder Elbow Surg 2008 Nov-Dec;17(6):e5–7.

30. Lederman E, Kweon C, Chhabra A. Late *Mycobacterium tuberculosis* infection in the shoulder of an immunocompromised host after hemiarthroplasty: a case report. J Bone Joint Surg Am 2011 Jun 15;93(12):e67(1-4).

Q. 17. What is the functional outcome after ATT in TB shoulder?

There is favorable response after ATT. Generally, heals with some loss of motion but no pain.

1. Tuli SM. Tuberculosis of the shoulder. In: Tuli SM, ed. Tuberculosis of the skeletal system. 3rd ed. New Delhi, India: Jaypee Brothers Medical Publishers (P) Ltd.; 2004:135–43.

2. Kapukaya A, Subasi M, Bukte Y, Gur A, Tuzuner T, Kilnc N. Tuberculosis of the shoulder joint. Joint Bone Spine 2006 Mar;73(2):177–81.

23. Martini M, BenkeddacheY, MedjaniY, Gottesman H. Tuberculosis of the upper limb joints. Int Orthop 1986;10:17–23.

11. Li JQ, Tang KL, Xu HT, Li QY, Zhang SX. Glenohumeral joint tuberculosis that mimics frozen shoulder: a retrospective analysis. J Shoulder Elbow Surg 2012 Sep;21(9):1207–12.

25. Longo UG, Marinozzi A, Cazzato L, Rabitti C, Maffulli N, Denaro V. Tuberculosis of the shoulder. J Shoulder Elbow Surg 2011 Jun;20(4):e19–21.

21. Nagaraj C, Singh S, Singh B, Trikha V, Rastogi S. Tuberculosis of the shoulder joint with impingement syndrome as initial presentation. J Microbiol Immunol Infect 2008 Jun;41(3):275–8.

14. Kizildag B, Sener A, Komurcu E, Karatag O, Kosar S. Glenohumeral joint tuberculosis with multiple cold abscesses: an uncommon cause of shoulder pain. BMJ Case Rep 2013 Aug 23;2013.

20. Mangwani J, Gupta AK, Yadav CS, Rao KS. Unusual presentation of shoulder joint tuberculosis: A case report. J Orthop Surg (Hong Kong) 2001 Jun;9(1):57–60.

ELBOW

Q. 1. What is the clinical presentation of TB elbow?

Tuberculosis of the elbow accounts for 2 to 5% of all osteo-articular tuberculosis. It can affect any age. The disease can present as synovitis, tenosynovitis, osteitis, arthritis, olecranon bursitis, myositis and abscess of brachialis and biceps brachii, bicipitoradial bursitis, epitrochlear lymphadenitis, ulnar nerve palsy, posterior ulnar nerve palsy, ulnar nerve tuberculoma, and/or non-healing ulcers.

The clinical features in **early disease are:** The onset of these symptoms is insidous. They present with:

1. Pain
2. Swelling (warm, red, swollen tender joint)
3. Synovial thickening (doughy/boggy on palpation)
4. Joint effusion
5. Fever (low grade, evening rise of temperature, night sweats)
6. Regional lymphadenopathy: Supratrochlear and axillary lymph nodes
7. Weight loss, anorexia
8. Restricted range of motion
9. Rarely, ulnar nerve palsy, posterior interosseous nerve palsy

In **advanced disease**, in addition to the above:

1. Wasting of arm and forearm muscles
2. Deformity (ranges from flexion/extension deformity to pathological posterior dislocation of elbow)
3. Discharging sinuses
4. Cold abscess

Classification of tuberculosis of elbow (Wilson 1953)

1. Synovial lesion (only 5%)
2. Extra-articular lesion
3. Coronoid lesion
4. Massive lesion involving all joint surfaces
5. Unclassified

Prognostic classification of TB elbow (Dhillon 2012 based on Martini 1986)

Stage 1. Synovial

Stage 2. Extra-articular away from joint

Stage 3A. Extra-articular lesions threatening to involve the joint

Stage 3B. Intra-articular lesions without gross destruction

Stage 4. Gross destruction.

Generally, cold abscess and subsequent sinuses which originates from the joint are located on lateral/posterolateral/ posterior aspect of the joint; while cold abscess and sinuses originating from supratrochlear lymph nodes are located in the medial side.

1. Tuli SM. Tuberculosis of the elbow joint. In: Tuli SM, ed. Tuberculosis of the skeletal system. 3rd ed. New Delhi, India: Jaypee Brothers Medical Publishers (P) Ltd.; 2004:144–52.

2. Chen WS, Wang CJ, Eng HL. Tuberculous arthritis of the elbow. Int Orthop 1997;21:367–70.

3. Aggarwal A, Dhammi I. Clinical and radiological presentation of tuberculosis of the elbow. Acta Orthop Belg 2006;72:282–7.

4. Agarwal A, Mumtaz I, Kumar P, Khan S, Qureshi NA. Tuberculosis of the elbow joint in children: A review of ten patients who were managed nonoperatively. J Bone Joint Surg Am 2010;92:436–41.

5. Wilson JN. Tuberculosis of the elbow; a study of thirty-one cases. J Bone Joint Surg Br 1953;35:551–60.

6. Dix-Peek SI, Vrettos BC, Hoffman EB. Tuberculosis of the elbow in children. J Shoulder Elbow Surg 2003;12:282–6.

7. Vohra R, Kang HS. Tuberculosis of the elbow. A report of 10 cases. Acta Orthop Scand 1995;66:57–8.

8. Martini M, Benkeddache Y, Medjani Y, Gottesman H. Tuberculosis of the upperlimb joints. Int Orthop 1986;10:17–23.

9. Parkinson RW, Hodgson SP, Noble J. Tuberculosis of the elbow: a report of five cases. J Bone Joint Surg Br 1990 May;72(3):523–4.

10. Dhillon MS, Goel A, Prabhakar S, Aggarwal S, Bachhal V. Tuberculosis of the elbow: A clinicoradiological analysis. Indian J Orthop 2012;46:200–5.

11. Lin YM, Tan TS, Lee TS. Tuberculous synovitis of the elbow joint. J Formos Med Assoc 2001 Aug;100(8):568–70.

12. Asaka T, Takizawa Y, Kariya T, Nitta E, Yasuda T, Fujita M, Sawasaki S, Naiki Y, Nakatani N, Doushita T, Miura T, Ueda F, Takamori M, Matsushima A. Tuberculous tenosynovitis in the elbow joint. Intern Med 1996 Feb;35(2):162-5.

13. Abdelwahab IF, Kenan S. Tuberculous abscess of the brachialis and biceps brachii muscles without osseous involvement. A case report. J Bone Joint Surg Am 1998 Oct;80(10):1521–4.

14. Seber S, Köse N. Tuberculous abscess of the brachialis and biceps brachii muscles without osseous involvement. A case report. J Bone Joint Surg Am 1999 Dec;81(12):1788.

15. Nishida J, Furumachi K, Ehara S, Satoh T, Okada K, Shimamura T. Tuberculous bicipitoradial bursitis: a case report. Skeletal Radiol 2007 May;36(5):445–8.

16. Singh AP, Chadha M, Singh AP, Mahajan S. Isolated tuberculous biceps tenosynovitis bicipitoradial bursitis: a case report. J Shoulder Elbow Surg 2009 Nov-Dec;18(6):e30–3.

17. Crum NF. Tuberculosis presenting as epitrochlear lymphadenitis. Scand J Infect Dis 2003;35(11-12):888–90.

18. Ramesh Chandra VV, Prasad BC, Varaprasad G. Ulnar nerve tuberculoma. J Neurosurg Pediatr. 2013 Jan;11(1):100–2.

19. Sinha GP. Tuberculoma of the ulnar nerve. J Bone Joint Surg Am 1975 Jan;57(1):131.

20. Wang CT, Sun JS, Hou SM. Mycobacterial infection of the upper extremities. J Formos Med Assoc 2000 Sep;99(9):710–5.

21. Ayhan S, Ozmen S, Uluoglu O, Demirtaþ Y, Boyacioglu M, Latifoglu O, Atabay K. Nonhealing ulcerative mass of the elbow: do not forget tuberculosis.Ann Plast Surg 2002 May;48(5):557–61.

22. Domingo A, Nomdedeu M, Tomás X, García S. Elbow tuberculosis: an unusual location and diagnostic problem. Arch Orthop Trauma Surg 2005 Feb;125(1):56–8.

Q. 2. What are the predominant manifestation of TB elbow?

Two types of clinical presentation are described:

a. Dry/stiff elbow

b. Exudative

Both the types of clinical presentations are seen depending on stage of disease and patient factors. Exudative stage is seen in the early to late disease. In exudative stage, pus draining sinus/sinuses with synovial swelling and limitation of movements is predominant. The dry type is more commonly seen in the later stage when the disease is close to healing by fibrous ankylosis. In dry type, the predominant feature is swelling and limitation of movements subject to duration of the disease to the extent of early ankylosis.

Q. 3. What are the findings on plain X-ray and in early and advanced disease?

The radiological findings are non-specific in the early stages and the initial lesions can be easily missed.

Radiographic features are usually noted 2 to 5 months after disease onset and only a joint effusion may be apparent in the very early stage.

1. *Synovitis stage*:
   a. Regional osteoporosis
   b. Increased soft tissue shadow (due to synovial hypertrophy, effusion)

2. *Early arthritis stage*:
   a. Loss of definition of articular surfaces
   b. **"Ice cream scoop"** appearance in the ulnar metaphyseal region in children
   c. Marginal erosions
   d. Diminution of joint space
   e. Destruction of joint space
   f. Periosteal reaction

3. *Advanced arthritis stage*:
   a. Marked diminution of joint space
   b. Gross destruction and deformation of joint
   c. Osteolytic cavities
   d. Sequestra **(coke-like)**
   e. Posterior dislocation of elbow
   f. Sclerosis, fibrous ankylosis
   g. Periosteal new bone formation

Classification of the radiological findings (Martini 1986)
- *Stage 1.* Localized osteoporosis, but no bony lesion

- *Stage 2.* One or more erosions or cavities in the bone and mild joint space narrowing
- *Stage 3.* Involvement of the entire joint without gross destruction including marked joint space narrowing
- *Stage 4.* Gross destruction

An "ice cream scoop" appearance in the ulnar metaphyseal region in children should raise one's suspicion of tuberculosis.

1. Tuli SM. Tuberculosis of the elbow joint. In: Tuli SM, ed. Tuberculosis of the skeletal system. 3rd ed. New Delhi, India: Jaypee Brothers Medical Publishers (P) Ltd.; 2004:144–52.

2. Chen WS, Wang CJ, Eng HL. Tuberculous arthritis of the elbow. Int Orthop 1997;21:367–70.

3. Aggarwal A, Dhammi I. Clinical and radiological presentation of tuberculosis of the elbow. Acta Orthop Belg 2006;72:282–7.

4. Agarwal A, Mumtaz I, Kumar P, Khan S, Qureshi NA. Tuberculosis of the elbow joint in children: A review of ten patients who were managed nonoperatively. J Bone Joint Surg Am 2010;92:436–41.

5. Wilson JN. Tuberculosis of the elbow; a study of thirty-one cases. J Bone Joint Surg Br 1953;35:551–60.

6. Dix-Peek SI, Vrettos BC, Hoffman EB. Tuberculosis of the elbow in children. J Shoulder Elbow Surg 2003;12:282–6.

7. Vohra R, Kang HS. Tuberculosis of the elbow. A report of 10 cases. Acta Orthop Scand 1995;66:57–8.

10. Dhillon MS, Goel A, Prabhakar S, Aggarwal S, Bachhal V. Tuberculosis of the elbow: A clinicoradiological analysis. Indian J Orthop 2012;46:200–5.

11. Martini M, Benkeddache Y, Medjani Y, Gottesman H. Tuberculosis of the upper limb joints. Int Orthop 1986;10:17–23.

Q. 4. What are the USG/CT/MRI findings of TB elbow in early and advanced disease?

Is there a role for contrast enhancement in CT/MRI?

On **ultrasound**, there are **no pathognomonic findings** of tuberculosis as such. It may also be helpful during aspiration of these effusions for microbiological and histopathological examination and molecular diagnosis (PCR). It may show:

1. Cold abscesses and joint effusions
2. Collections in bursae

3. Synovial hypertrophy
4. Lymphadenopathy

CT scan findings are **non-specific** for elbow tuberculosis. Findings include:

1. Erosions and lytic areas of destruction in the involved bone (geographical extent of lesion can be delineated)
2. Cavitation
3. Narrowing of joint
4. Sequestra(coke-like sequestra)
5. Soft tissue extension can be delineated
6. Contrast enhancement of swollen lymph nodes

CT scan has been used for CT-guided biopsy from lesions. The use of contrast has not been mentioned but uniform enhancement of abscess wall has been reported in other foci of osteoarticular TB.

On MRI, nonspecific features suggestive of TB elbow include:

1. Low signal on T1-weighted images and high signal on T2-weighted images suggestive of marrow edema
2. Regions of necrosis seen as intermediate signal intensity on T2-weighted images
3. Thickening of synovium
4. Tenosynovitis
5. Soft tissue abscesses
6. Intraosseous abscess and cavitation
7. Joint effusion
8. Contrast enhancement of hypertrophic synovium, swollen lymph nodes and abscesses
9. Intraneural tuberculoma occasionally.

23. De Backer AI, Mortelé KJ, Vanhoenacker FM, Parizel PM. Imaging of extraspinal musculoskeletal tuberculosis. Eur J Radiol 2006;57:119–30.

24. De Backer AI, Vanhoenacker FM, Sanghvi DA. Imaging features of extraaxial musculoskeletal tuberculosis. Indian J Radiol Imaging 2009 Jul-Sep;19(3):176–86.

25. Ding YS, Wei TS, Liu SY, Ho SY, Liang WC, Yang CP. Early-stage tuberculous arthritis of the elbow presenting as lateral epicondylitis: diagnosis with sonography. J Ultrasound Med 2008 Feb;27(2):293–7.

2. Chen WS, Wang CJ, Eng HL. Tuberculous arthritis of the elbow. Int Orthop 1997;21:367–70.

12. Asaka T, Takizawa Y, Kariya T, Nitta E, Yasuda T, Fujita M, Sawasaki S, Naiki Y, Nakatani N, Doushita T, Miura T, Ueda F, Takamori M, Matsushima A. Tuberculous tenosynovitis in the elbow joint. Intern Med 1996 Feb;35(2):162–5.

Q. 5. Is there any role of biopsy (open or percutaneous)?

The elbow being a superficial joint, which is easily accessible for aspiration biopsy. Aspiration cytology may be performed from joint effusion, cold abscess, epitrochlear lymph nodes. A core biopsy may be taken from the bony lesion. Open biopsies are rarely required, however, it may be combined with joint debridement.

Q. 6. Is there any role of elbow arthroscopy—assessment/ biopsy/drainage of pus?

Arthroscopic technique can be used, with the advantage of being minimally invasive, to allow direct visualization of joint and hence allow for excision of tubercular synovium, granulation tissue and pannus over cartilage. In view of superficial location of lesion, use of arthroscopic techniques usually is not practiced.

26. Schubert T, Dubuc JE, Barbier O. A review of 24 cases of elbow arthroscopy using the DASH questionnaire. Acta Orthop Belg 2007 Dec;73(6):700–3.

27. Titov AG, Nakonechniy GD, Santavirta S, Serdobintzev MS, Mazurenko SI, Konttinen YT. Arthroscopic operations in joint tuberculosis. Knee 2004 Feb;11(1):57–62.

Q. 7. What is the role of epitrochlear/axillary LN biopsy in establishing diagnosis?

Epitrochlear lymph node biopsy/FNAC has been used to diagnose suspected cases of TB elbow in many studies. Supratrochlear lymph nodes may not be enlarged in all cases, but in cases where they are, the tissue may be taken (by FNAC) is supportive for the diagnoses of TB.

"Supratrochlear and/or axillary lymph nodes were found in 10 out of 48 patients (20.8%). Tuli reported enlarged lymph nodes in

nearly one-third of his patients. Patel found enlarged supratrochlear lymph nodes in nearly all his patients."But series shown by Aggarwal et al. had no patient with enlarged lymph node."

28. Patel DA. The supratrochlear lymph nodes: their diagnostic significance in aswollen elbow joint. Ann R Coll Surg Engl 2001;83:425–6.

17. Crum NF. Tuberculosis presenting as epitrochlear lymphadenitis. Scand J Infect Dis 2003;35(11-12):888–90.

3. Aggarwal A, Dhammi I. Clinical and radiological presentation of tuberculosis of the elbow. Acta Orthop Belg 2006;72:282–7.

4. Agarwal A, Mumtaz I, Kumar P, Khan S, Qureshi NA. Tuberculosis of the elbow joint in children: A review of ten patients who were managed nonoperatively. J Bone Joint Surg Am 2010;92:436–41.

5. Wilson JN. Tuberculosis of the elbow; a study of thirty-one cases. J Bone Joint Surg Br 1953;35:551–60.

6. Dix-Peek SI, Vrettos BC, Hoffman EB. Tuberculosis of the elbow in children. J Shoulder Elbow Surg 2003;12:282–6.

7. Vohra R, Kang HS. Tuberculosis of the elbow. A report of 10 cases. Acta Orthop Scand 1995;66:57–8.

9. Parkinson RW, Hodgson SP, Noble J. Tuberculosis of the elbow: a report of five cases. J Bone Joint Surg Br 1990 May;72(3):523–4.

10. Dhillon MS, Goel A, Prabhakar S, Aggarwal S, Bachhal V. Tuberculosis of the elbow: A clinicoradiological analysis. Indian J Orthop 2012;46:200–5.

Q. 8. What are the differential diagnoses and when can the patient be started on ATT?

The differential diagnosis in patients with elbow involvement should include pyogenic arthritis, gout, pigmented villonodular synovitis, haemophilic arthropathy, rheumatoid arthritis, synovial osteochondromatosis and neoplasm.

The diagnosis is established on the following criteria:

1. Clinical and hematological parameters (raised ESR, relative lymphocytosis and monocytosis)
2. Radiological evidence (as above)
3. Imaging evidence (as above)
4. Needle/CT-guided/USG guided/open biopsy
5. Microbiological—smear for AFB/culture/BACTEC
6. Molecular—PCR/GeneXpert

In early disease in the stage of synovitis, when clinico-radiological evidence is nonspecific, a tissue biopsy is required to establish a diagnosis. In an endemic region with classical clinicoradiological diagnosis of arthritis/advances arthritis, the ATT may be initiated. It is almost always possible to ascertain diagnosis in a tubercular elbow by cytology/biopsy, as elbow is a superficial joint. However, wherever possible tissue should be procured by needle biopsy/aspiration and sent for histopathological, microbiological and molecular tests for confirmation.

3. Aggarwal A, Dhammi I. Clinical and radiological presentation of tuberculosis of the elbow. Acta Orthop Belg 2006;72:282–7.

4. Agarwal A, Mumtaz I, Kumar P, Khan S, Qureshi NA. Tuberculosis of the elbow joint in children: A review of ten patients who were managed nonoperatively. J Bone Joint Surg Am 2010;92:436–41.

5. Wilson JN. Tuberculosis of the elbow; a study of thirty-one cases. J Bone Joint Surg Br 1953;35:551–60.

6. Dix-Peek SI, Vrettos BC, Hoffman EB. Tuberculosis of the elbow in children. J Shoulder Elbow Surg 2003;12:282–6.

7. Vohra R, Kang HS. Tuberculosis of the elbow. A report of 10 cases. Acta Orthop Scand 1995;66:57–8.

9. Parkinson RW, Hodgson SP, Noble J. Tuberculosis of the elbow: a report of five cases. J Bone Joint Surg Br 1990 May;72(3):523–4.

10. Dhillon MS, Goel A, Prabhakar S, Aggarwal S, Bachhal V. Tuberculosis of the elbow: A clinicoradiological analysis. Indian J Orthop 2012;46:200–5.

Q. 9. What is the end point of treatment? Which are the definitive markers of healing/response—X-ray/CT/MRI/PET?

Studies have reported a variable treatment duration ranging from 9 to 18 months. No definitive cardinal signs of healing have been reported. The following markers can be taken as supportive evidence.

1. Healing of sinuses
2. Resolution of swelling, tenderness
3. Normalization of ESR
4. On X-ray, remineralization of bone and sharpening of articular margins.

5. On MRI, resolution of abscesses, resolution of marrow edema and low signal intensity in STIR images (fatty replacement of diseased area on T1WI and T2 WI).

6. On PET, no uptake of 18F-FDG in the lesion (data on PET is still under evolution).

Q. 10. What splintage is to be given and for how long? When to go for mobilization and CPM? Role of functional cast brace?

The elbow needs to be splinted with an above elbow plaster slab for 4–8 weeks to alleviate pain and spasm and give rest to the joint. After the pain subsides with ATT, elbow should be mobilized with gradual CPM along with cast brace at night time or during rest. Alternatively, an appropriate hinged brace can also be used. The brace should continue for 3–9 months during rest periods.

29. Dahl CS. Physical therapist management of tuberculous arthritis of the elbow. Phys Ther 2001 Jun;81(6):1253–9.

10. Dhillon MS, Goel A, Prabhakar S, Aggarwal S, Bachhal V. Tuberculosis of the elbow: A clinicoradiological analysis. Indian J Orthop 2012;46:200–5.

3. Aggarwal A, Dhammi I. Clinical and radiological presentation of tuberculosis of the elbow. Acta Orthop Belg 2006;72:282–7.

4. Agarwal A, Mumtaz I, Kumar P, Khan S, Qureshi NA. Tuberculosis of the elbow joint in children: A review of ten patients who were managed nonoperatively. J Bone Joint Surg Am 2010;92:436–41.

5. Wilson JN. Tuberculosis of the elbow; a study of thirty-one cases. J Bone Joint Surg Br 1953;35:551–60.

6. Dix-Peek SI, Vrettos BC, Hoffman EB. Tuberculosis of the elbow in children. J Shoulder Elbow Surg 2003;12:282–6.

7. Vohra R, Kang HS. Tuberculosis of the elbow. A report of 10 cases. Acta Orthop Scand 1995;66:57–8.

9. Parkinson RW, Hodgson SP, Noble J. Tuberculosis of the elbow: A report of five cases. J Bone Joint Surg Br 1990 May;72(3):523–4.

1. Tuli SM. Tuberculosis of the elbow joint. In: Tuli SM, ed. Tuberculosis of the skeletal system. 3rd ed. New Delhi, India: Jaypee Brothers Medical Publishers (P) Ltd.; 2004:144–52.

Q. 11. What are the indications for surgery in tuberculosis of elbow—synovectomy, debridement, arthrotomy?

Nonoperative treatment with ATT (2 IIRZE । 10 HRE) for at least 12 months (may be up to 18 months), rest to the joint in functional position (using plaster or brace for 6–8 weeks) and gentle mobilization thereafter, as tolerated, should be instituted as first-line treatment in all cases. A majority of patients heal with good functional outcome. Surgery is rarely indicated.

Indications for surgery include:
1. To obtain tissue for diagnosis when ATT is started based on clinicoradiological diagnosis and patient fails to show adequate clinicoradiological response.
2. To obtain tissue for drug sensitivity testing when drug resistance is suspected and the response to ATT is suboptimal.
3. Drainage of large abscess (arthrotomy and joint lavage).
4. Joint debridement (synovectomy, removal of loose bodies, rice bodies and pannus).
5. Juxta-articular lesion (impending joint involvement).
6. Expanding lesion.
7. Nerve entrapment.
8. Impending collapse of bone.
9. Arthrodesis in a healed tubercular elbow with painful fibrous ankylosis.
10. Correction of deformity in healed elbow.

Indications for tissue diagnosis are:
1. To establish a definitive diagnosis when clinicoradiological picture is ambiguous especially when a patient is from a non-endemic region.
2. To establish a diagnosis when ATT is started on clinicoradiological diagnosis (presumptive TB elbow) but shows no improvement in signs/symptoms despite ATT taken for 30–45 days.
3. To rule out malignancy, when suspected.
4. To obtain tissue for culture and drug sensitivity testing when the response to ATT is suboptimal and drug resistance is suspected.

3. Aggarwal A, Dhammi I. Clinical and radiological presentation of tuberculosis of the elbow. Acta Orthop Belg 2006;72:282–7.

4. Agarwal A, Mumtaz I, Kumar P, Khan S, Qureshi NA. Tuberculosis of the elbow joint in children: A review of ten patients who were managed nonoperatively. J Bone Joint Surg Am 2010;92:436–41.

5. Wilson JN. Tuberculosis of the elbow; a study of thirty-one cases. J Bone Joint Surg Br 1953;35:551–60.

6. Dix-Peek SI, Vrettos BC, Hoffman EB. Tuberculosis of the elbow in children. J Shoulder Elbow Surg 2003;12:282–6.

7. Vohra R, Kang HS. Tuberculosis of the elbow. A report of 10 cases. Acta Orthop Scand 1995;66:57–8.

9. Parkinson RW, Hodgson SP, Noble J. Tuberculosis of the elbow: a report of five cases. J Bone Joint Surg Br 1990 May;72(3):523–4.

10. Dhillon MS, Goel A, Prabhakar S, Aggarwal S, Bachhal V. Tuberculosis of the elbow: A clinicoradiological analysis. Indian J Orthop 2012;46:200–5.

Ref 4: *"Antitubercular chemotherapy is highly effective for the treatment of elbow tuberculosis in children and obviated the need for surgical synovectomy in the present series. There is no osseous barrier or gradient to the penetration of antitubercular drugs. Previous studies have shown similar results in association with nonoperative treatment when compared with surgical synovectomy and debridement. Wilson excised a focal lesion in the medial epicondyle in one case and performed arthrodesis of the elbow in three other cases. However, he reported that excision of the focus was unnecessary and that the lesion could well be treated nonoperatively. Vohra and Kang reported on a series of ten cases of elbow tuberculosis in adults who were managed non-operatively with antitubercular medication without a hospital stay. Generally, the extra-articular lesions have a good prognosis and that the result of treatment of intra-articular lesions depends on the amount of involvement of the joint."*

Q. 12. What is the role of elbow arthrodesis, resection/ interposition arthroplasty?

Excisional/interposition arthroplasty is indicated after completion of growth potential. After excisional arthroplasty, the elbow may be relatively mobile and stable. However, a PVC orthosis may be required, if unstable or for overhead work.

1. When elbow heals in an unsound position
2. When there is painful fibrous ankylosis

3. Patient desires a mobile elbow

4. As a precursor first stage when a 2-stage total elbow arthroplasty is contemplated in a healed disease.

Elbow arthrodesis is rarely indicated. It is considered for patients who desires a stable elbow for heavy manual labor.

30. Todd TW.IX. The end result of excision of the elbow for tuberculosis. Ann Surg 1913 Mar;57(3):430–3.

31. De Amezaga G.XIII. Tuberculosis of the elbow, arthroplasty. Ann Surg 1907 Oct;46(4):617–622.5.

32. Bao YC, Li YL, Ning GZ, Wu Q, Feng SQ. Forked osteotomy arthroplasty for elbow tuberculosis: six years of follow-up. Eur J Orthop Surg Traumatol 2014 Aug;24(6):857–62.

33. Asopa V, Wallace AL. Case report: Management of occult tuberculosis infection by 2-stage arthroplasty of the elbow. J Shoulder Elbow Surg 2004 May-Jun;13(3):364–5.

 1. Tuli SM. Tuberculosis of the elbow joint. In: Tuli SM, ed. Tuberculosis of the skeletal system. 3rd ed. New Delhi, India: Jaypee Brothers Medical Publishers (P) Ltd.; 2004:144–52.

Q. 13. What is the role of total elbow arthroplasty in active disease/healed disease?

There is only one report in recent literature mentioning the use of replacement arthroplasty for TB elbow. Large scale studies are needed to generate a recommendation. There is no report of replacement of arthroplasty for healed tuberculosis with painful fibrous ankylosis of elbow.

Asopa et al managed a patient who had previously undergone total elbow arthroplasty for severe osteoarthritis and was later diagnosed with an occult tubercular infection with a 2-stage arthroplasty which involved removal of implant, ATT for 6 months and revision elbow arthroplasty after one year of implant removal. Patient had no recurrence at 6-month follow-up.

33. Asopa V, Wallace AL. Case report: Management of occult tuberculosis infection by 2-stage arthroplasty of the elbow. J Shoulder Elbow Surg 2004 May-Jun;13(3):364–5.

Q. 14. How to prognosticate the outcome in a case of TB elbow?

There is usually a favorable response to ATT. The disease heals with good functional outcome, if treatment is started in synovitis or early arthritis stage. The functional outcome is poor in cases which present in or progresses to advanced arthritis and excision/fusion procedure may be necessary to obtain a painless joint.

3. Aggarwal A, Dhammi I. Clinical and radiological presentation of tuberculosis of the elbow. Acta Orthop Belg 2006;72:282–7.

4. Agarwal A, Mumtaz I, Kumar P, Khan S, Qureshi NA. Tuberculosis of the elbow joint in children: A review of ten patients who were managed nonoperatively. J Bone Joint Surg Am 2010;92:436–41.

5. Wilson JN. Tuberculosis of the elbow; a study of thirty-one cases. J Bone Joint Surg Br 1953;35:551–60.

6. Dix-Peek SI, Vrettos BC, Hoffman EB. Tuberculosis of the elbow in children. J Shoulder Elbow Surg 2003;12:282–6.

7. Vohra R, Kang HS. Tuberculosis of the elbow. A report of 10 cases. Acta Orthop Scand 1995;66:57–8.

9. Parkinson RW, Hodgson SP, Noble J. Tuberculosis of the elbow: a report of five cases. J Bone Joint Surg Br 1990 May;72(3):523–4.

10. Dhillon MS, Goel A, Prabhakar S, Aggarwal S, Bachhal V. Tuberculosis of the elbow: A clinicoradiological analysis. Indian J Orthop 2012;46:200–5.

Ref 10: *"The mainstay of treatments is uninterrupted multidrug antituberculous chemotherapy, splinting, and active mobilization once pain and spasm subside. Surgical synovectomy, curettage of periarticular erosions and joint debridement are not always necessary. Conservative treatment leads to satisfactory results in a large majority of cases, with retention of a good range of motion."*

"Debridement, curettage and arthrolysis, followed by vigorous physiotherapy, are essential to achieve a better range of movement."

HAND AND WRIST

Q. 1. What is the clinical presentation of TB wrist? What is the clinical presentation of TB dactylitis (TB hand)/TB tenosynovitis? What is the common age of presentation of TB dactylitis?

Tuberculosis of wrist and hand can affect any age although tubercular dactylitis is more commonly seen in children less than 5 years of age. The disease can present as synovitis, tenosynovitis, osteitis, arthritis, bursitis, carpal tunnel syndrome, non-healing ulcers (botryomycosis like picture) and paronychia.

The patients present with in **early disease**:
1. Pain (occasionally painless)
2. Swelling (warm, red, swollen tender joint)
3. Synovial thickening (doughy/boggy on palpation)
4. Joint effusion
5. Fever (low grade, evening rise of temperature, night sweats)
6. Regional lymphadenopathy (supratrochlear and/or axillary)
7. Weight loss, anorexia may occur.
8. Restricted range of motion
9. Rarely, median nerve palsy (carpal tunnel syndrome)
10. Rarely, paronychia, nail dystrophy

In **advanced disease**, in addition to the above:
1. Wasting of forearm muscles, thenar and hypothenar eminences are found.
2. Deformity (ranges from dorsiflexion/volar flexion deformity of wrist/MCP/interphalangeal joints to pathological subluxation or dislocation or fractures) may occur.
3. Enlargement of digit (sausage finger)/metacarpal (spina ventosa) is other presentation.
4. Discharging sinuses
5. Cold abscess, compound palmar ganglion are the other presentations.
   There is usually delay in the diagnosis of hand tuberculosis, which frequently leads to more morbidity and a worse outcome.

1. Tuli SM. Tuberculosis of the wrist. In: Tuli SM, ed. Tuberculosis of the skeletal system. 3rd ed. New Delhi, India: Jaypee Brothers Medical Publishers (P) Ltd.; 2004:153–58.

2. Tuli SM. Tuberculosis of short tubular bones. In: Tuli SM, ed. Tuberculosis of the skeletal system. 3rd ed. New Delhi, India: Jaypee Brothers Medical Publishers (P) Ltd.; 2004:159–61.

3. Al-Qattan MM, Al-Namla A, Al-Thunayan A, Al-Omawi M. Tuberculosis of the hand. J Hand Surg Am 2011 Aug;36(8):1413–21; quiz 1422.

4. Al-Qattan MM, Helmi AA. Chronic hand infections. J Hand Surg Am 2014 Aug;39(8):1636–45.

5. Subasi M, Bukte Y, Kapukaya A, Gurkan F. Tuberculosis of the metacarpals and phalanges of the hand. Ann Plast Surg 2004 Nov;53(5):469–72.

6. Kotwal PP, Khan SA.Tuberculosis of the hand: clinical presentation and functional outcome in 32 patients. J Bone Joint Surg Br 2009 Aug;91(8):1054–7.

7. Agarwal A, Qureshi NA, Kumar P, Khan S. Tubercular osteomyelitis of metacarpals and phalanges in children. Hand Surg 2011;16(1):19–27.

8. Tsai MS, Liu JW, Chen WS, de Villa VH. Tuberculous wrist in the era of effective chemotherapy: an eleven-year experience. Int J Tuberc Lung Dis 2003 Jul;7(7):690–4.

9. Leung PC. Tuberculosis of the hand. Hand 1978 Oct;10(3):285–91.

10. Lau JH, Chow SP, Stroebel AB, Collins RJ. Mycobacterial infection of the hand: clinical features and functional results. Hand 1983 Jun;15(2):192–200.

11. Al-Qattan MM, Bowen V, Manktelow RT. Tuberculosis of the hand. J Hand Surg Br 1994 Apr;19(2):234–7.

12. Regnard PJ, Barry P, Isselin J. Mycobacterial tenosynovitis of the flexor tendons of the hand. A report of five cases. J Hand Surg Br 1996 Jun;21(3):351–4.

13. Agarwal A, Khan SA, Qureshi NA. Multifocal osteoarticular tuberculosis in children. J Orthop Surg (Hong Kong) 2011 Dec;19(3):336–40.

14. Agarwal A, Kant KS, Kumar A, Shaharyar A, Verma I, Suri T. Lytic lesions of distal radius in children: a rare tubercular presentation. Hand Surg 2014;19(3):369–74.

15. Sreekanth R, Pallapati SC, Thomas BP. Tuberculous botryomycosis of the hand: case report. J Hand Surg Am 2014 Sep;39(9):1810–2.

16. Krapohl BD, Kömürcü F, Stöckl-Hiesleitner S, Deutinger M. Flexor tendon synovitis of the hand as first manifestation of atypical tuberculosis. Acta Orthop Belg 2007 Feb;73(1):111–3.

17. Woon CY, Phoon ES, Lee JY, Puhaindran ME, Peng YP, Teoh LC.Rice bodies, millet seeds, and melon seeds in tuberculous tenosynovitis of the hand and wrist. Ann Plast Surg 2011 Jun;66(6):610–7.

18. Ebrahimzadeh MH, Jupiter JB. Isolated tuberculosis of a metacarpal bone in a 2-year-old child. J Hand Surg Eur Vol 2007 Feb;32(1):109.

19. Khanna D, Chakravarty P, Agarwal A, Gupta R. Tuberculous dactylitis presenting as paronychia with pseudopterygium and nail dystrophy. Pediatr Dermatol 2013 Nov-Dec;30(6):e172–6.

20. Kang HJ, Jung SH, Yoon HK, Hahn SB, Kim SJ. Carpal tunnel syndrome caused by space occupying lesions. Yonsei Med J 2009 Apr 30;50(2):257–61.

21. Ritz N, Connell TG, Tebruegge M, Johnstone BR, Curtis N. Tuberculous dactylitis—an easily missed diagnosis. Eur J Clin Microbiol Infect Dis 2011 Nov;30(11):1303–10.

22. Martini M, Benkeddache Y, Medjani Y, Gottesman H. Tuberculosis of the upper limb joints. Int Orthop 1986;10:17–23.

Q. 2. What is the predominant manifestation of TB wrist/ hand?

Exudative manifestation is more common. Tubercular dactylitis often presents as ballooning of metacarpals (spina ventosa) and phalanges (sausage fingers) in tuberculosis.

3. Al-Qattan MM, Al-Namla A, Al-Thunayan A, Al-Omawi M. Tuberculosis of the hand. J Hand Surg Am 2011 Aug;36(8):1413–21; quiz 1422.

4. Al-Qattan MM, Helmi AA. Chronic hand infections. J Hand Surg Am 2014 Aug;39(8):1636–45.

5. Subasi M, Bukte Y, Kapukaya A, Gurkan F. Tuberculosis of the metacarpals and phalanges of the hand. Ann Plast Surg 2004 Nov;53(5):469–72.

6. Kotwal PP, Khan SA. Tuberculosis of the hand: clinical presentation and functional outcome in 32 patients. J Bone Joint Surg Br 2009 Aug;91(8):1054–7.

7. Agarwal A, Qureshi NA, Kumar P, Khan S. Tubercular osteomyelitis of metacarpals and phalanges in children. Hand Surg 2011;16(1): 19–27.

8. Tsai MS, Liu JW, Chen WS, de Villa VH. Tuberculous wrist in the era of effective chemotherapy: an eleven-year experience. Int J Tuberc Lung Dis 2003 Jul;7(7):690–4.

9. Leung PC. Tuberculosis of the hand. Hand 1978 Oct;10(3):285-91.

10. Lau JH, Chow SP, Stroebel AB, Collins RJ. Mycobacterial infection of the hand: clinical features and functional results. Hand 1983 Jun;15(2):192–200.

11. Al-Qattan MM, Bowen V, Manktelow RT. Tuberculosis of the hand. J Hand Surg Br 1994 Apr;19(2):234–7.

12. Regnard PJ, Barry P, Isselin J. Mycobacterial tenosynovitis of the flexor tendons of the hand. A report of five cases. J Hand Surg Br 1996 Jun;21(3):351–4.

13. Agarwal A, Khan SA, Qureshi NA. Multifocal osteoarticular tuber-culosis in children. J Orthop Surg (Hong Kong). 2011 Dec;19(3):336–40.

14. Agarwal A, Kant KS, Kumar A, Shaharyar A, Verma I, Suri T. Lytic lesions of distal radius in children: a rare tubercular presentation. Hand Surg 2014;19(3):369–74.

Q. 3. What are the findings on plain X-ray in early and advanced disease?

Plain radiographs may not show any findings in very early stage of the disease. However, it may show in:

1. *Synovitis stage*:
  a. Regional osteoporosis
  b. Increased soft tissue shadow (due to synovial hypertrophy, effusion)

2. *Early arthritis stage*:
  a. Loss of definition of articular surfaces
  b. Marginal erosions
  c. Enlargement of epiphysis in children
  d. Ballooning of cortex of metacarpals **(spina ventosa)**
  e. Diminution of joint space
  f. Destruction of joint space
  h. Periosteal reaction

3. *Advanced arthritis stage*:
  a. Marked diminution of joint space
  b. Gross destruction and deformation of joint
  c. Osteolytic cavities*
  d. Sequestra [**coke-like**]
  e. Sclerosis, fibrous ankylosis

f. Soft tissue calcific foci (**periosteal new bone formation**)

g. Honey-combing in shafts of metacarpals and phalanges

*Patterns of osteolysis seen in tuberculosis of hand (Al-Qattan 2011) are described as:

1. *Geographic well-defined cyst* similar to simple bone cyst

2. *Honeycomb pattern* similar to giant cell tumor

3. *Mixed lytic-sclerotic pattern* similar to Ewing's sarcoma, chronic fungal infections

4. *Diaphyseal lytic lesion extending into the epiphysis* seen in children

5. Spina ventosa lesion. (It is seen as massive spindle-shaped expansion of phalanx or metacarpal. (Latin: spina is "short bone," and ventosa is "filled with air").

   In children, it is associated with subperiosteal hyperplasia.

6. *Osteolysis pattern similar to chronic bacterial osteomyelitis* with a sclerotic rim and sinuses.

Classification of the radiological findings (Martini 1986)

- *Stage 1.* Localized osteoporosis, but no bony lesion

- *Stage 2.* One or more erosions or cavities in the bone and mild joint space narrowing

- *Stage 3.* Involvement of the entire joint without gross destruction including marked joint space narrowing

- *Stage 4.* Gross destruction

3. Al-Qattan MM, Al-Namla A, Al-Thunayan A, Al-Omawi M. Tuberculosis of the hand. J Hand Surg Am 2011 Aug;36(8):1413–21.

23. Sunderamoorthy D1, Gupta V, Bleetman A. TB or not TB: an unusual sore finger. Emerg Med J 2001 Nov;18(6):490–1.

9. Leung PC. Tuberculosis of the hand. Hand 1978 Oct;10(3):285–91.

24. Hsu CY, Lu HC, Shih TT. Tuberculous infection of the wrist: MRI features. AJR Am J Roentgenol 2004 Sep;183(3):623–8.

25. Jaovisidha S, Chen C, Ryu KN, Siriwongpairat P, Pekanan P, Sartoris DJ, Resnick D. Tuberculous tenosynovitis and bursitis: imaging findings in 21 cases. Radiology 1996 Nov;201(2):507–13.

26. De Backer AI, Mortelé KJ, Vanhoenacker FM, Parizel PM. Imaging of extraspinal musculoskeletal tuberculosis. Eur J Radiol 2006;57:119–30.

27. De Backer AI, Vanhoenacker FM, Sanghvi DA. Imaging features of extraaxial musculoskeletal tuberculosis. Indian J Radiol Imaging 2009 Jul-Sep;19(3):176–86.

"The diagnosis should always be considered in cases of unexplained swelling of a finger or toe—particularly in those at a higher risk of having tuberculosis. The radiological changes may be grouped in four broad categories:

- *Soft tissue swelling, which is often marked and fusiform with no apparent change in neighboring bones or joints.*
- *The earliest evidence of bony involvement is periosteitis indicated by linear deposition of new bone with increasing cortical thickness and involucrum formation. Gradual destruction with sequestration of the bone then occurs while the involucrum thickens. If much of the involucrum's internal aspect is absorbed a cyst-like cavity remains, which appears to ballooned out or injected with air, the so-called spina ventousa.*
- *Diffuse uniform infiltration's with "honeycombing"—The affected phalanx may show minimal or moderate expansion and appear infiltrated throughout with honeycombed or lace-like appearance.*
- *Localized destruction with reactive osteitis—the phalanx shows small areas of cortical or cancellous destruction with no apparent change in the other parts of the bone. Diaphyseal sequestration and pathological fractures can also occur."*

Q. 4. What are the USG/CT/MRI findings of TB wrist/hand in early and advanced disease?

Is there a role for contrast enhancement in CT/MRI?

On **ultrasound**, there are **no pathognomonic findings** as such. It may also be helpful during aspiration of these effusions for microbiological and histopathological examination and molecular diagnosis. It may show:

1. Cold abscesses and joint effusions
2. Collections in bursae (compound palmar ganglion)
3. Hyperechoic contents in cystic masses or rice bodies.
4. Synovial hypertrophy
5. Lymphadenopathy

   CT scan may be performed for TB of wrist. The findings are **non-specific** which include:

1. Erosions and lytic areas of destruction in the involved bone (geographical extent of lesion can be delineated).
2. Cavitation.
3. Narrowing of joint.
4. Sequestra.

5. Soft tissue extension can be delineated.
6. Contrast enhancement of swollen lymph nodes.

CT scan has been used for CT-guided biopsy from lesions. Contrast-enhanced radiographic studies (i.e. arthrography, tenography, or bursography) have been used and are useful in the detection of communication between the diseased tendon sheaths or bursae and adjacent organs and in verification of the extent of infection.

On MRI, nonspecific features suggestive of TB include:

1. Low signal on T1-weighted images and high signal on T2-weighted images suggestive of marrow edema.
2. Regions of necrosis seen as intermediate signal intensity on T2-weighted images.
3. Thickening of synovium.
4. Tenosynovitis with fluid seen within the tendon sheath.
5. Rice bodies, millet seeds, and melon seeds represented by multiple nodules or small, low-signal dots scattered in the synovial fluid on T2WI.
6. Encasement of median nerve.
7. Soft tissue abscesses.
8. Intraosseous abscess and cavitation.
9. Joint effusion.
10. Contrast enhancement of hypertrophic synovium, swollen lymph nodes and abscesses.

17. Woon CY, Phoon ES, Lee JY, Puhaindran ME, Peng YP, Teoh LC. Rice bodies, millet seeds, and melon seeds in tuberculous tenosynovitis of the hand and wrist. Ann Plast Surg 2011 Jun;66(6):610–7.

24. Hsu CY, Lu HC, Shih TT.Tuberculous infection of the wrist: MRI features. AJR Am J Roentgenol 2004 Sep;183(3):623–8.

25. Jaovisidha S, Chen C, Ryu KN, Siriwongpairat P, Pekanan P, Sartoris DJ, Resnick D. Tuberculous tenosynovitis and bursitis: imaging findings in 21 cases. Radiology 1996 Nov;201(2):507–13.

26. De Backer AI, Mortelé KJ, Vanhoenacker FM, Parizel PM. Imaging of extraspinal musculoskeletal tuberculosis. Eur J Radiol 2006;57: 119–30.

27. De Backer AI, Vanhoenacker FM, Sanghvi DA. Imaging features of extraaxial musculoskeletal tuberculosis. Indian J Radiol Imaging 2009 Jul-Sep;19(3):176–86.

"The diagnosis of tuberculous infection of the wrist should be considered when T2 low-signal synovial thickening around the flexor and extensor tendons is present and the synovial fluid collection contains low-signal and nonenhanced foci in the tendon sheath. In addition, bone erosion, osteomyelitis, and median nerve encasement are also frequently present."

Q. 5. Is there any role of wrist arthroscopy—assessment/biopsy/drainage of pus?

Arthroscopic technique can offer the advantage of direct visualization of joint and hence allow for excision of tubercular synovium, granulation tissue and pannus over cartilage, but should be done only by experienced surgeon. A good open biopsy is preferred over bad arthroscopic biopsy.

6. Kotwal PP, Khan SA. Tuberculosis of the hand: clinical presentation and functional outcome in 32 patients. J Bone Joint Surg Br 2009 Aug;91(8):1054–7.

Q. 6. What is the role of epitrochlear/axillary LN biopsy in establishing diagnosis?

Epitrochlear lymph node biopsy/FNAC has been used to diagnose suspected cases of TB in many studies. Supratrochlear lymph nodes may not be enlarged in all cases, but in cases where they are, the tissue taken is diagnostic for TB.

28. Patel DA. The supratrochlear lymph nodes: their diagnostic significance in a swollen elbow joint. Ann R Coll Surg Engl 2001; 83:425–6.

7. Agarwal A, Qureshi NA, Kumar P, Khan S. Tubercular osteomyelitis of metacarpals and phalanges in children. Hand Surg 2011;16(1): 19–27.

13. Agarwal A, Khan SA, Qureshi NA. Multifocal osteoarticular tuberculosis in children. J Orthop Surg (Hong Kong) 2011 Dec;19(3):336–40.

Q. 7. When to start treatment and what is the duration of treatment?

The differential diagnosis in patients with wrist and hand involvement should include pyogenic arthritis, fungal arthritis, gout, pigmented villonodular synovitis, hemophilic arthropathy, rheumatoid arthritis, deQuervain's tenosynovitis, sarcoidosis, sickle cell disease, synovial osteochondromatosis and neoplasm (enchondroma, giant cell tumor, Ewing's sarcoma, chondroblastoma).

The diagnosis is established on the following criteria:
1. Clinical and hematological parameters (raised ESR, relative lymphocytosis and monocytosis)
2. Radiological evidence (as above)
3. Imaging evidence (as above)
4. Needle/CT-guided/USG guided/arthroscopic/open biopsy
   a. Microbiological—Smear for AFB/culture/BACTEC
   b. Molecular—PCR/GeneXpert/Line Probe Assay
   c Histopathological examination

In early disease in the stage of synovitis, when clinico-radiological evidence is nonspecific, a tissue biopsy is needed to establish a diagnosis.

In a region where facilities are lacking in, a patient coming from an endemic region with classical clinicoradiological evidence of advanced arthritis can be diagnosed on the same and ATT can be instituted.

However, wherever possible tissue should be procured by needle biopsy/aspiration and sent for histopathological, microbiological and molecular tests for confirmation. The duration of TB wrist and hand is variable as describe in literature (from 9 to 18 months). It is recommended to prescribe ATT (2 HZRE + 10 HRE) which may be extended to 18 months depending on case-to-case basis.

3. Al-Qattan MM, Al-Namla A, Al-Thunayan A, Al-Omawi M. Tuberculosis of the hand. J Hand Surg Am 2011 Aug;36(8):1413–21; quiz 1422.

4. Al-Qattan MM, Helmi AA.Chronic hand infections. J Hand Surg Am 2014 Aug;39(8):1636–45.

5. Subasi M, Bukte Y, Kapukaya A, Gurkan F. Tuberculosis of the metacarpals and phalanges of the hand. Ann Plast Surg 2004 Nov;53(5):469–72.

6. Kotwal PP, Khan SA. Tuberculosis of the hand: clinical presentation and functional outcome in 32 patients. J Bone Joint Surg Br 2009 Aug;91(8):1054–7.

7. Agarwal A, Qureshi NA, Kumar P, Khan S. Tubercular osteomyelitis of metacarpals and phalanges in children. Hand Surg 2011;16(1): 19–27.

8. Tsai MS, Liu JW, Chen WS, de Villa VH. Tuberculous wrist in the era of effective chemotherapy: an eleven-year experience. Int J Tuberc Lung Dis 2003 Jul;7(7):690–4.

9. Leung PC. Tuberculosis of the hand. Hand 1978 Oct;10(3):285–91.

10. Lau JH, Chow SP, Stroebel AB, Collins RJ. Mycobacterial infection of the hand: clinical features and functional results. Hand 1983 Jun;15(2):192–200.

11. Al-Qattan MM, Bowen V, Manktelow RT. Tuberculosis of the hand. J Hand Surg Br 1994 Apr;19(2):234–7.

12. Regnard PJ, Barry P, Isselin J. Mycobacterial tenosynovitis of the flexor tendons of the hand. A report of five cases. J Hand Surg Br 1996 Jun;21(3):351–4.

13. Agarwal A, Khan SA, Qureshi NA. Multifocal osteoarticular tuberculosis in children. J Orthop Surg (Hong Kong) 2011 Dec;19(3):336–40.

14. Agarwal A, Kant KS, Kumar A, Shaharyar A, Verma I, Suri T. Lytic lesions of distal radius in children: a rare tubercular presentation. Hand Surg 2014;19(3):369–74.

Q. 8. What is the end point of treatment? Which is the definitive marker of healing—X-ray/CT/MRI/PET?

Various studies have reported a treatment duration ranging from 9 to 18 months. No definitive cardinal signs of healing have been reported. But for clinical use, markers of healing are same as all other joints.

The following markers can be taken as supportive evidence of a responding/healing lesion.

1. Healing of sinuses
2. Resolution of swelling, tenderness
3. Normalization of ESR
4. On X-ray, remineralization of bone, sharpening of articular margins
5. On MRI, resolution of abscesses, resolution of marrow edema, low signal intensity in STIR images
6. On PET, no uptake of 18F-FDG in the lesion (data is evolving).

Q. 9. What splintage is to be given and for how long?

The wrist needs to be splinted with an above elbow plaster slab with the wrist in 15° dorsiflexion and forearm in midprone position for 2–4 weeks to alleviate pain and spasm and give rest to the joint. After the pain subsides with ATT, wrist should be mobilized with gradual continuous passive motion (CPM), cast brace or appropriate hinged brace. The brace should be worn in between mobilization for 18 months to prevent collapse of small bones of the wrist.

A scaphoid cast for 6–8 weeks is indicated, if the first carpometacarpal, metacarpophalangeal, interphalangeal joints are involved or the first metacarpal, trapezium are involved.

1. Tuli SM. Tuberculosis of the wrist. In: Tuli SM, ed. Tuberculosis of the skeletal system. 3rd ed. New Delhi, India: Jaypee Brothers Medical Publishers (P) Ltd.; 2004:153–58.

2. Tuli SM. Tuberculosis of short tubular bones. In: Tuli SM, ed. Tuberculosis of the skeletal system. 3rd ed. New Delhi, India: Jaypee Brothers Medical Publishers (P) Ltd.; 2004:159–61.

3. Al-Qattan MM, Al-Namla A, Al-Thunayan A, Al-Omawi M. Tuberculosis of the hand. J Hand Surg Am 2011 Aug;36(8):1413–21; quiz 1422.

7. Agarwal A, Qureshi NA, Kumar P, Khan S. Tubercular osteomyelitis of metacarpals and phalanges in children. Hand Surg 2011;16(1): 19–27.

Q. 10. What are the indications for surgery in tuberculosis of wrist and hand?

Nonoperative treatment with ATT (2 HRZE and 10 HRE) for at least 12 months (may be 18 months), rest to the joint in functional position (using plaster or brace for 6–8 weeks) and gentle mobilization thereafter, as tolerated, should be instituted as first-line treatment in all cases. A majority of patients heal with good functional outcome. Surgery is rarely indicated.

Indications for surgery include:

1. Expanding lesion
2. Nerve entrapment (carpal tunnel release and debridement)
3. Impending collapse of bone

4. Drainage of large abscess (arthrotomy and joint lavage)
5. Joint debridement (synovectomy, removal of loose bodies, rice bodies and pannus)
6. To obtain tissue for diagnosis when ATT started based on clinicoradiological diagnosis fails to show clinicoradiological response
7. To obtain tissue for drug sensitivity testing when drug resistance is suspected and the response to ATT is suboptimal (failure of conservative treatment)
8. Correction of deformity in healed disease
9. Arthrodesis in a healed tubercular wrist with painful fibrous ankylosis.

Indications for tissue diagnosis are:

1. To establish a definitive diagnosis when clinicoradiological picture is ambiguous especially when a patient is from a non-endemic region.
2. To establish a diagnosis when ATT given on clinico-radiological diagnosis for 30 to 45 days shows no improvement in signs/symptoms.
3. To rule out malignancy when suspected (diagnostic dilemma).
4. To obtain tissue for culture and drug sensitivity testing when the response to ATT is suboptimal.

3. Al-Qattan MM, Al-Namla A, Al-Thunayan A, Al-Omawi M. Tuberculosis of the hand. J Hand Surg Am 2011 Aug;36(8):1413–21; quiz 1422.

4. Al-Qattan MM, Helmi AA. Chronic hand infections. J Hand Surg Am 2014 Aug;39(8):1636–45.

5. Subasi M, Bukte Y, Kapukaya A, Gurkan F. Tuberculosis of the metacarpals and phalanges of the hand. Ann Plast Surg 2004 Nov;53(5):469–72.

6. Kotwal PP, Khan SA. Tuberculosis of the hand: clinical presentation and functional outcome in 32 patients. J Bone Joint Surg Br 2009 Aug;91(8):1054–7.

7. Agarwal A, Qureshi NA, Kumar P, Khan S. Tubercular osteomyelitis of metacarpals and phalanges in children. Hand Surg 2011;16(1): 19–27.

8. Tsai MS, Liu JW, Chen WS, de Villa VH. Tuberculous wrist in the era of effective chemotherapy: an eleven-year experience. Int J Tuberc Lung Dis 2003 Jul;7(7):690–4.

9. Leung PC. Tuberculosis of the hand. Hand 1978 Oct;10(3):285–91.

10. Lau JH, Chow SP, Stroebel AB, Collins RJ. Mycobacterial infection of the hand: clinical features and functional results. Hand 1983 Jun;15(2):192–200.

11. Al-Qattan MM, Bowen V, Manktelow RT. Tuberculosis of the hand. J Hand Surg Br 1994 Apr;19(2):234–7.

12. Regnard PJ, Barry P, Isselin J. Mycobacterial tenosynovitis of the flexor tendons of the hand. A report of five cases. J Hand Surg Br 1996 Jun;21(3):351–4.

13. Agarwal A, Khan SA, Qureshi NA. Multifocal osteoarticular tuberculosis in children. J OrthopSurg (Hong Kong) 2011 Dec;19(3):336–40.

14. Agarwal A, Kant KS, Kumar A, Shaharyar A, Verma I, Suri T. Lytic lesions of distal radius in children: a rare tubercular presentation. Hand Surg 2014;19(3):369–74.

Q. 11. What is the role of wrist arthrodesis?

Arthrodesis is to be used as the treatment of last resort in cases:

1. Where conservative management or surgical debridement heals with a painful fibrous ankylosis

2. Where there is complete collapse of multiple carpal bones leading to a painful arthritic joint.

"The good functional results are produced in the metacarpals and phalanges by conservative management and rehabilitation. Despite the extent of joint destruction, the arthrodesis usually is never needed. Arthrodesis can be suggested as a final method in the management of TB. The pathology in TB lends itself to the debridement of infective tissue and hand being a non-weight-bearing joints, more joint irregularity is acceptable."

---

5. Subasi M, Bukte Y, Kapukaya A, Gurkan F. Tuberculosis of the metacarpals and phalanges of the hand. Ann Plast Surg 2004 Nov;53(5):469–72.

8. Tsai MS, Liu JW, Chen WS, de Villa VH. Tuberculous wrist in the era of effective chemotherapy: an eleven-year experience. Int J Tuberc Lung Dis. 2003 Jul;7(7):690–4.

Q. 12. How to prognosticate a case?

Generally there is favourable response to ATT. The disease heals with good functional outcome, if treatment is started in synovitis or early arthritis stage.

The functional outcome is poor in cases which present in or progress to advanced arthritis and a fusion procedure may be necessary to obtain a painless joint.

1. Al-Qattan MM, Al-Namla A, Al-Thunayan A, Al-Omawi M. Tuberculosis of the hand. J Hand Surg Am 2011 Aug;36(8):1413–21; quiz 1422.
2. Al-Qattan MM, Helmi AA. Chronic hand infections. J Hand Surg Am 2014 Aug;39(8):1636–45.
3. Subasi M, Bukte Y, Kapukaya A, Gurkan F. Tuberculosis of the metacarpals and phalanges of the hand. Ann Plast Surg 2004 Nov;53(5):469–72.
4. Kotwal PP, Khan SA. Tuberculosis of the hand: clinical presentation and functional outcome in 32 patients. J Bone Joint Surg Br 2009 Aug;91(8):1054–7.
5. Agarwal A, Qureshi NA, Kumar P, Khan S. Tubercular osteomyelitis of metacarpals and phalanges in children. Hand Surg 2011;16(1): 19–27.
6. Tsai MS, Liu JW, Chen WS, de Villa VH. Tuberculous wrist in the era of effective chemotherapy: an eleven-year experience. Int J Tuberc Lung Dis 2003 Jul;7(7):690–4.
7. Leung PC. Tuberculosis of the hand. Hand 1978 Oct;10(3):285–91.
8. Lau JH, Chow SP, Stroebel AB, Collins RJ. Mycobacterial infection of the hand: clinical features and functional results. Hand 1983 Jun;15(2):192–200.
9. Al-Qattan MM, Bowen V, Manktelow RT. Tuberculosis of the hand. J Hand Surg Br 1994 Apr;19(2):234–7.
10. Regnard PJ, Barry P, Isselin J. Mycobacterial tenosynovitis of the flexor tendons of the hand. A report of five cases. J Hand Surg Br 1996 Jun;21(3):351–4.
11. Agarwal A, Khan SA, Qureshi NA. Multifocal osteoarticular tuberculosis in children. J OrthopSurg (Hong Kong) 2011 Dec;19(3):336–40.
12. Agarwal A, Kant KS, Kumar A, Shaharyar A, Verma I, Suri T. Lytic lesions of distal radius in children: a rare tubercular presentation. Hand Surg 2014;19(3):369–74.

Chapter 7

Clinical Case Scenarios

Case 1: Diagnostic dilemma

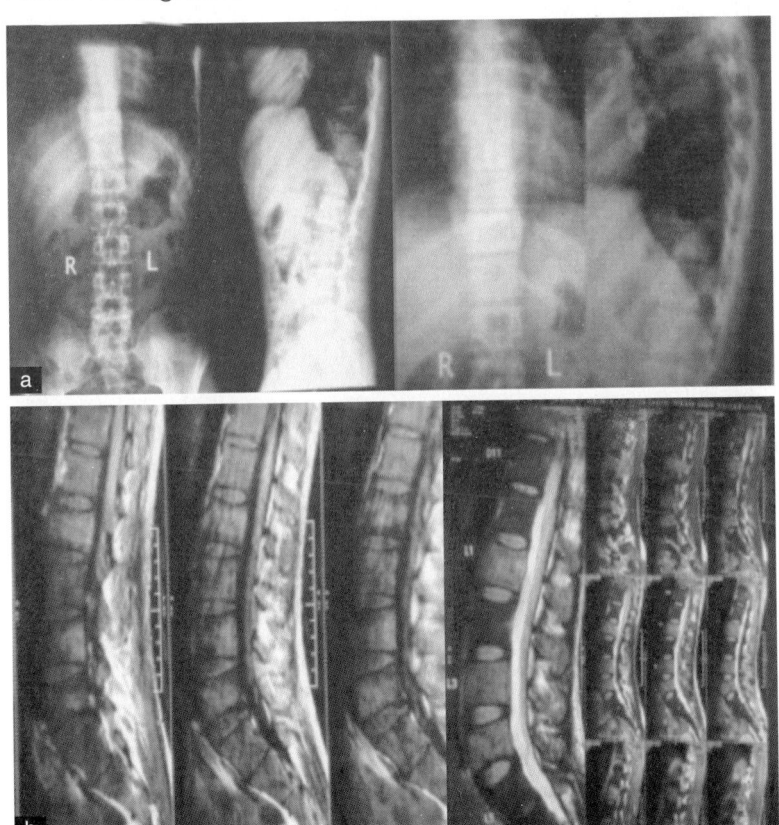

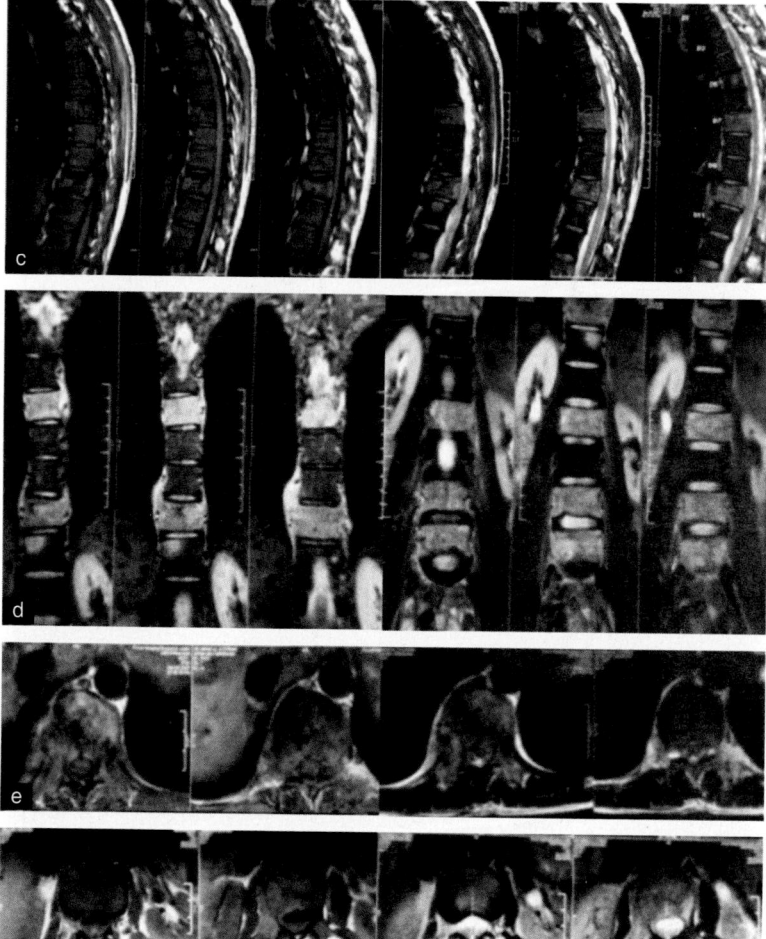

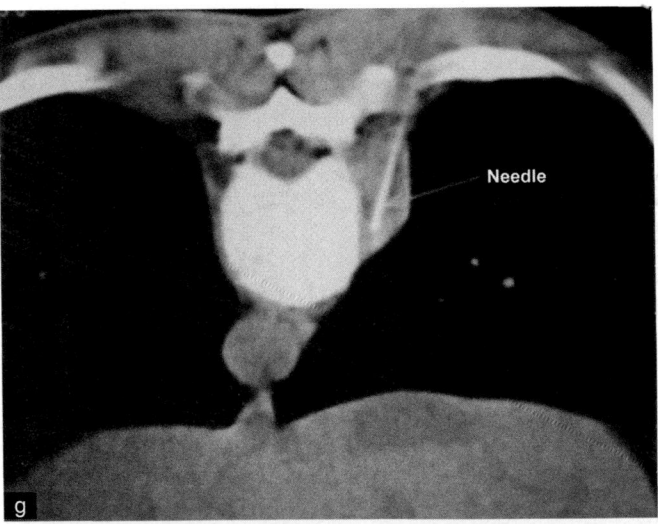

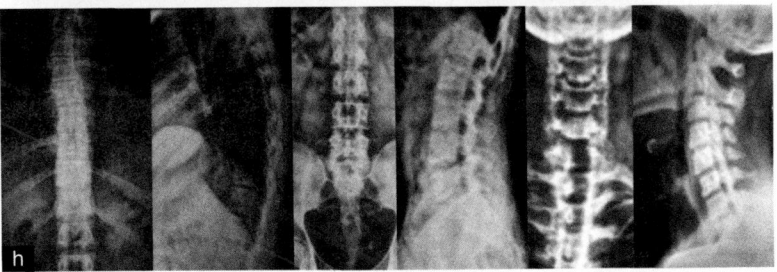

A 33-year-old male, computer operator by profession, presented with mid-back pain for past 3 months with associated decreased appetite. He had history of weight loss (15 kg) in 3 months on reporting. Patient was taking only analgesics for the pain. On general examination, no abnormality was seen. Diffuse tenderness was present in the dorsolumbar spine with associated paravertebral spasm. There was no spinal deformity or psoas fullness and no neural deficit. X-rays (Fig. a) of whole spine showed no abnormal fingings. His blood picture with serum alkaline phosphatase (ALP) was with normal limits with only raised ESR (86 mm/hr). MRI (Figs b–f) showed diffuse alteration of signal intensity involving multiple dorsal and lumbar vertebral bodies (D7, D10, L1, L3, L4) (Figs e, f). Similar changes were also noted in the posterior elements of D10, L1, L3 and L4 (Figs a to d). A differential diagnoses of myeloinfiltrative pathology (metastases/lymphoma/leukemia) and multifocal tuberculosis were considered. A CT-guided biopsy (Fig. g) was done which on TB-PCR and histology ascertained the diagnosis of tuberculosis. He was treated with ATT for 18 months and had an uneventful recovery. Fig. (h) shows X-rays after 8 years follow-up.

Comments: If clinicoradiological presentation and MRI findings are not classical for tuberculosis, every effort should be made to establish tissue diagnosis. No place for empirical treatment.

Case 2: Diagnostic dilemma

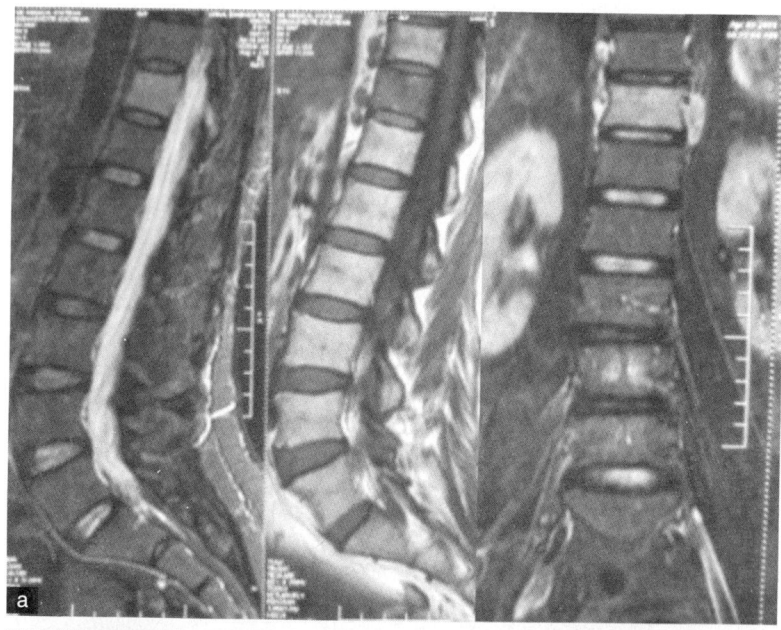

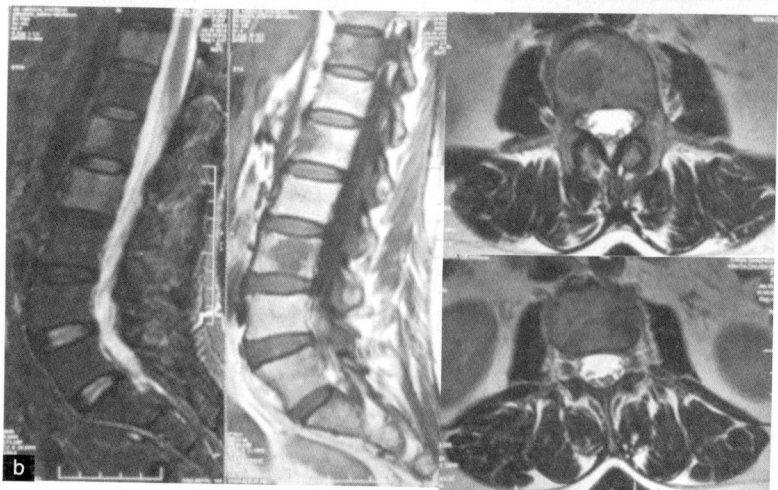

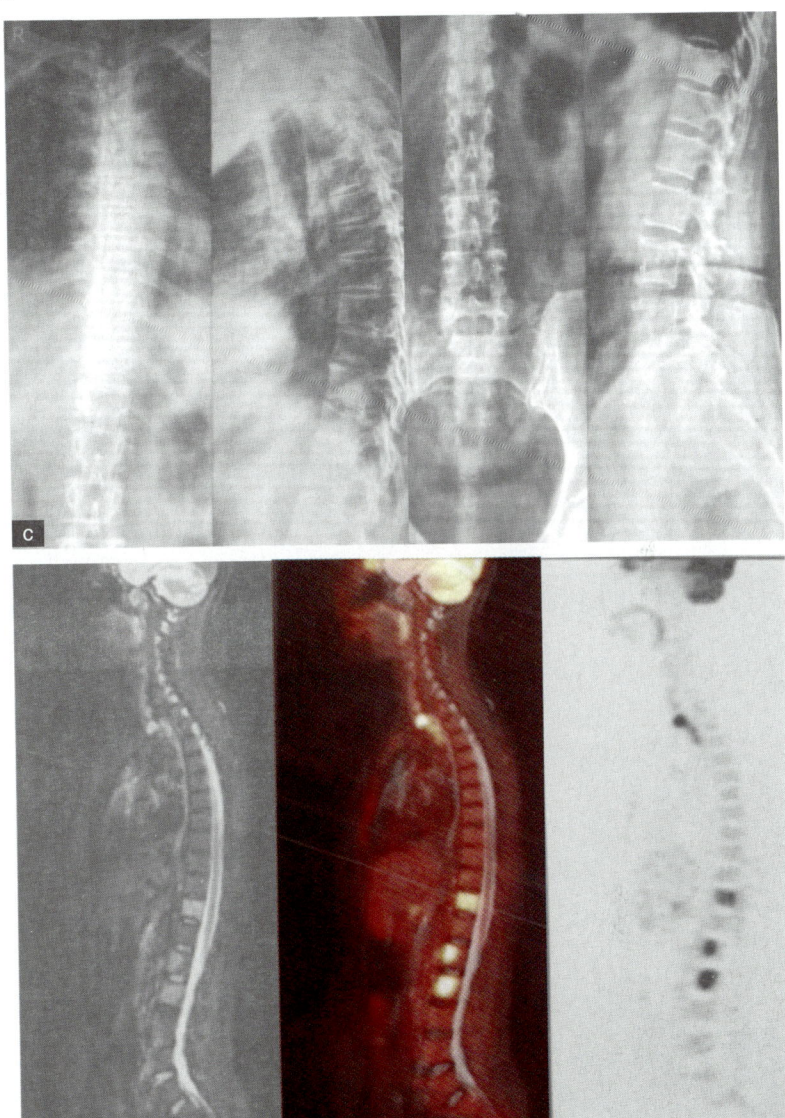

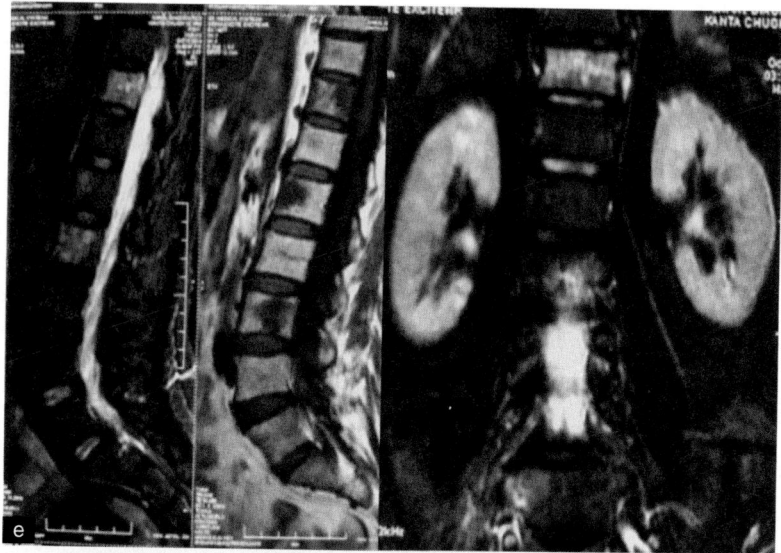

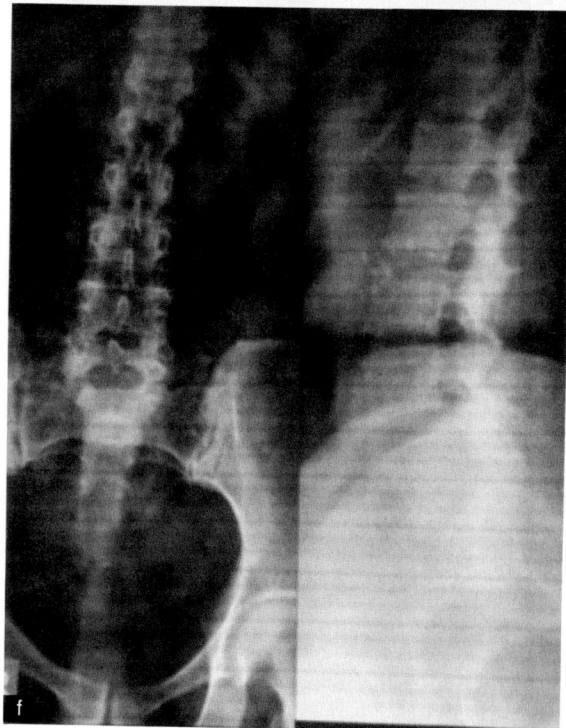

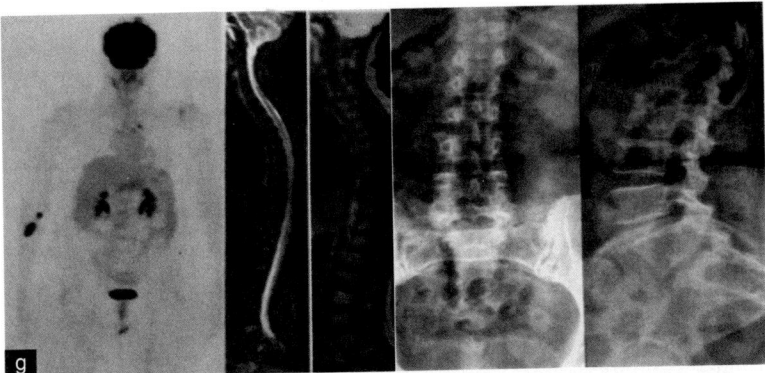

A 58-year-old female presented with complaints of low back pain for past 6 months. It was more at nights, increased with activity and partially relieved with rest. There was associated loss of weight present (8 kg in 3 months). Patient had no history of trauma or any comorbidities. After 3 months of back pain, patient was advised MRI and bed rest by some other orthopedic surgeon. MRI (Fig. a) showed altered signal intensity in D11 (hypointense on T1WI and isointense on T2WI) with no pre- or paravertebral collection. Patient got a repeat MRI just before presenting at GTBH (after 6 months of back pain). The new MRI (Fig. b) showed altered signals at multiple levels (D11, L1–L3 and L5) with minimal soft tissue collection. On examination, other systems were found to be normal. There was diffuse moderate tenderness in the lumbar spine, but no associated deformity or neural deficit. X-rays (Fig. c) had no significant findings apart from degenerative changes in spine. Montaux test was positive. With a differential diagnosis of myeloproliferative disease like lymphoma, and multiple myeloma; metastases and multifocal tuberculosis patient underwent PET-MRI (Fig. d) which showed multiple FDG avid lesions with increased uptake in D11, L1–L5 with multiple enlarged lymph nodes of supra-clavicular region, mediastinum and retroperitoneum. Patient underwent supra-clavicular lymph node biopsy, which showed epithelioid granulomas suggestive of tuberculosis. Patient was started on ATT. After 9 months, MRI and X-rays (Figs e, f) showed features of decrease in the signal intensity and healing. At 12 months, PET-MRI (Fig. g) showed absence of any FDG avid lesion, suggesting healing. The ATT was stopped at 12 months. She is still under follow-up for past 3 years with no new symptoms.

Case 3: TB spine with neurological deficit in pregnancy

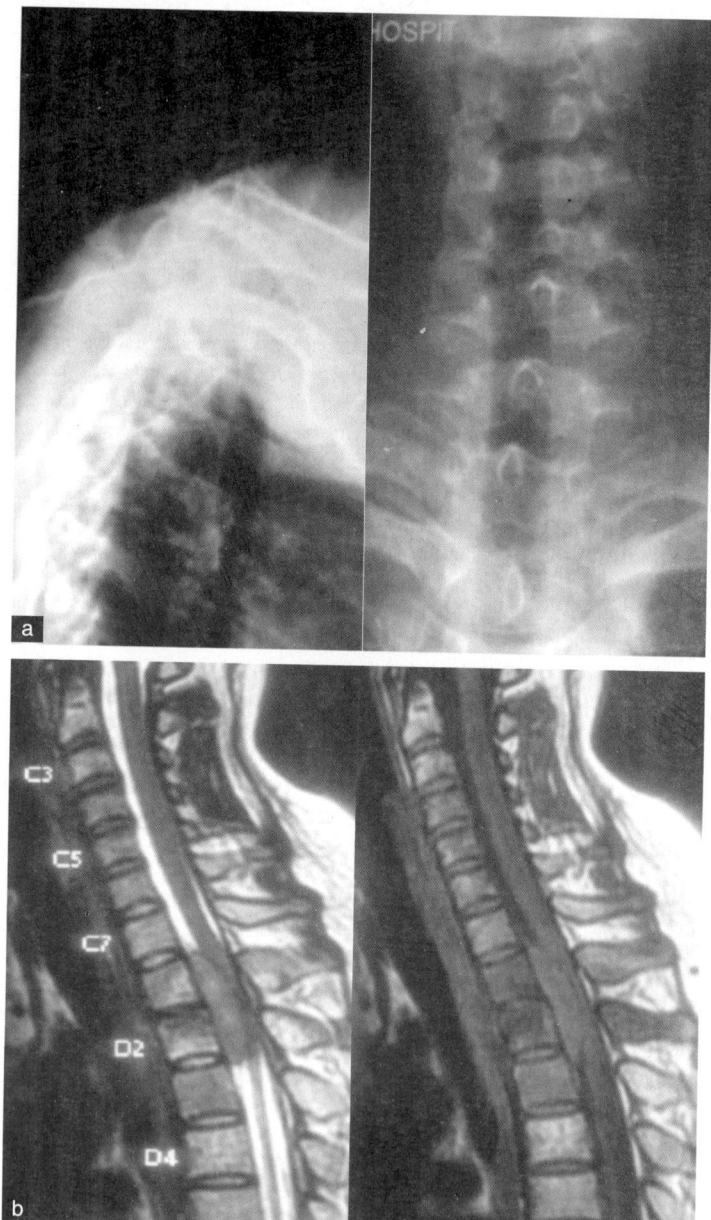

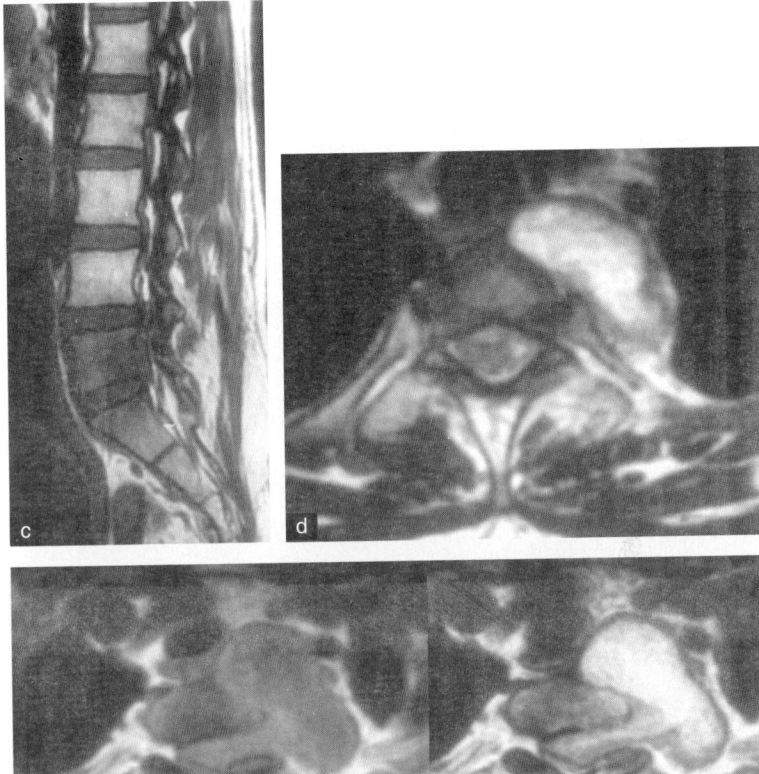

A 23-year-old female presented with 32 weeks of pregnancy and insidious onset pain in cervicodorsal (CD) spine with grade IV paraplegia developing over 3 weeks. The X-rays (Fig. a) lateral and AP view, were not helpful in diagnosis. T2WI and T1W, (Fig. b) MRI showed hyper- (T2WI) and hypointense (T1WI) signal respectively, from D1–D4 with intraspinal compression. T1WI (Fig. c) MRI of LS spine also showed a skip lesion of L5–S1. The axial scan T2WI and T1WI (Figs d, e) showed bright signal in T2WI and low signal in T1WI suggestive of liquid collection at CD spine. Intraspinal liquid compression is also noted. She was started on bed rest and ATT based on MRI diagnosis. The patient underwent lower segment cesarean section (LSCS) and a healthy baby was delivered. The patient started showing neural improvement in a short span after ceserean section delivery.

Comments: Sometime these patients report for the first time during pregnancy with spinal tubercular disease and neurological deficit. The liquid compression is likely to resolve on ATT, bed rest and after delivery patient may start showing neural improvement.

Case 4: TB spine with paraplegia

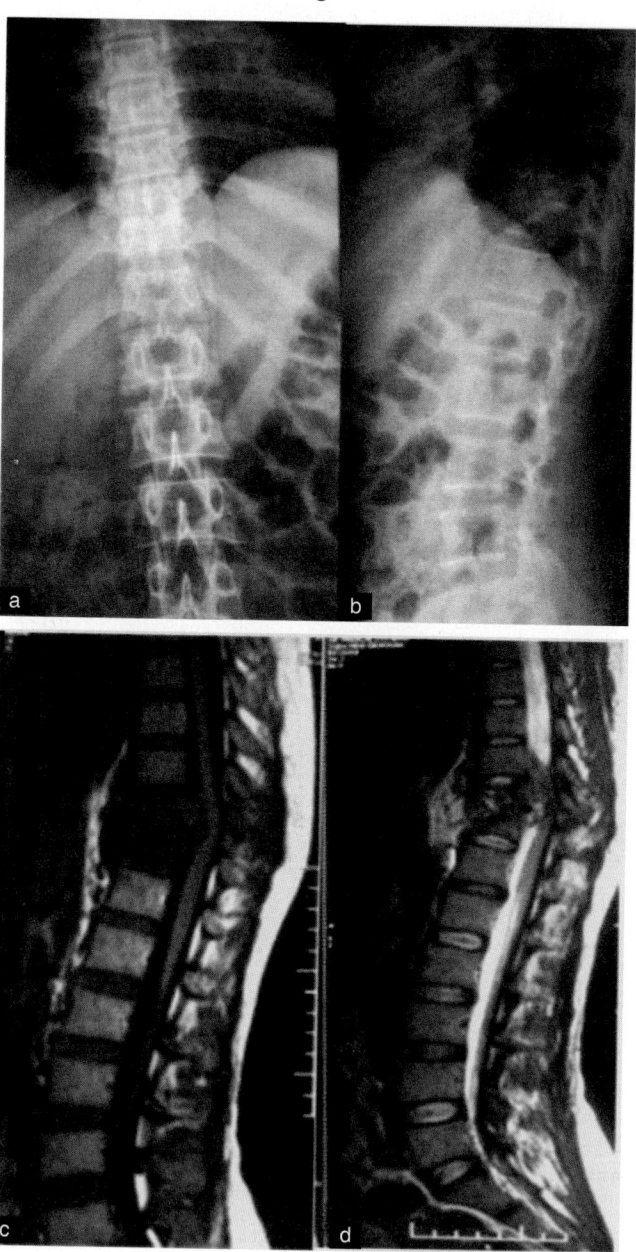

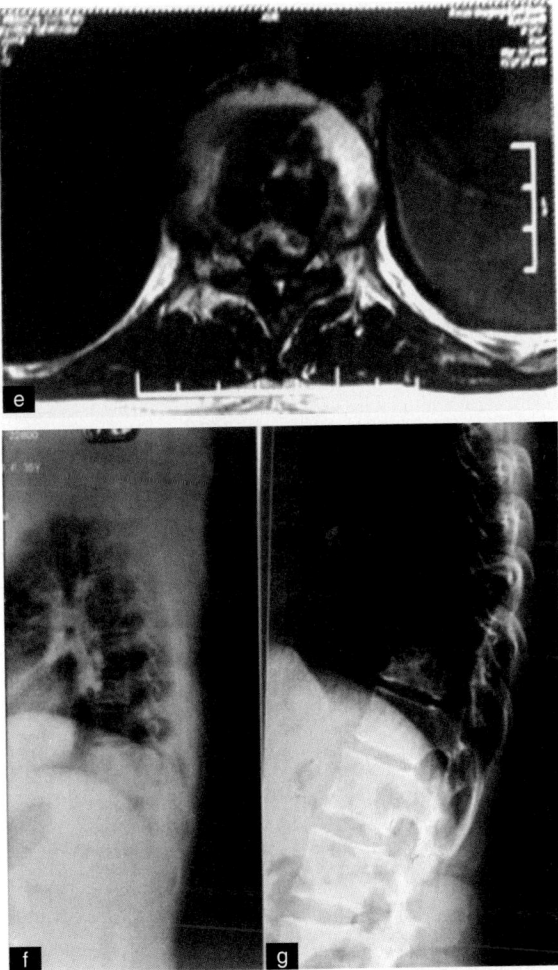

A 38-year-old female of spinal TB D10–D11 with grade III paraplegia. AP and lateral radiographs (Figs a, b) show involvement of D10 and D11 vertebrae with fuzziness of end plates and obliteration of D10–D11 disc space. T1WI and T2WI mid-sagittal scan (Figs c, d) shows hypointense signal on T1WI and hyperintense signal on T2WI, with destruction of D10 and D11 vertebrae. Axial image (Fig. e) shows hyperintense paravertebral collection. Extrapleural anterolateral decompression with bone grafting was performed, following which patient improved neurologically. Immediate postoperative radiograph (Fig. f) and radiograph (Fig. g) at three and half years follow-up showing bony fusion of D10 and D11 vertebrae. Patient had complete neurological recovery.

Case 5: TB spine with neural deficit

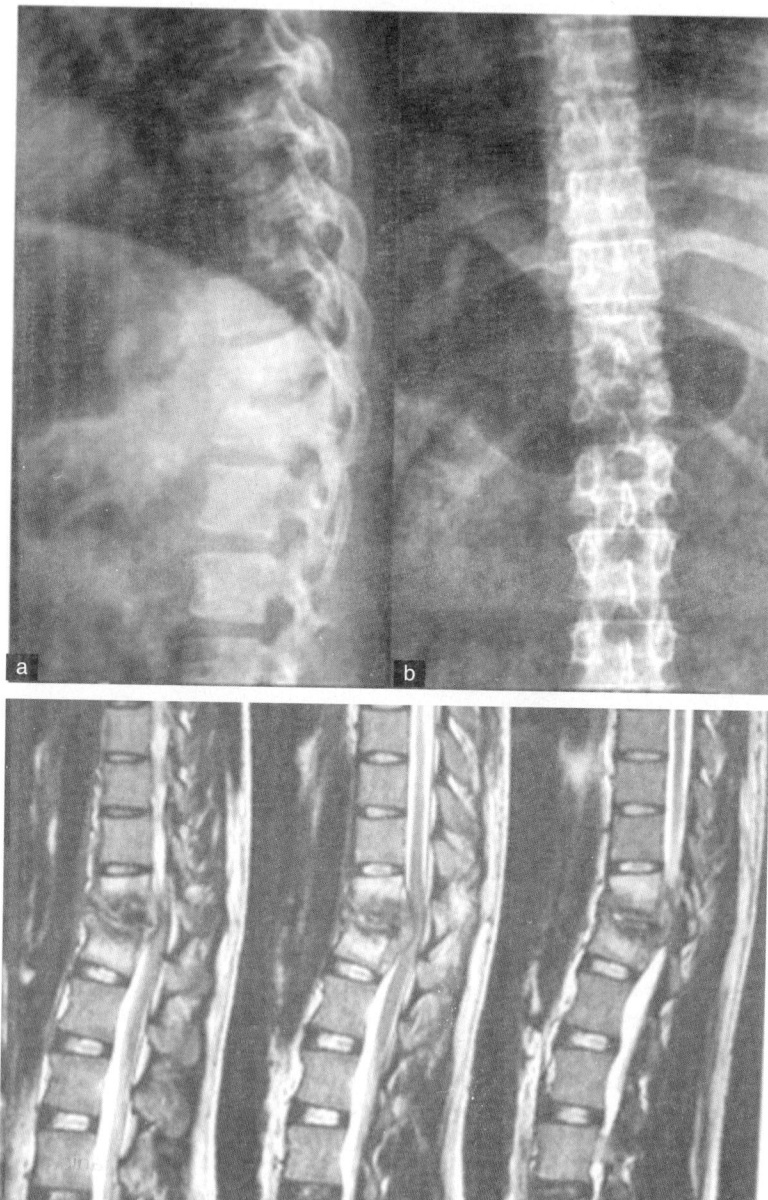

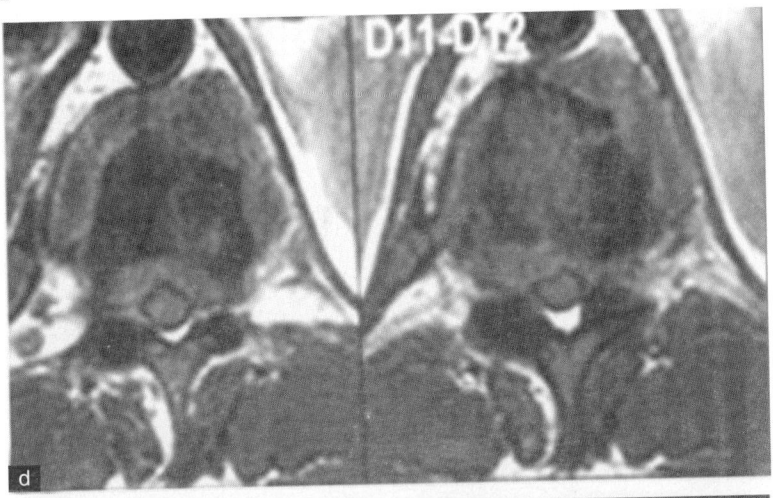

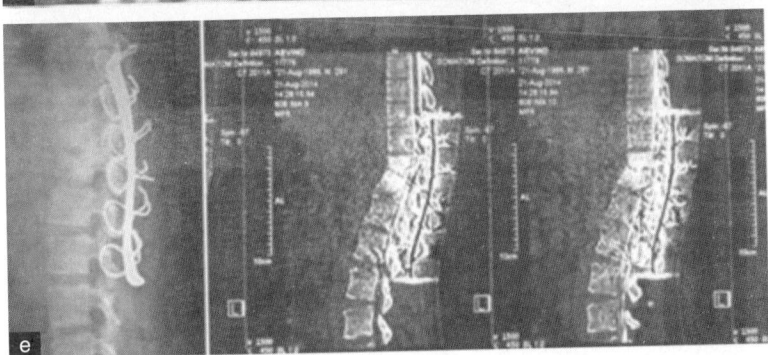

A 26-year-old patient of spinal tuberculosis of D11–D12 with grade IV paraplegia of one year duration. Preoperative radiographs (Figs a, b) depicting end plate destruction of D11 and D12 vertebrae with reduced disc space between D11 and D12. T2WI mid-sagittal scan (Fig. c) and axial T1WI scan (Fig. d) show destruction of affected D11 and D12 vertebrae and significant spinal cord compression leading to complete paraplegia below this level (Fig. d). Extrapleural anterolateral decompression along with posterior Hartshill instrumentation and bone grafting was performed as single stage surgery by "T incision". But patient did not show any neurological recovery. CT myelogram (Fig. e) was then performed which showed uninterrupted flow of dye across the lesion, suggesting adequate spinal cord decompression. Patient showed signs of good neurological recovery within 6 months.

Case 6: TB spine in a junctional (D-L junction) area

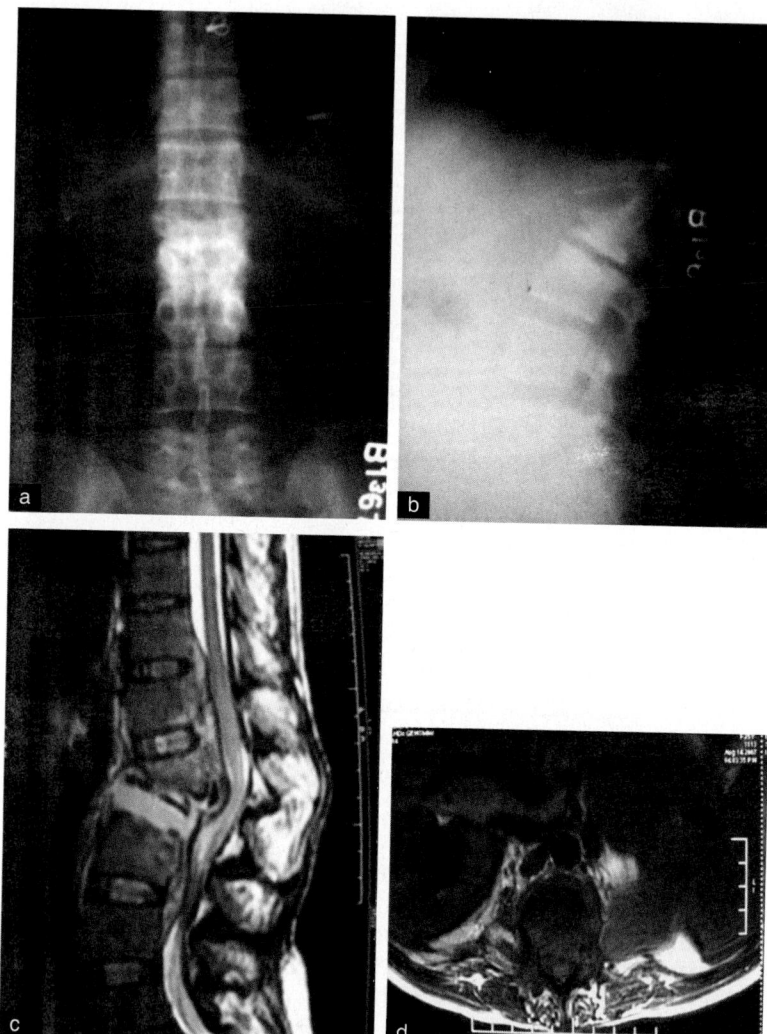

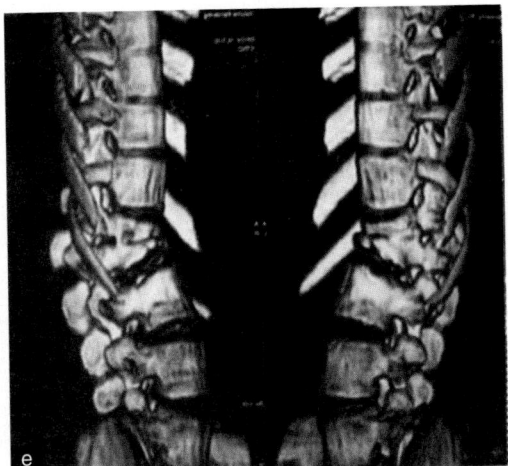

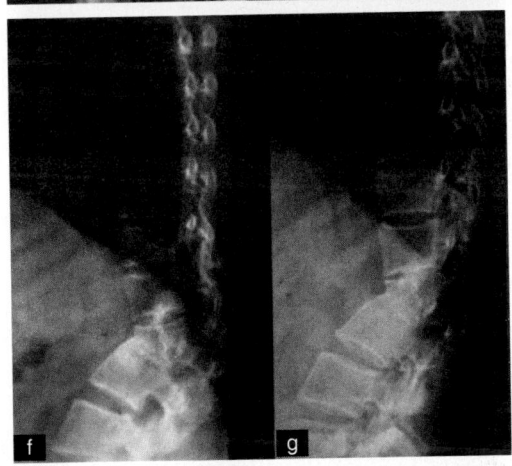

A 33-year-old female of spinal tuberculosis with grade I paraplegia of 6 months duration. IAP and lateral radiographs (Figs a, b) show collapse of L1 and L2 vertebrae with loss of disk space in between and gibbus deformity. T2WI mid-sagittal scan (Fig. c) shows destruction of L1 and L2 vertebrae with hyperintense signal and compression of spinal cord. T1WI axial image (Fig. d) shows para-vertebral pus collection. The CT scan (Fig. e) shows involvement and collapse of L1 and L2 vertebrae. Extrapleural anterolateral decompression (*see* Fig. 5.13A–C) with anterior bone grafting done following which patient had complete neurological recovery. The follow-up radiographs (Figs f, g) at 4 years and 7 years showing fusion of L1 and L2 vertebrae with healed kyphosis with no active lesion. Now this patient has 10 years follow-up available. The instrumentation was not performed due to nonavailability of implant, however, in this present time posterior column shortening and posterior instrumentation could have corrected the spinal deformity as well.

Case 7: Intraspinal tuberculoma

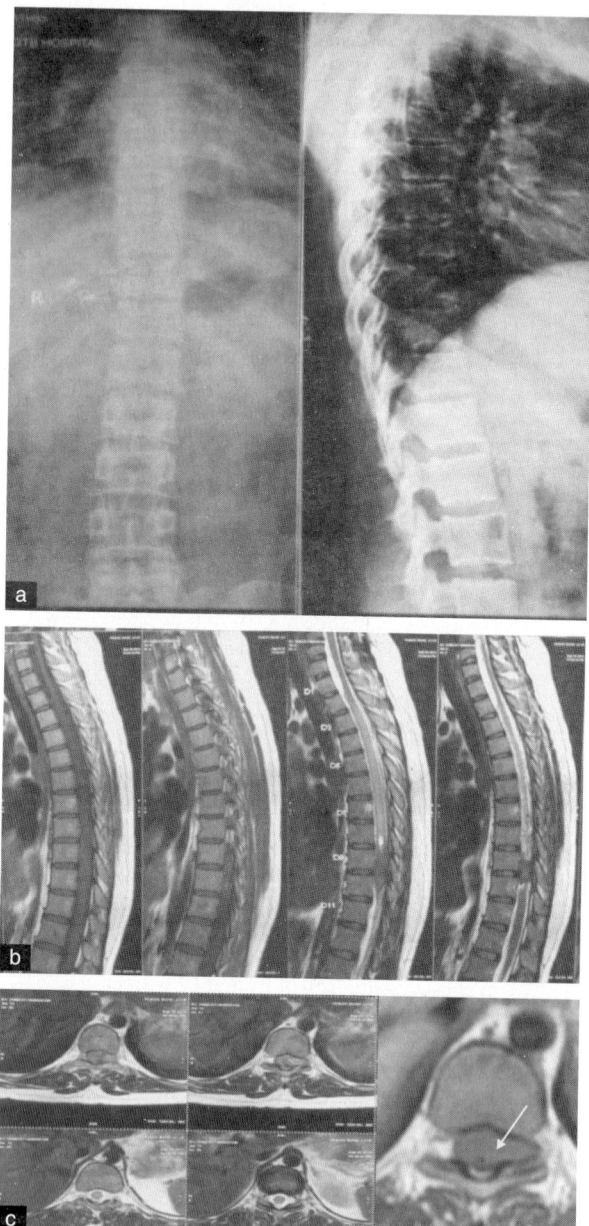

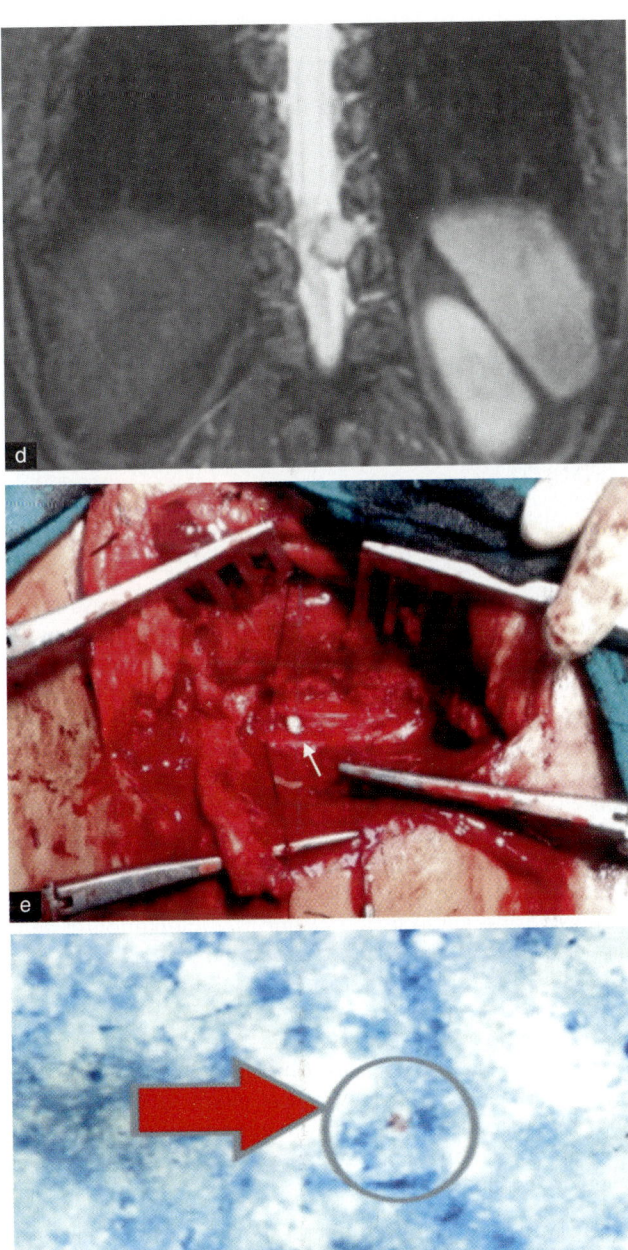

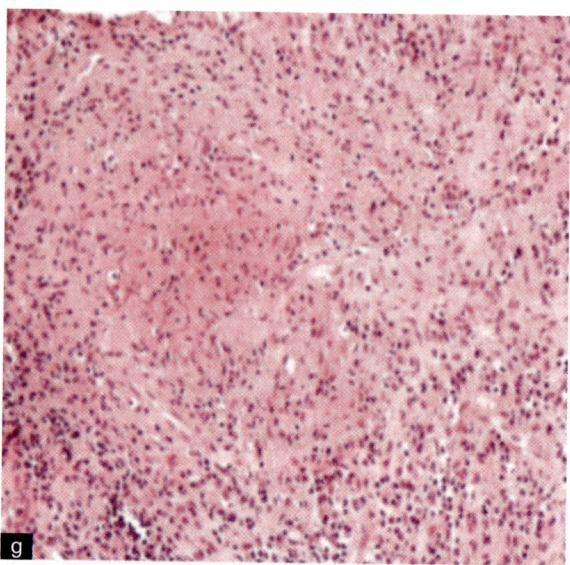

A 19-year-old female presented with complaints of weakness and sensory loss in both lower limbs for past 1 month. There was no bowel/bladder complaints. She had history of tubercular meningitis 4 years ago treated with category I ATT for 6 months. On examination, she had non-tender spine with no deformity. She had clasp knife spasticity with power of 3/5 in all muscle groups of lower limb. Deep tendon reflexes were exaggerated with presence of ankle clonus. The sensation below L1 dermatome was decreased. Plain radiographs (Fig. a) were essentially normal. Mid-sagittal sections T1WI and T2WI of MRI (Fig. b) show hypointense lesion in the spinal canal at the level of D10. Axial section (Fig. c) shows dumbell-shaped lesion exiting through intervertebral canal. Coronal sections (Fig. d) showing the same lesion exiting the intervertebral canal. The differential diagnosis of spinal tumor syndrome was considered. In view of compressive lesion, surgical decompression was performed by laminectomy and durotomy (Fig. e). Intraoperative photograph shows a nodular dirty looking lesion. On both sides of meninges, a bead of pus was seen (arrow). Pus was collected with associated granulation tissue. Figs f and g showed AFB on cytological examination and necrotizing granuloma on histopathological examination. Hence a diagnosis of intradural/extradural granuloma was made. The patient was treated by ATT and showed uneventful neural recovery.

Comments: One-third cases of spinal tumor syndrome where D/D is intraspinal tumors (neurofibroma, meningioma and others) would turn out to be intraspinal TB granuloma in endemic regions for TB.

Case 8: TB of lumbar spine with panvertebral involvement

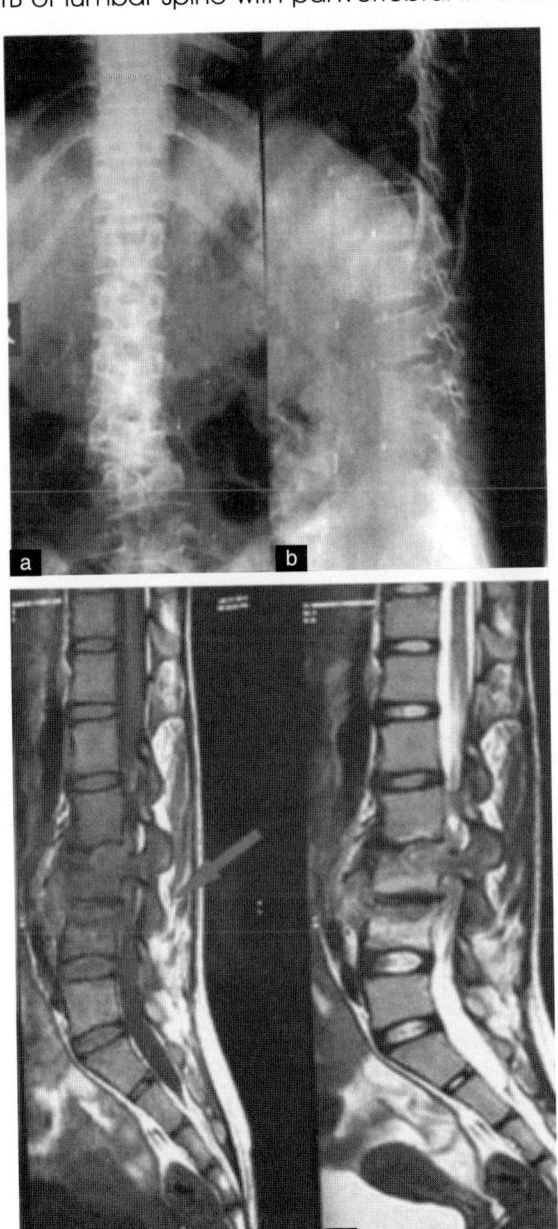

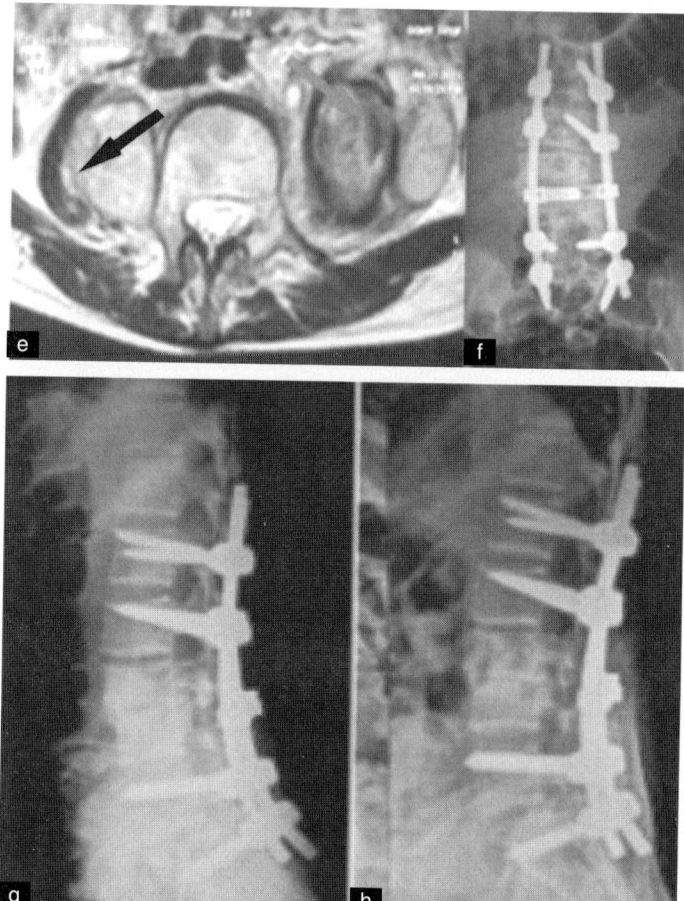

An 18-year-old female of spinal tuberculosis L3–L4 with kyphosis without neurological deficit. Preoperative AP (Fig. a) and lateral (Fig. b) radiographs of lumbar spine show destruction of L3 and L4 vertebral bodies, reduced L3 and L4 disk space with mild scoliosis (panvertebral disease). Mid-sagittal T1WI and T2WI (Figs c, d) show involvement of L3 and L4 vertebral bodies being hypointense on T1WI and hyperintense on T2WI with prevertebral collection. The arrow shows involvement of pedicle and posterior column as well. Axial T2WI MRI (Fig. e) shows involvement of posterior elements with bilateral psoas abscesses. Patient was taken for posterior instrumen-tation and transpedicular debridement of lesion. AP and lateral radiographs (Figs f, g) show correction of kyphosis. 12 months follow-up X-ray (Fig. h) showing fusion of disease segment.

Case 9: TB spine with paraplegia (panvertebral involvement)

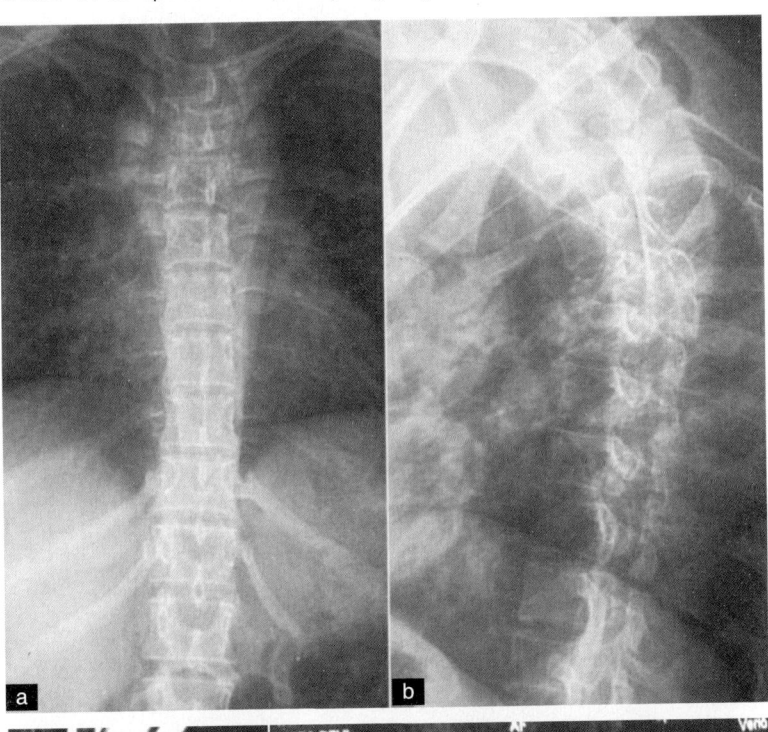

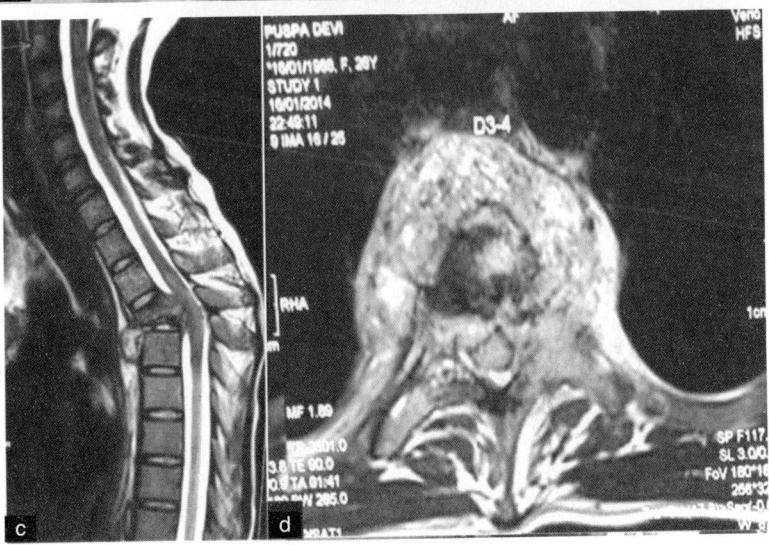

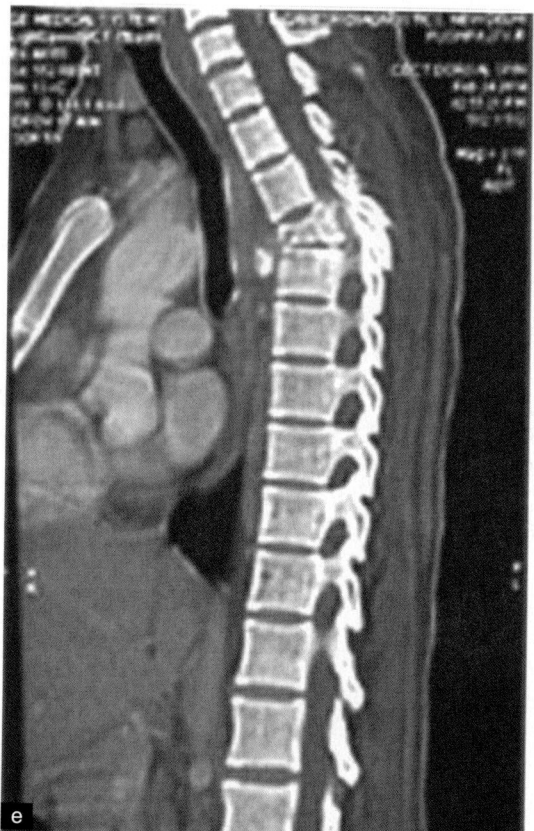

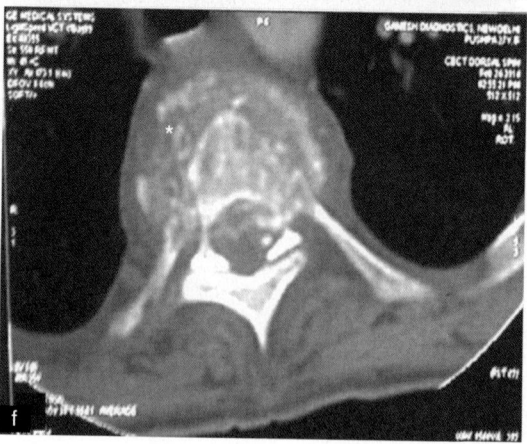

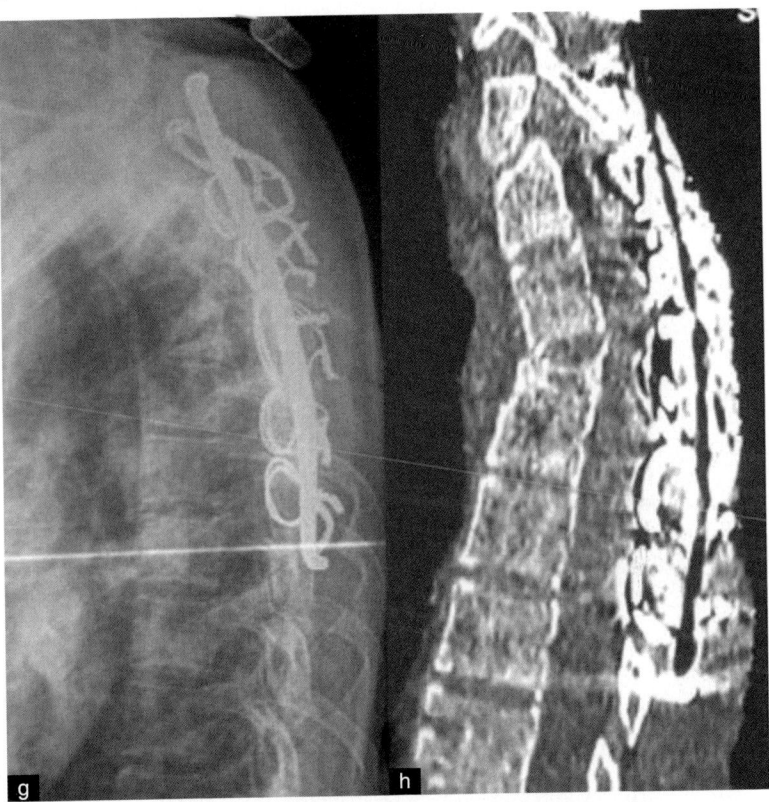

A 27-year-old female of spinal tuberculosis D3–D4 with grade IV paraplegia of 6 months duration. AP and lateral radiographs (Figs a, b) show panvertebral destruction of D3 vertebra (absence of pedicle shadow of right D3 vertebra) with decreased D2–D3 and D3–D4 disk space with end plate destruction. Mid-sagittal T2WI and axial MRI (Figs c, d) show complete destruction of D3 with paravertebral collection and spinal cord compression. Sagittal reconstructed image and axial section (Figs e, f) show fragmented D4 with calcific collection outside vertebtal body(*). Patient was kept on bed rest and category 1 ATT. Anterolateral decompression with posterior Hartshill instrumentation was performed. Lateral radiograph (Fig. g) and CT scan (Fig. h) at 6 months follow-up show aligned spine. Patient recovered to grade II paraplegia at final follow-up.

Case 10: TB spine with panvertebral involvement

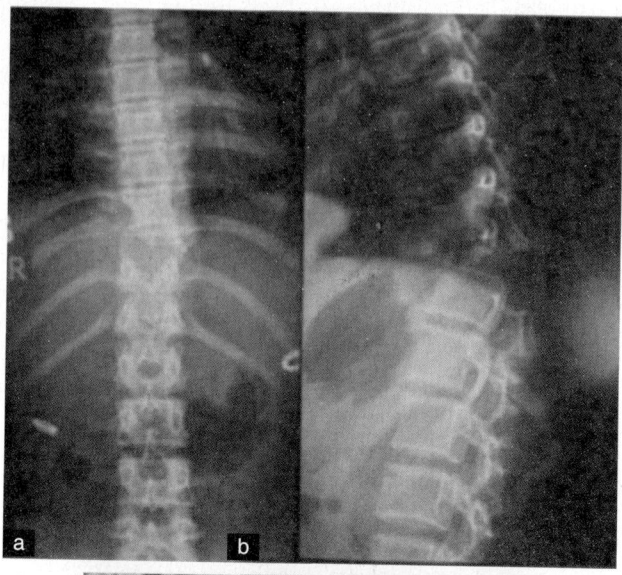

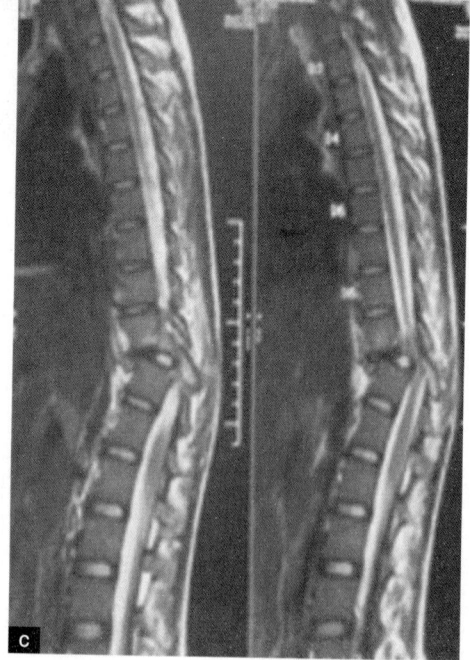

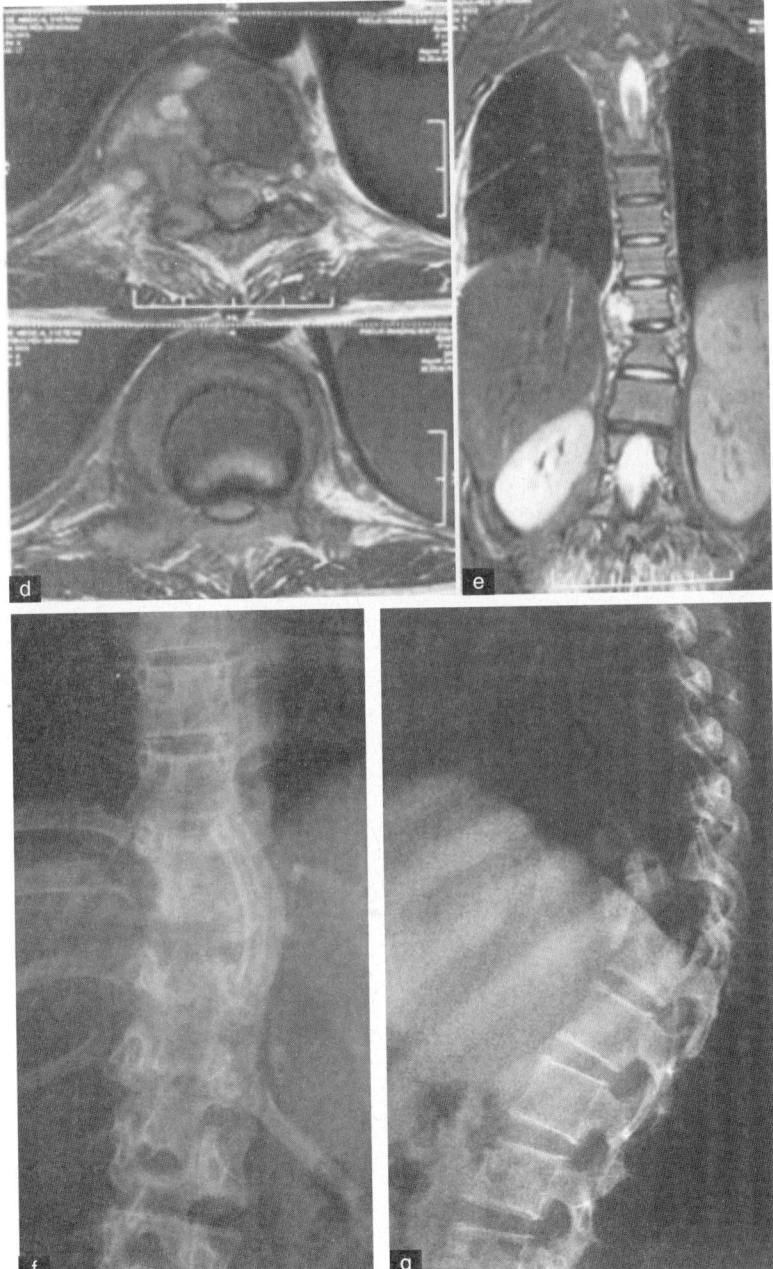

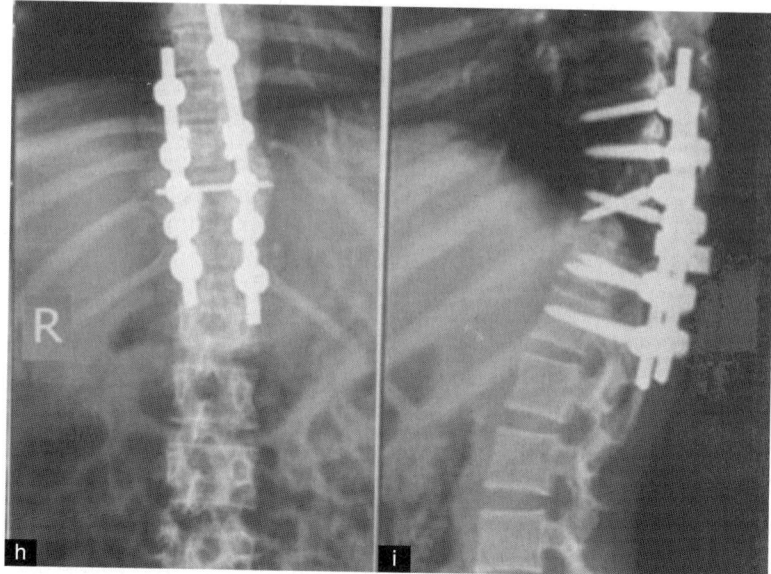

An 11-year-old female of spinal TB D9–D10 with pathological subuxation of D10 over D11 vertebra and grade IV paraplegia of 3 months duration. AP and lateral radiographs (Figs a, b) show involvement of D9 and D10 vertebrae with pathological subluxation of D10 over D11 vertebra. T2WI mid-sagittal MRI scan (Fig. c) showing significant spinal cord compression due to D10 vertebra leading to grade IV paraplegia. Axial images (Fig. d) show prevertebral and paravertebral collection of pus and destruction of right facets of proximal vertebrae. Coronal image (Fig. e) showing paravertebral pus collection bilaterally. These findings were missed by surgeon who treated her first and operated her by anterolateral decompression by extrapleural approach with rib bone graft on the left side. At this stage, patient reported to us. Follow-up radiographs lateral and AP view (Figs f, g) at the time of referral to us showed translation of proximal spine over distal D10–D11 and rib graft on left side. The patient was taken up for spinal stabilization by pedicle screw instrumentation and posterior spinal fusion (Figs h and i). Although she started showing neurological recovery but had persistent neurological deficit inspite of sound posterior fusion.

Comment: The panvertebral disease should be appreciated at first instance and instrumentated stabilization should be performed.

Case 11: TB spine with instability (panvertebral involvement)

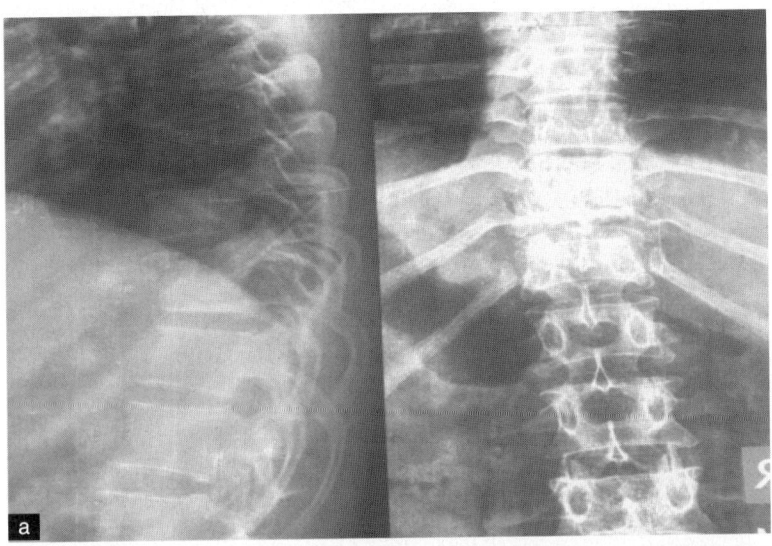

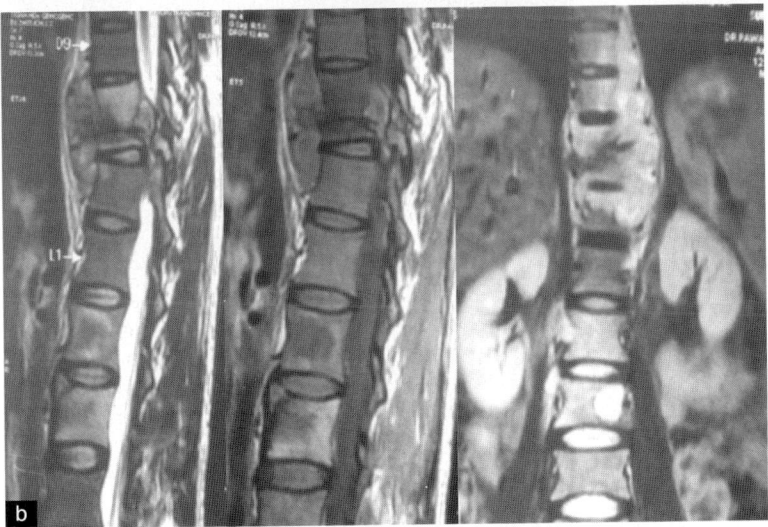

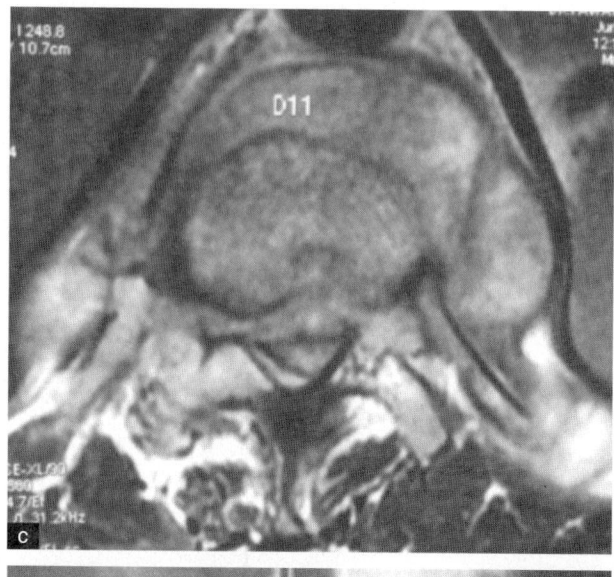

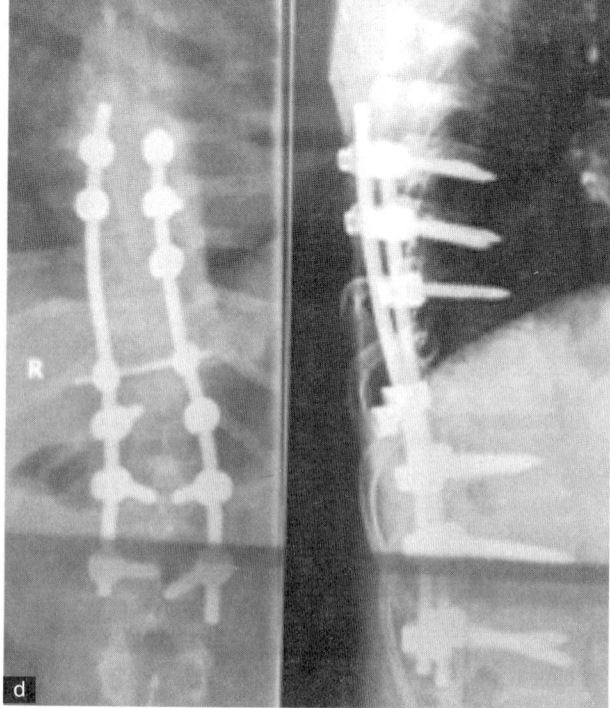

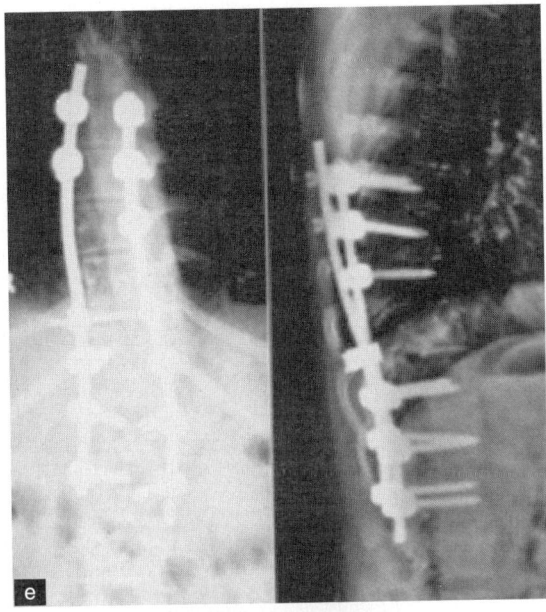

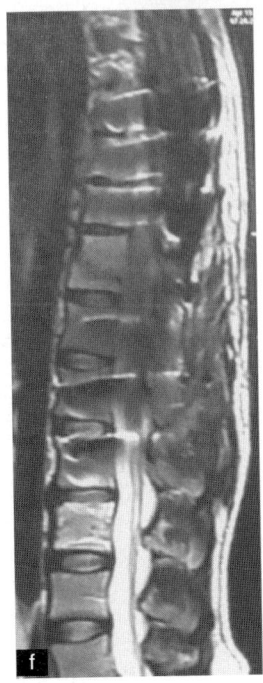

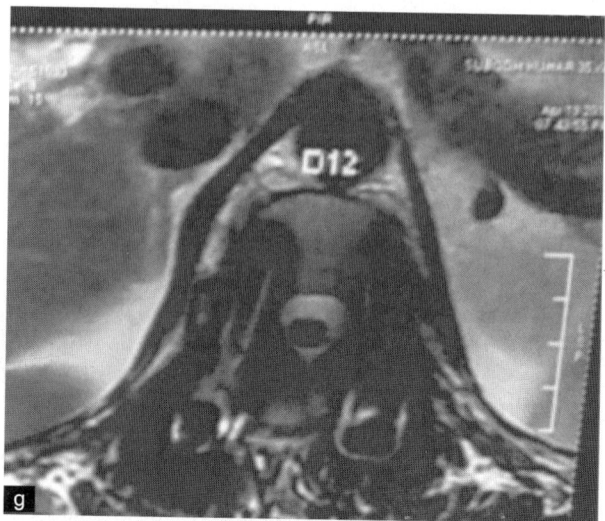

A 34-year-old male presented with complaints of pain in lower back for 1.5 years and weakness in bilateral lower limbs for 4 months. Low grade fever with constitutional symptoms were also present. On examination, patient had kyphotic deformity present at level of D10–D12, with tenderness over D10–D12 level. Tone was increased in bilateral lower limbs with exaggerated deep tendon reflexes. With fair power in muscle of hip, knee and ankle and poor in EHL and FHL. There was sensory loss of more than 50% below D10. There was no bladder or bowel involvement. Plain X-rays (Fig. a) showed reduced disk space between D10 and D11 with near total loss of vertebral body of D11, with inconspicuous pedicles of the same vertebra. The AP X-rays show a mild scoliosis and lateral X-rays show a translation of proximal vertebrae in comparison to distal, suggesting panvertebral involvement. MRI mid-sagittal T2WI and T1WI and coronal section T2WI (Fig. b) showed loculated pre- and paravertebral collection with destruction of D11 with cord compression. The disk between D10 and D11 was preserved and the collection was hypointense of T1WI and hyperintense on T2WI. Axial sections (Fig. c) showed the disease to be involving posterior complex more on the left side, making it a panvertebral disease. Patient was started on ATT and strict bed rest. Since, patient had neural deficit with an unstable spine, he was taken for instrumented stabilization by pedicle screws and decompression by costotransversectomy (Fig. d) at D10. Patient showed complete neural recovery in postoperative course. At one year follow-up, the X-rays (Fig. e) showed features of healing and MRI (Figs f, g) showed complete resolution of marrow edema and loss of all collections. ATT was stopped after the scan.

Comments: The panvertebral lesion needs to be appreciated early lest the neural deficit appears as a result of pathological subluxation/dislocation. Even on clinical grounds, this patient had more sensory loss than motor raising suspicion for global compression.

Case 12: TB spine with pathological subluxation at lumbar spine (missed panvertebral Involvement at first instance)

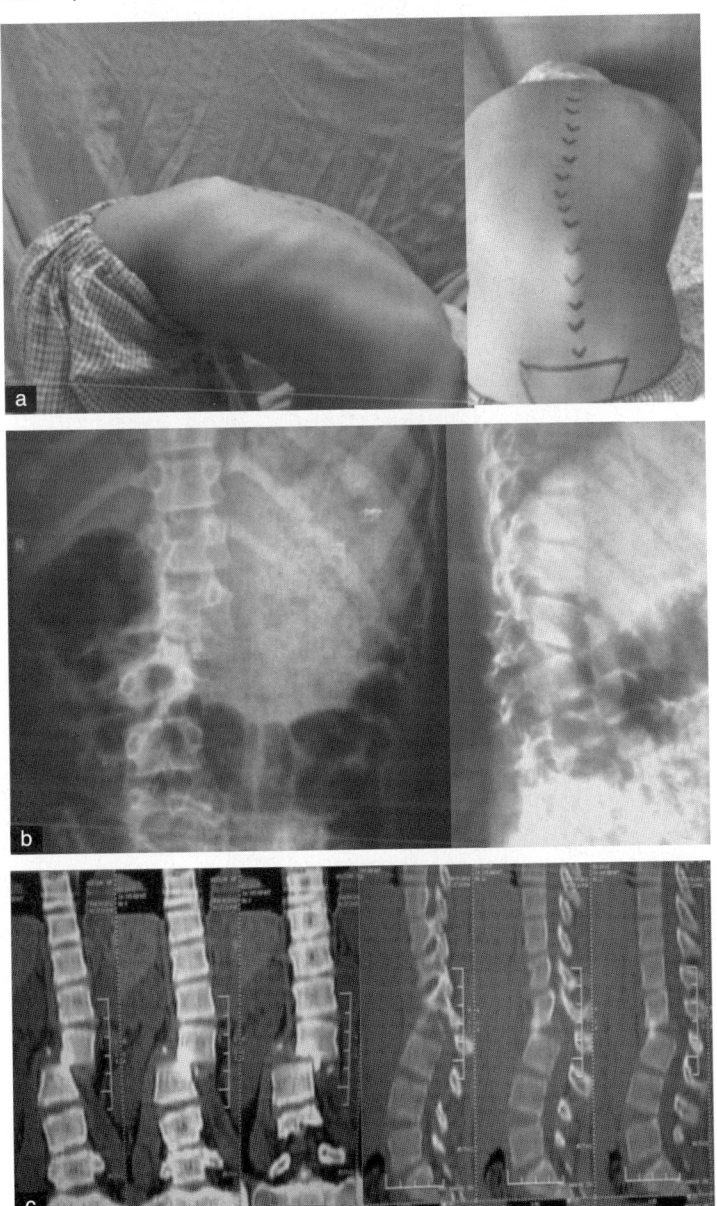

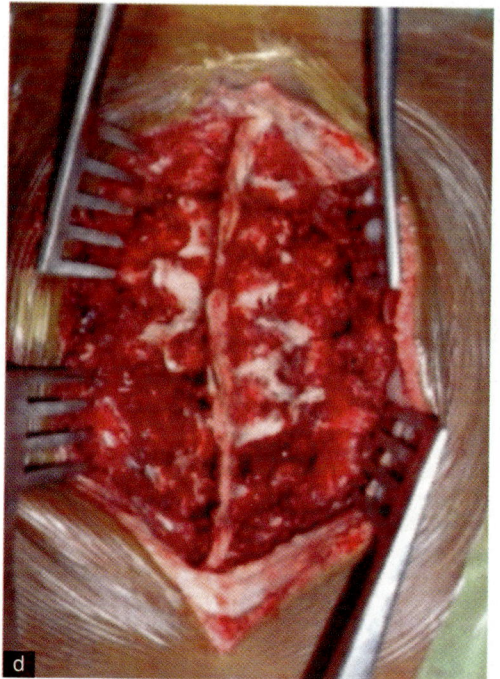

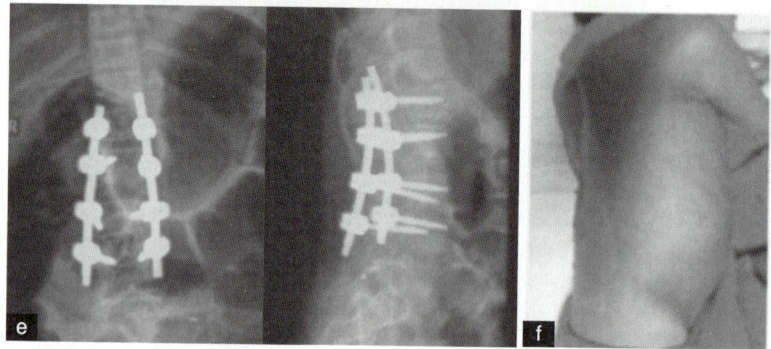

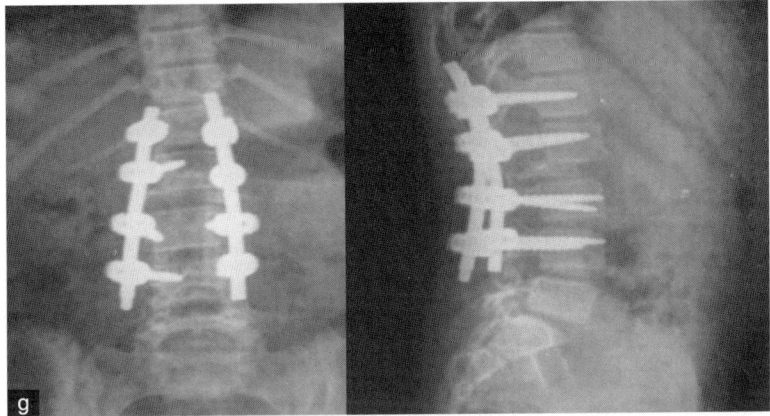

g

A 9-year-old female child came to the OPD with complaints of low back ache with on and off fever for past 9 months. Her parents had noticed deformity in spine for last 5 months. On examination (Fig. a), there was a kyphoscoliotic deformity with apex of kyphus at L1–L3, but there was no neural deficit. Plain radiographs (Fig. b) showed near total loss of body of L2 with complete facet joint dislocation with associated rotation and translation of L1 over L3 vertebra. Plain reconstructed image on CT (Fig. c) confirmed these findings. The ESR was 49 mm/hr with other blood investigations were within normal limits. Patient was receiving ATT from primary health center with a presumptive diagnosis of TB spine. Chemotherapy was continued and she was kept on complete bed rest. In view of the deformity (Fig. d), patient was taken up for surgery, i.e. posterior stabilization and derotation of vertebra using pedicle screw system. Tissue was sent for histopathology and culture which confirmed the diagnosis of tuberculosis (Fig. e). Postoperatively patient had no neural deficit and there was complete correction of the deformity. Patient is now disease-free and able to do all her routine activities. Postoperative clinical photo (Fig. f), and post-operative X-ray (Fig. g) at 5 months follow-up show corrected kyphotic deformity.

Comments: Complete rotational translation of vertebra is usually due to severe trauma. It is rare to see such deformities due to infective pathology. Since the disease affected L2–3 level, hence the neural deficit was minimal inspite of gross translation and rotation vertebrae. These lesions should be diagnosed before the vertebrae subluxate/dislocate.

Case 13: TB spine with severe lumbar kyphosis

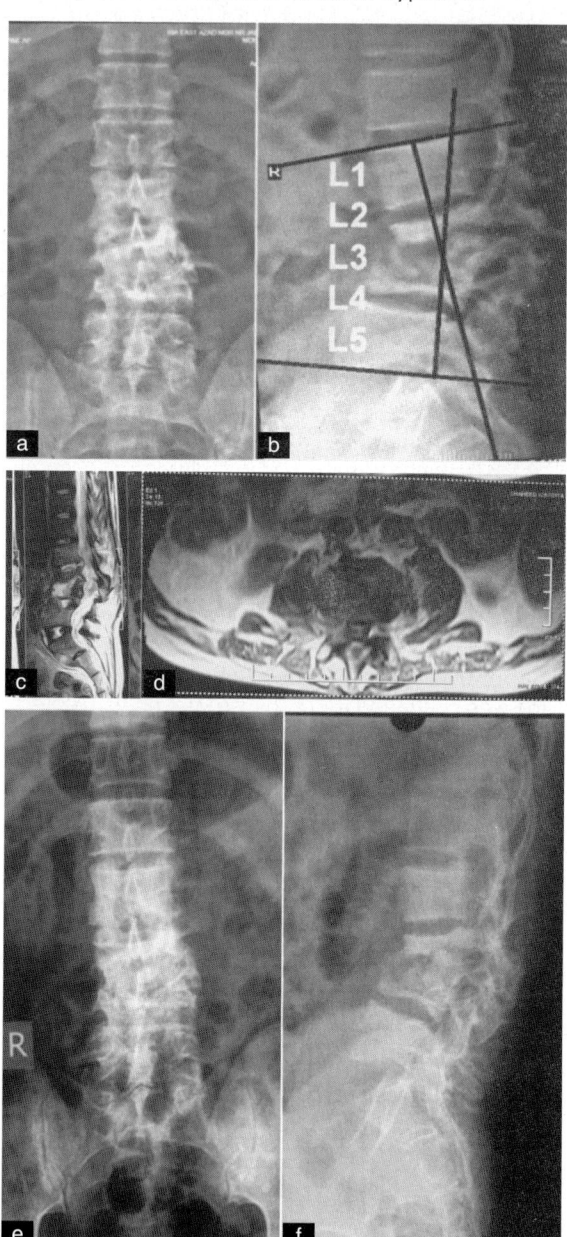

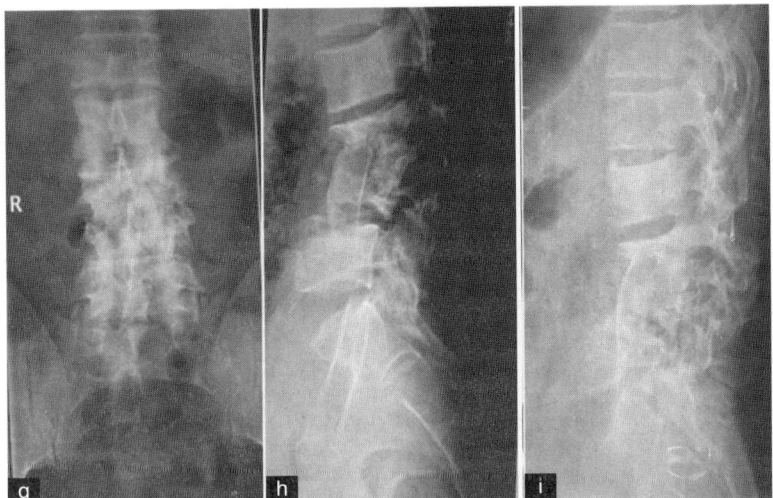

A 35-year-old male patient of tuberculosis of L2–L5 spine with no neurological deficit of one and half year duration. Patient took category I (6 months) and category II (3 months) treatment from private hospital. AP and lateral radiographs (Figs a and b) show panvertebral involvement of lumbar spine with destruction of L2 to L4 vertebrae. The kyphotic deformity was severe, however, was corrected by 10° by cephalocaudal traction. The L3 vertebral body is completely destroyed. T2WI mid-sagittal scan and axial scan (Figs c, d) show hyperintense signal with gross destruction. Patient was taken for posterior pedicle instrumentation and posterior column shortening. Pus was draining from multiple pedicle holes after probing. The spontaneous posterior fusion of L2–L4 was observed in view of long-standing disease, therefore, pedicle fixation was abandoned. The patient was put on cephalocaudal traction by head and halter traction and bilateral upper tibial steinmann pins. AP and lateral X-rays (Figs e, f) of patient before anterior bone grafting shows some correction of kyphotic deformity. AP and lateral X-rays (Figs g, h) after anterior decompression show iliac crest bone graft placed in gap. One year follow-up (Fig. i) shows fusion of bone and healing of lesion with maintained correction of kyphosis.

Case 14: TB spine of dorsolumbar junction

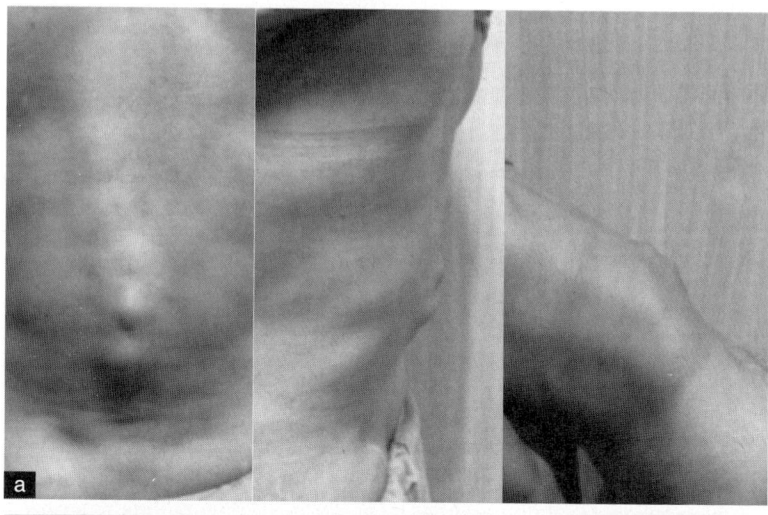

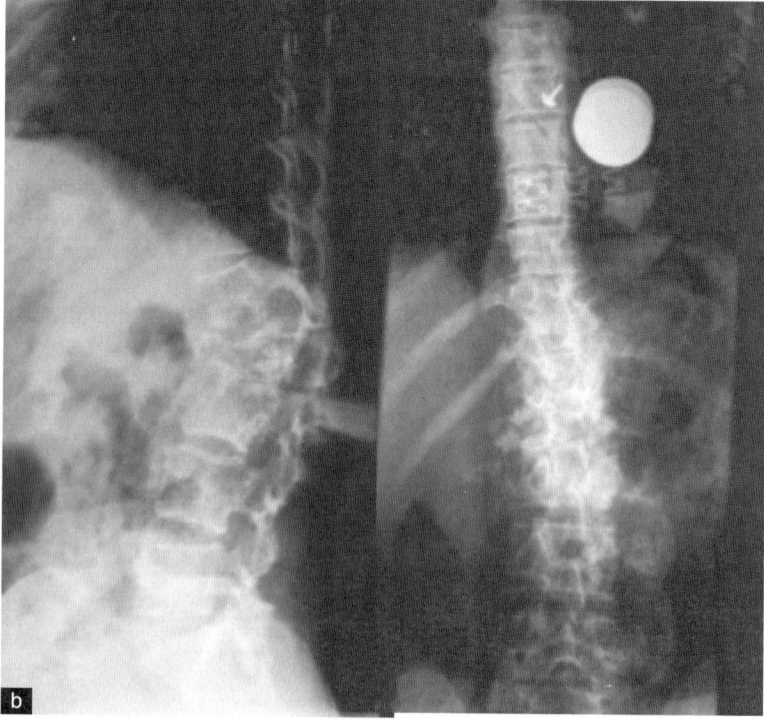

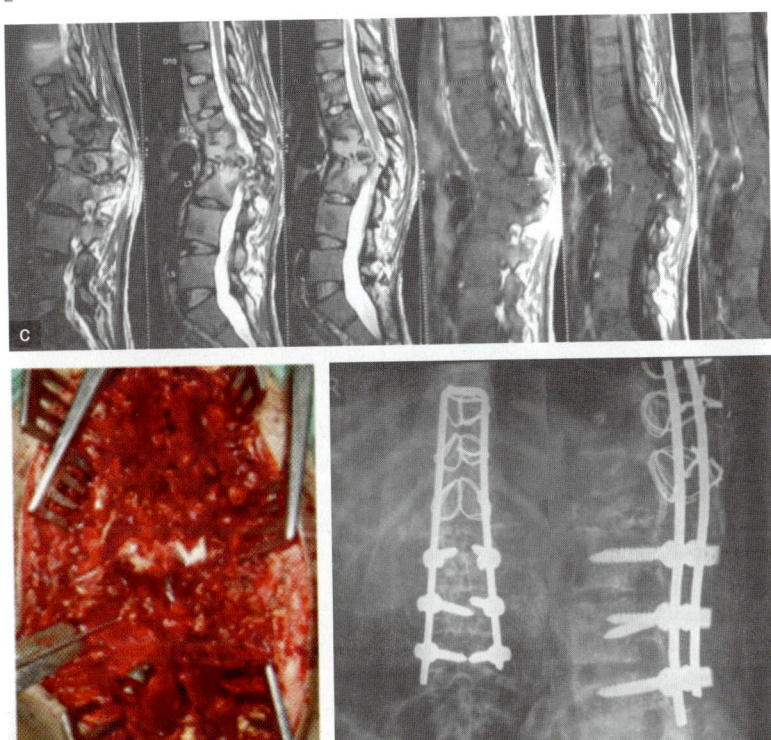

A 25-year-old lady presented with complaints of pain in back for past three and half years. She had noticed a deformity since last 3 yrs. There was associated history of loss of weight. Examination of the spine revealed tender kyphotic deformity at D11–L2 with no neural deficit (Fig. a). Plain radiographs (Fig. b) showed loss of body of L1 and L2 with regional osteopenia and kyphotic deformity. There was reduced disk space between the vertebral bodies. T1WI sagittal section of MRI (Fig. c) shows hypointense signal and T2WI showed hyperintense signal in destroyed vertebral bodies of D11–L2. There was prevertebral collection with reduction of canal diameter and cord compression. Patient was taken for surgical decompression and instrumented stabilization with kyphotic deformity correction by midline posterior approach (Fig. d). But on accessing the pedicle in D11 to L2 pedicle there was pus (arrow) coming out from pedicle holes. There was no hold of pedicle screw in vertebral bodies. Hence a hybrid fixation using pedicle screws (L3–L5) and Hartshill rectangle and sublaminar wires (D11,12 L1) (Fig. e). The kyphotic deformity is corrected and spine is well aligned.

Case 15: TB spine in a child with kyphotic deformity

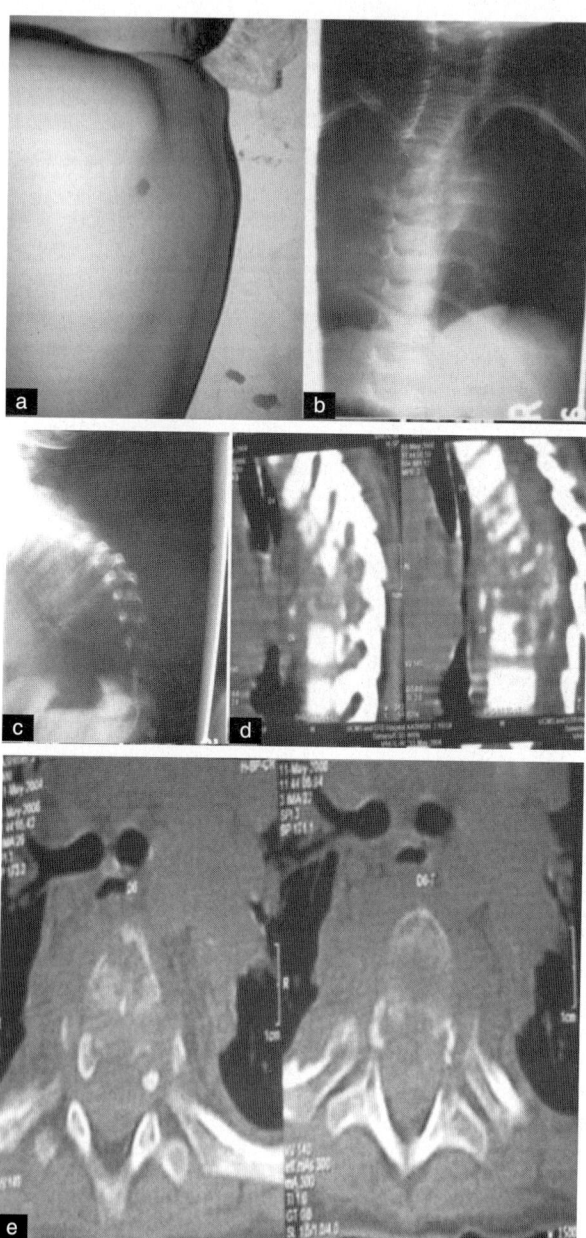

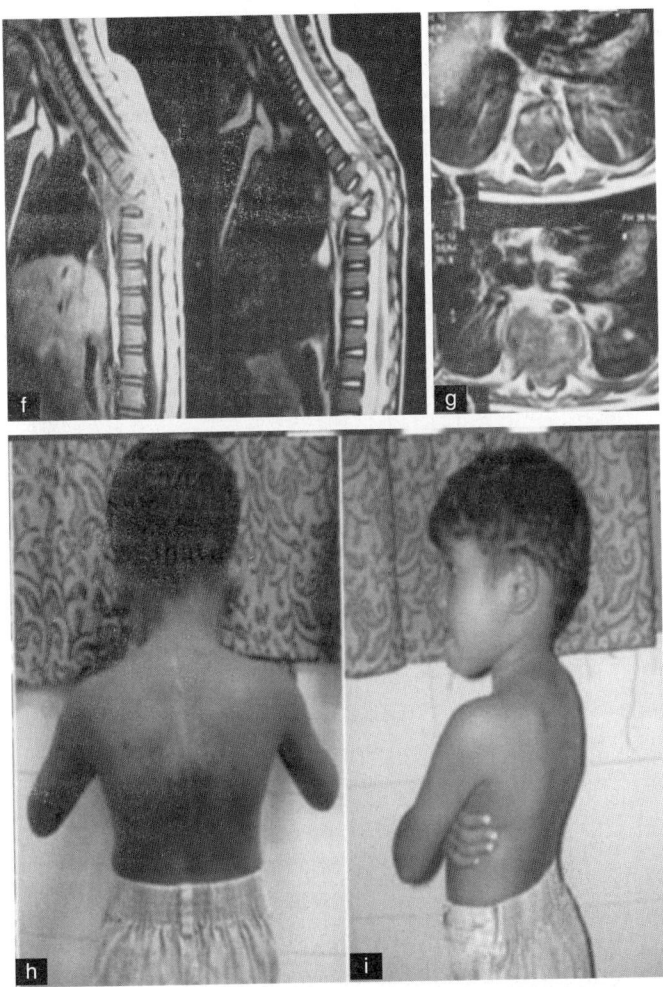

A 3-year-old female of spinal TB of D4–D8 with kyphosis. Preoperative clinical photograph (Fig. a) shows kyphosis of mid-dorsal spine. AP and lateral radiographs (Figs b, c) show involvement of multiple vertebrae at dorsal region. CT scan (mid-sagittal reconstructed image) and axial images (Figs d, e) show complete destruction of D5–D8 vertebrae with fragmentation of vertebral body. T1WI and T2WI sagittal scan (Fig. f) show paravertebral liquid collection of pus. T2WI and spinal cord compression. Axial images (Fig. g) show paravertebral pus collection. The patient was operated with anterolateral decompression and posterior Hartshill instrumentation and deformity correction. The follow-up postoperative clinical photographs (Figs h, i) showing correction of deformity and surgical scar mark.

Case 16: TB spine in a child with kyphotic deformity

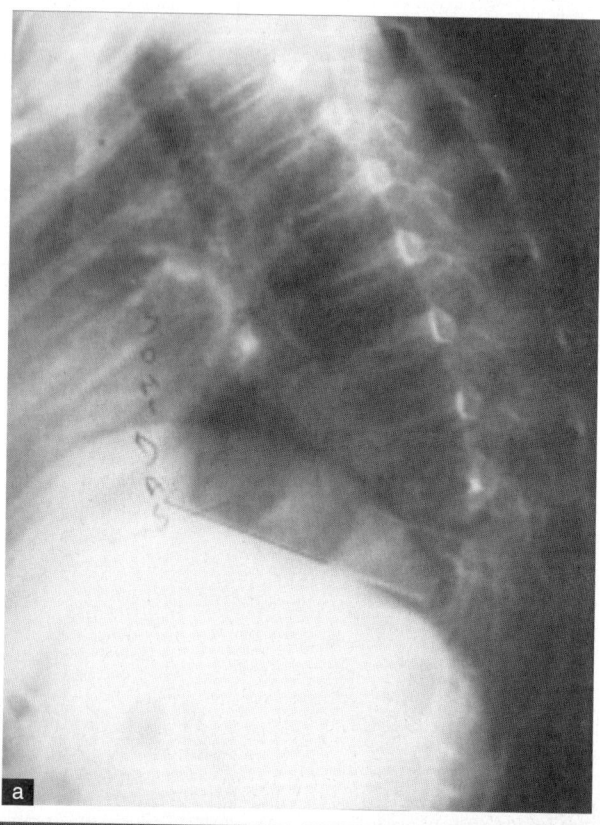

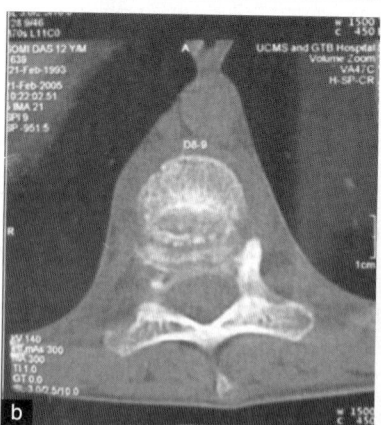

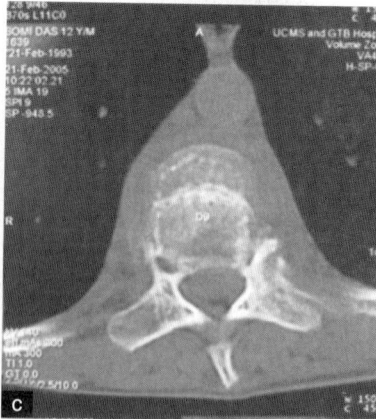

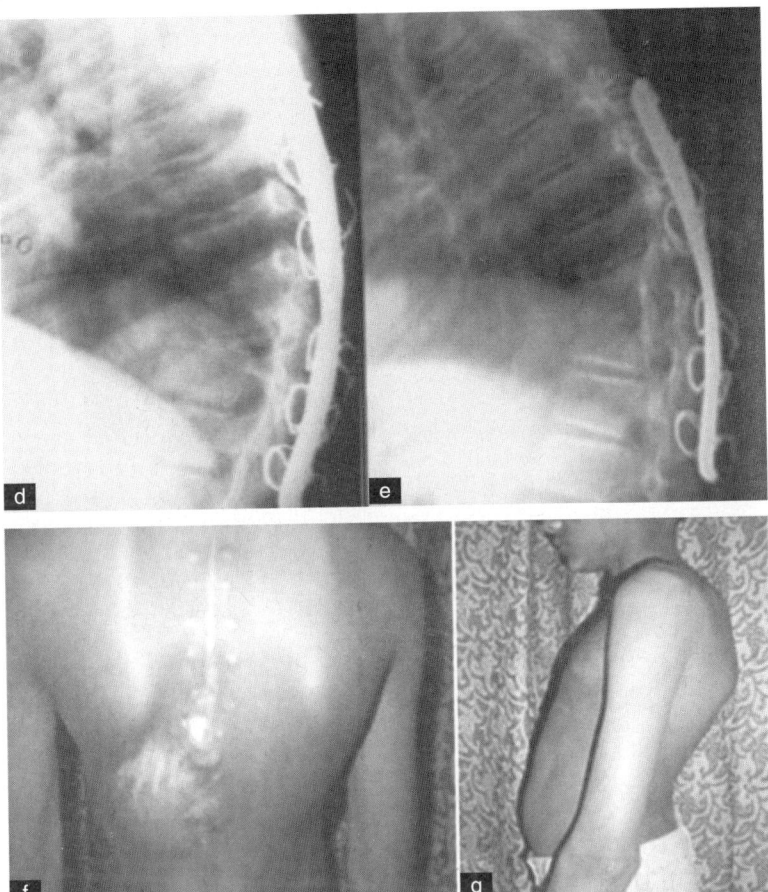

A 13-year-old male presented with spinal tuberculosis D8–D9 with angular kphosis and no neurological deficit. Lateral radiograph (Fig. a) shows collapse of D8 vertebra with angular kyphosis at dorsal region. The axial images (Figs b, c) show involvement of D8 and D9 vertebrae. Patient was operated for deformity correction by extrapleural anterolateral decompression, and posterior Hartshill instrumentation. The immediate postoperative and 2 years follow-up radiographs (Figs d, e) show correction of deformity and fusion of affected vertebrae. The clinical photographs (Figs f, g) show surgical scar mark and correction of deformity.

Case 17: TB spine in a child with kyphotic deformity

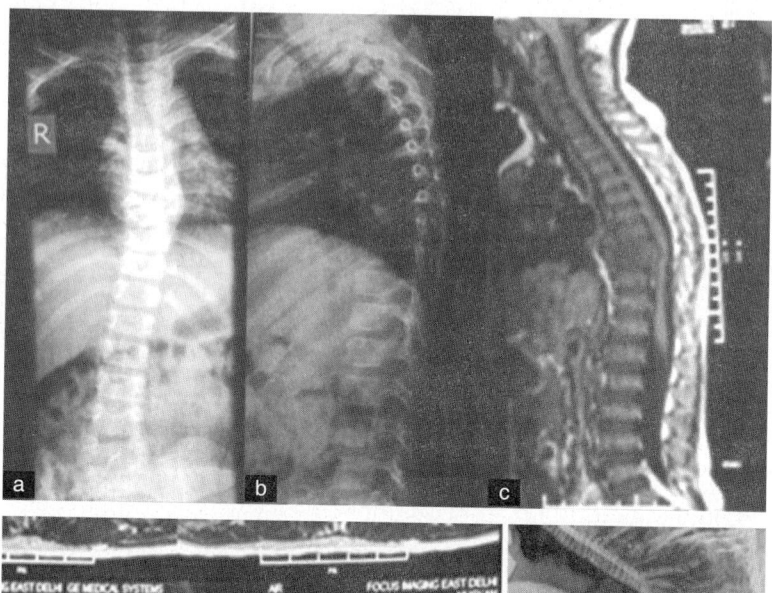

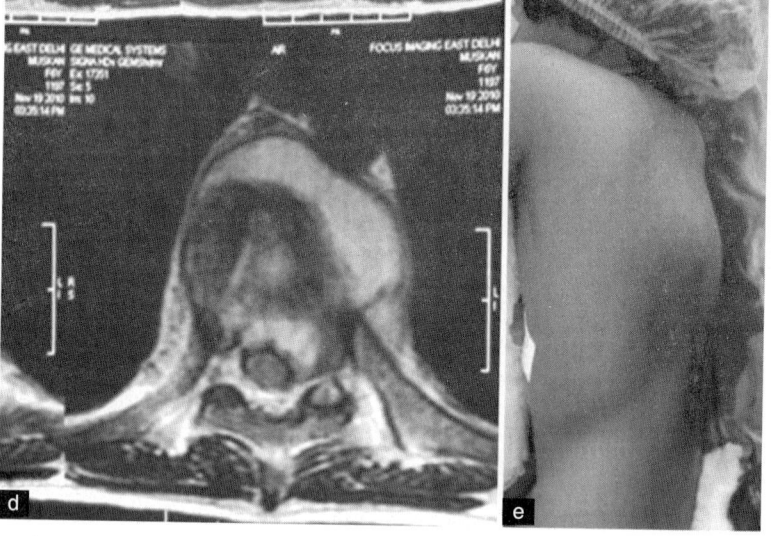

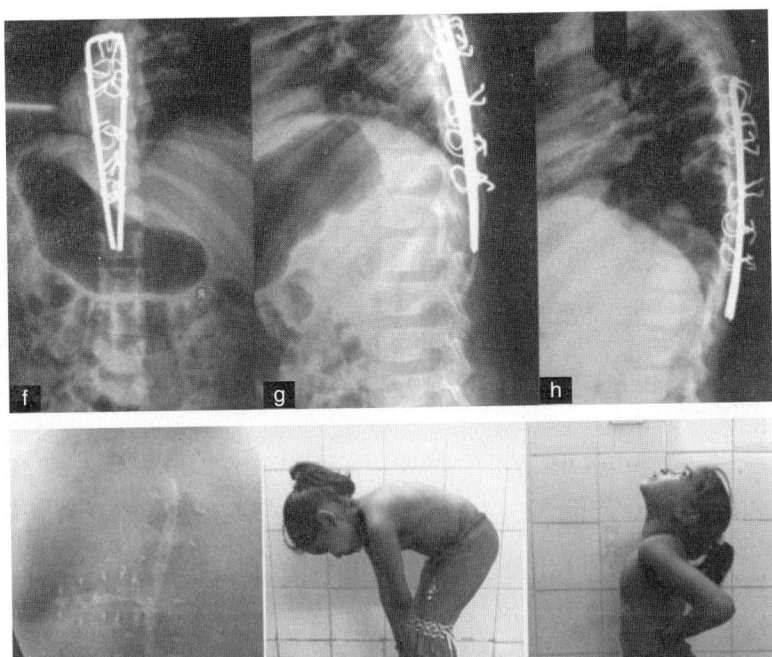

A 6-year-old female, of spinal TB D7–D9 with kyphotic defomity and no neurological deficit. AP and lateral radiographs (Figs a, b) show destruction of D8 vertebra with reduced disc space between D7–D8 and D8–D9 vertebrae. T1WI mid-sagittal and T2WI axial scan (Figs c, d) show destruction of D8 vertebra with pre- and paravertebral collection showing hypointense signal in T1WI and bright signal in T2WI. Preoperative clinical photograph (Figs e) showing kyphotic deformity. Patient was operated for deformity correction by extrapleural anterolateral approach and posterior Hartshill instrumentation. Postoperative AP and lateral radiographs (Figs f, g) lateral radiograph (Fig. h) at one year followup showing correction of kyphosis. Post-operative clinical photographs (Figs i–k) at one year follow-up show healed scar and well-corrected kyphotic deformity

Case 18: TB cervical spine with severe kyphotic deformity in a child

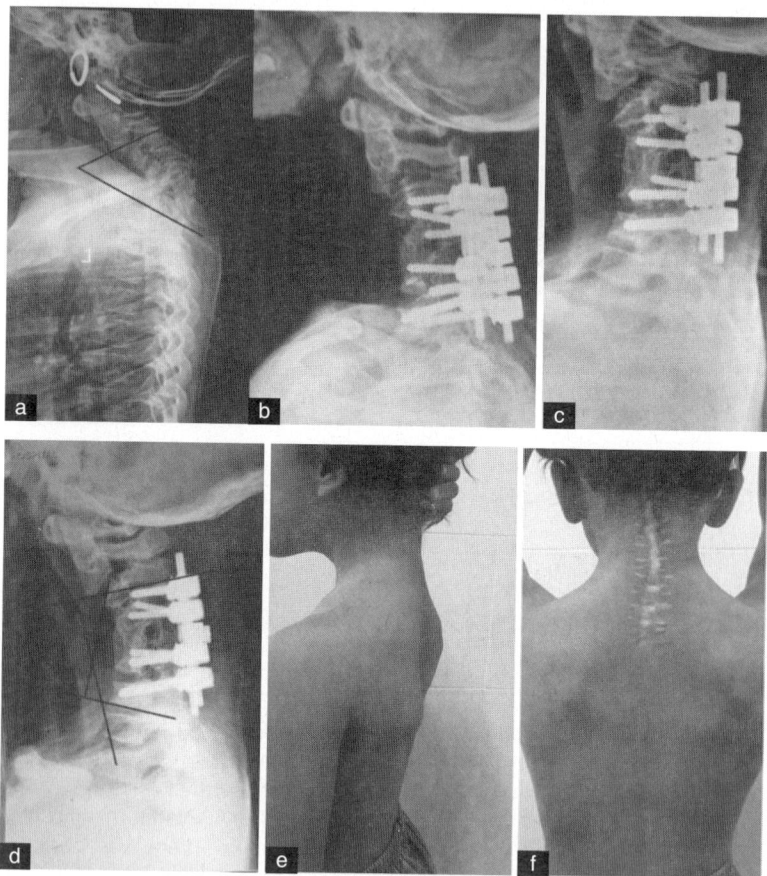

Case of spinal TB C4–C7 in a 7-year-old child. Figure (a) shows lateral radiograph of cervical spine showing involvement of C3–C7 vertebrae with complete destruction of C5 and C6 vertebral bodies with modified Konstam angle of 45°. The patient was placed on head halter traction for 2 weeks which corrected kyphotic deformity to some degree. Patient was taken for lateral mass fixation as first stage followed by second stage anterior bone grafting. Figs (b–d) show postoperative X-rays at 3 months, 6 months and 21 months showing fusion of bone graft and modified Konstam angle of 25° at final follow-up. The clinical photographs (Figs e, f) at 21 months follow-up show scar and well-corrected deformity.

Case 19: TB spine with severe lumbar kyphosis

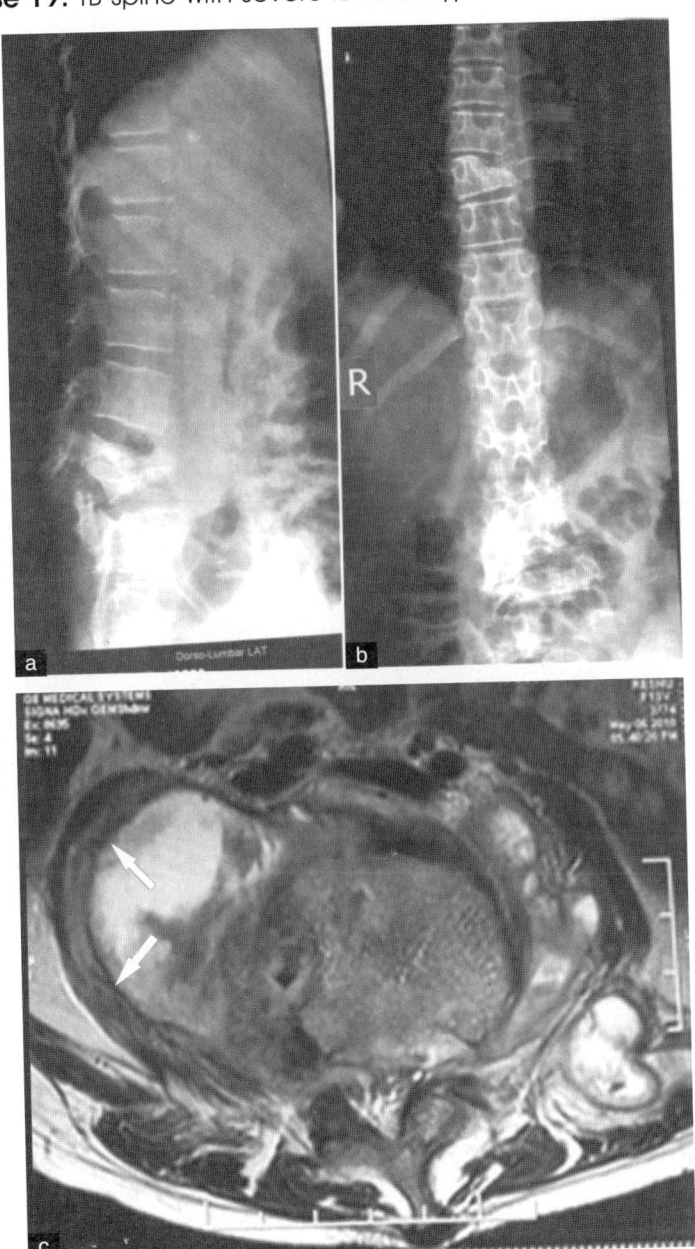

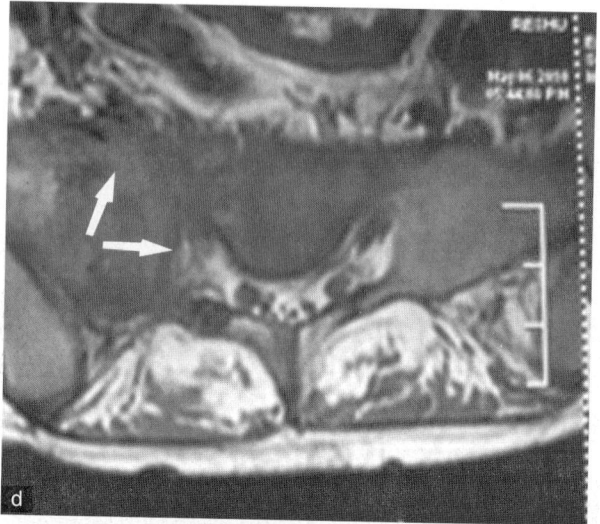

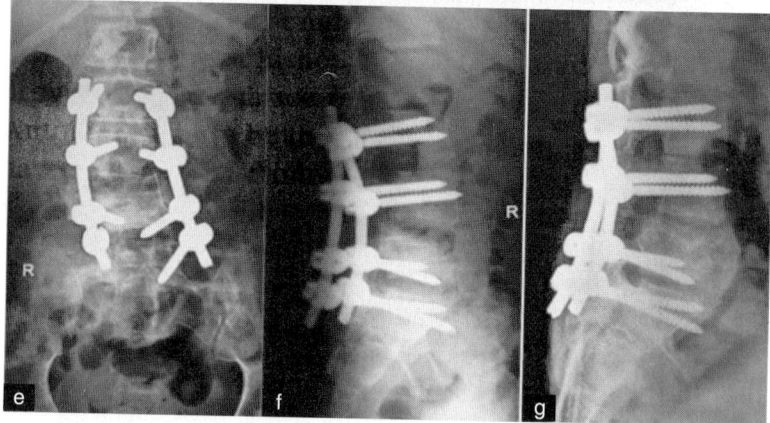

A 13-year-old female presented with history of low backache and lumbar kyphosis with no neurological deficit of 6 months duration. Lateral and AP radiographs (Figs a, b) showing destruction of L4 and L5 vertebrae with severe lumbar kyphosis. T2WI and T1WI axial scan (Figs c, d) show wet lesion (bright signal in T2WI and low signal in T1WI) depicting prevertebral collection of pus and right psoas abscess. The patient was operated by midline posterior approach, transpedicular debridement of anterior lesion along with kyphotic deformity correction and stabilization by pedicle instrumentation. Immediate postoperative radiographs (Figs e, f) show correction of lumbar kyphosis. Two-year follow-up X-ray (Fig. g) shows bony fusion of L4 and L5 vertebrae. The lumbar kyphosis is corrected and well preserved.

Case 20: TB spine in a child with kyphotic deformity

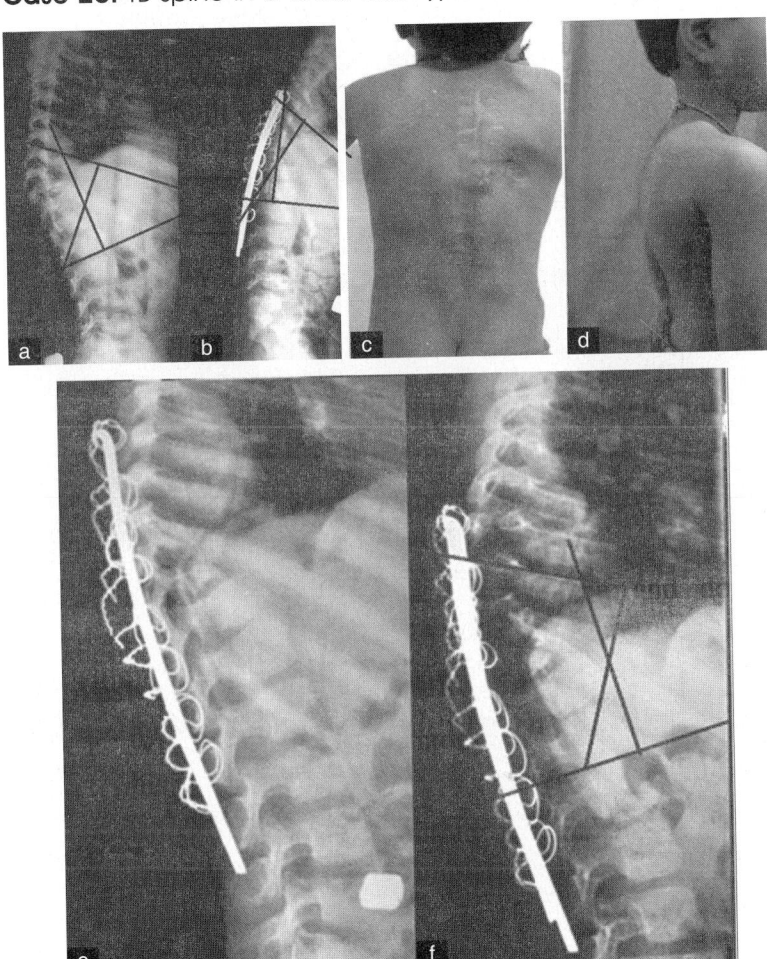

Case of spinal TB D8–D10 with kyphosis in 4-year-old male child showing (Fig. a) preoperative lateral radiograph with destruction of D8–D10 vertebral bodies and modified Konstam angle of 40°. Patient was taken for anterior decompression and deformity correction by extrapleural anterolateral approach and posterior instrumentation by Hartshill sub-laminar wiring. (Fig. b) Immediate postoperative lateral radiograph with modified Konstam angle of 22°. Postoperative clinical photograph (Figs c, d) showing 'T' shaped incision and corrected deformity. Lateral radiographs (Figs e, f) at 12 and 24 months follow-up with final angle of 30°.

Case 21: TB spine with severe kyphotic deformity with neural deficit

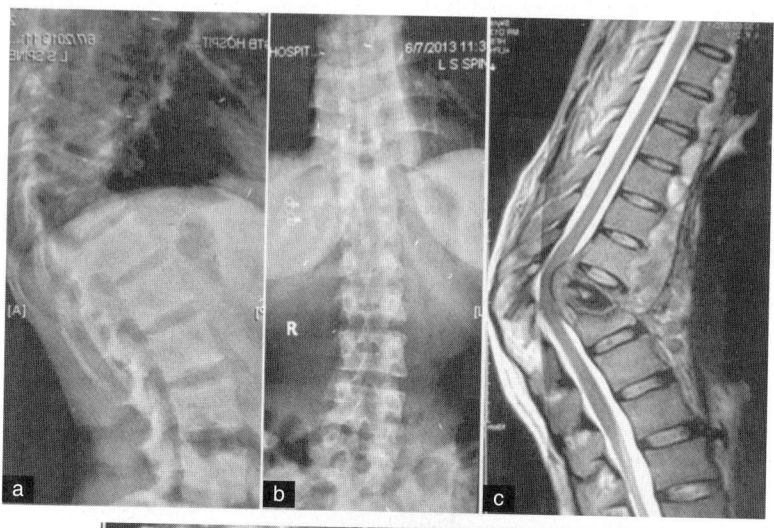

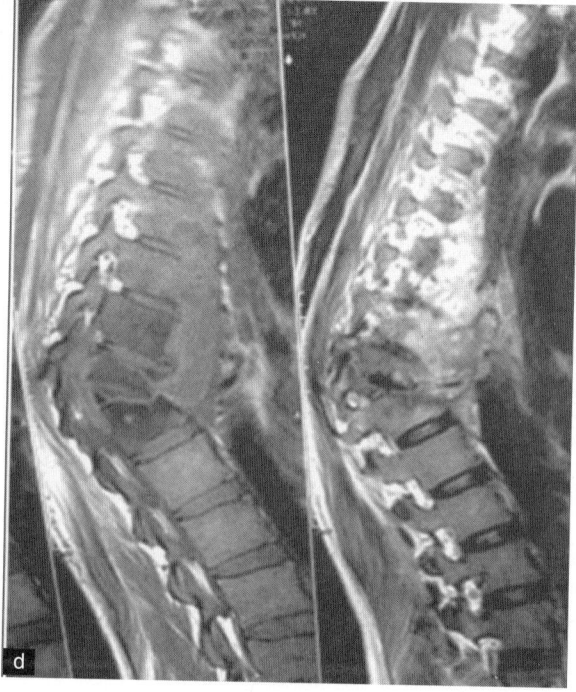

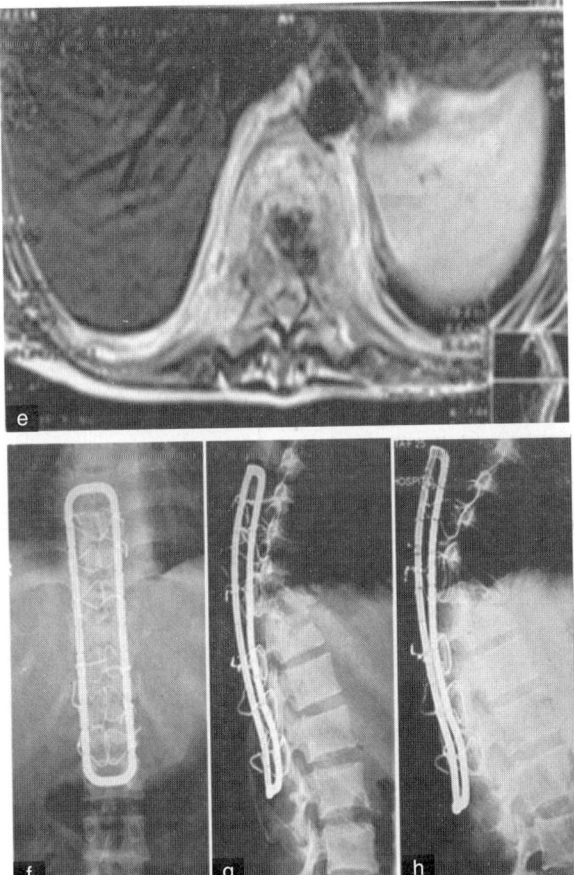

A 25-year-old female of tuberculosis of spine D8–D11 with grade II para-plegia of one year duration. Lateral and AP radiographs (Figs a, b) show destruction of D8 to D11 vertebrae with angular kyphosis. T2WI and T1WI sagittal scan (Figs c, d) show complete destruction of D9 vertebra with significant compression of spinal cord. The prevertebral collection (liquid) can be appreciated in front of at least 6 vertebral bodies above the D10 level. Axial scan (Fig. e) shows collection in paravertebral and in psoas and compromised neural arch. The anterior decompression, posterior column shortening, Hartshill instrumentation with anterior and posterior bone grafting was performed by extrapleural anterolateral approach and patient started on category I ATT. Postoperative radiographs (Figs f, g) with deformity correction. One year follow-up radiograph (Fig. h) shows bony fusion. Patient had complete neurological recovery.

Case 22: TB spine with kyphotic deformity

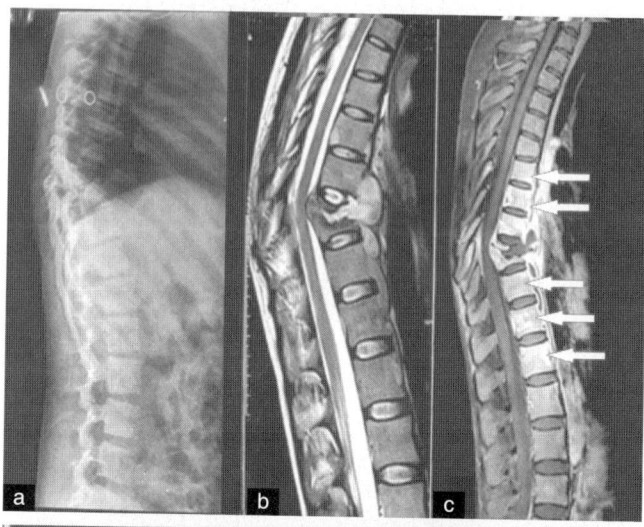

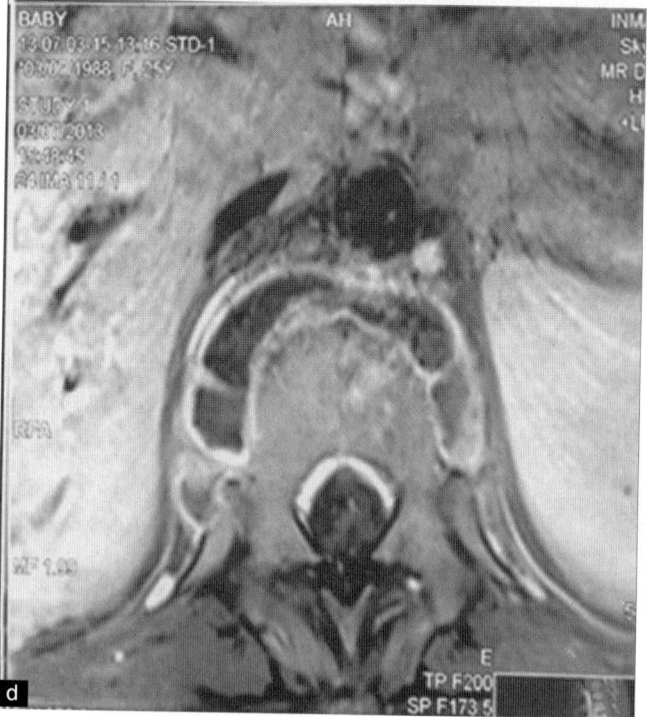

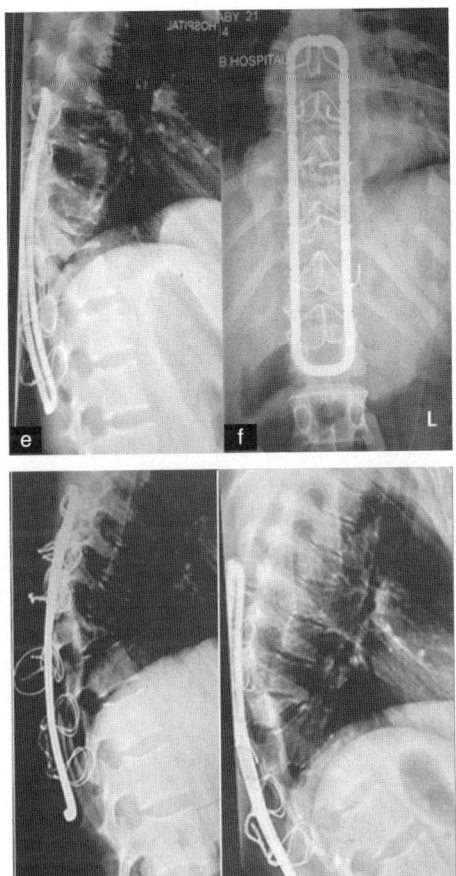

A 21-year-old female with complaints of pain and deformity in dorsolumbar region with angular kyphosis and grade I paraplegia. Lateral radiograph (Fig. a) shows destruction of D9 and D10 vertebrae with obliterated disk space. T2WI mid-sagittal scan (Fig. b) shows destruction of two vertebral bodies with prevertebral collection (bright signal) and compression of spinal cord by retropulsed granulation tissue. T1WI mid-sagittal contrast enhanced image (Fig. c) shows enhancement of 3 vertebral bodies on each side of D9 and D10 verebrae suggesting a long segment disease. The axial scan (Fig. d) shows septate pre- and paravertebral collection with rim enhancement. Anterolateral decompression with posterior instrumentation with Hartshill and bone grafting was performed. Immediate postoperative radiographs (Figs e, f) and follow-up at 6 months (Fig. g) and one year (Fig. h) show healing of the lesion.

Case 23: TB spine in a child with severe kyphotic deformity

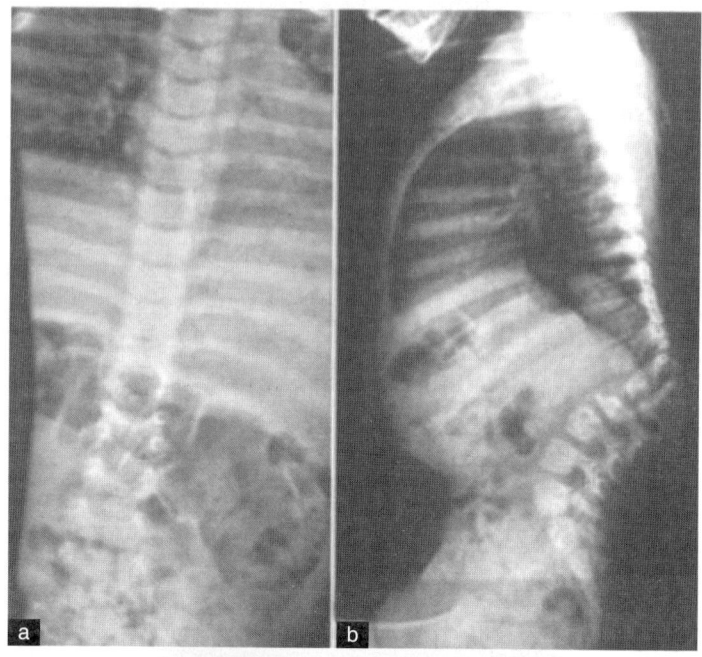

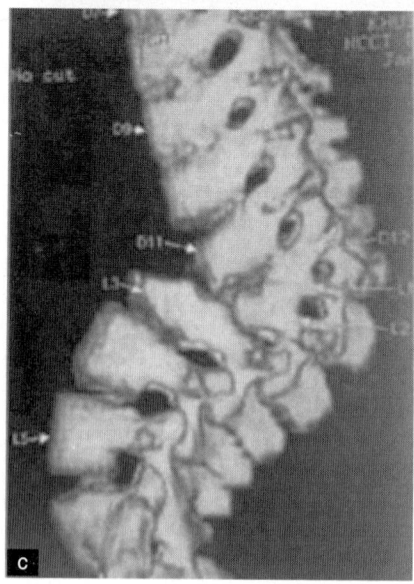

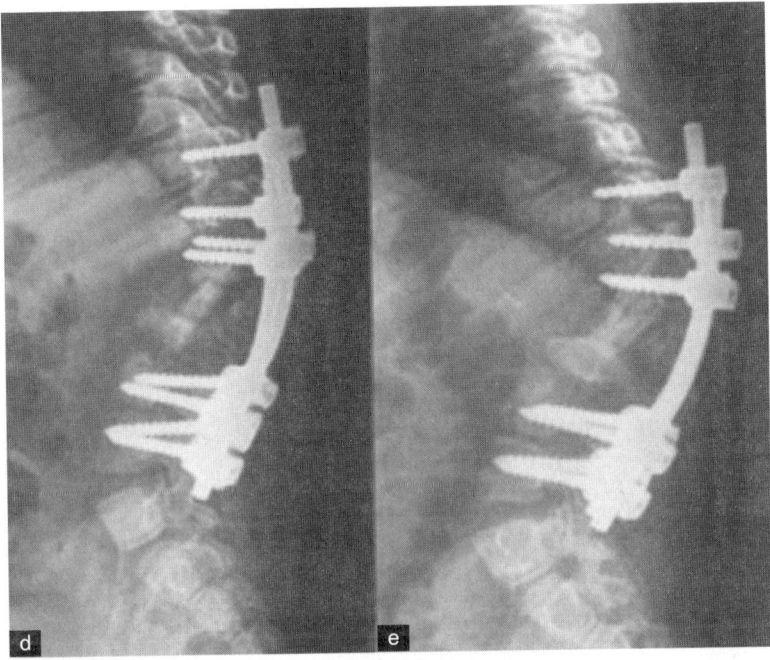

A 9-year-old female presented with diagnosis of spinal tuberculosis and rounded kyphosis of dorsolumbar junction without neurological deficit. AP and lateral radiographs (Figs a, b) show severe kyphotic deformity at dorsolumbar junction with involvement of multiple vertebrae (D11–L3). 3D reconstructed CT scan (Fig. c) sagittal image shows destruction and fusion of D11–L2 and partly L3 vertebral bodies leading to kyphosis. Patient was operated for deformity correction and posterior instrumentation and fusion with iliac crest bone graft. 2 weeks later, anterior gap grafting was performed by extrapleural anterolateral approach. The fibular graft was used to bridge the gap. Lateral radiographs at 6 and 18 months (Figs d, e) follow-up show correction of kyphosis with fusion of graft. Although the screw backout at highest level was appreciated, the patient was nursed in lateral position in immediate postoperative period as lying supine was painful due to pedicle prominence in a thin child. The minerva jacket was given for 3 months after anterior bone grafting.

Case 24: TB spine in a child with kyphotic deformity

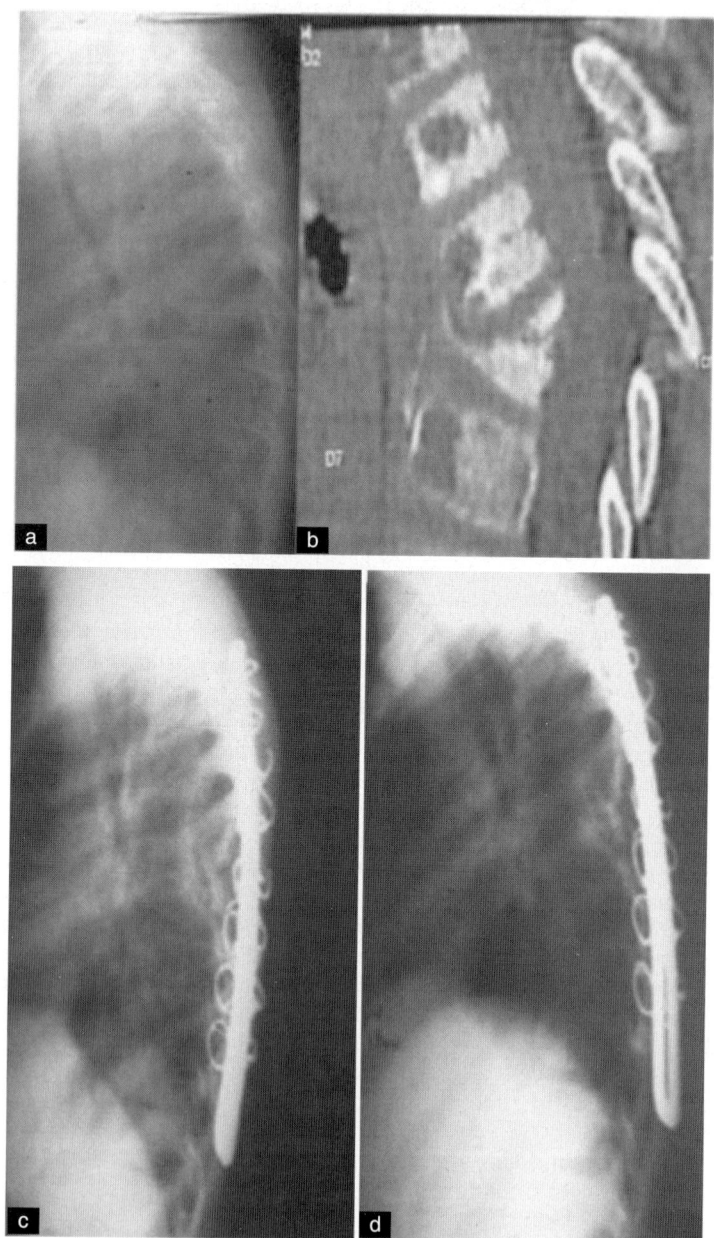

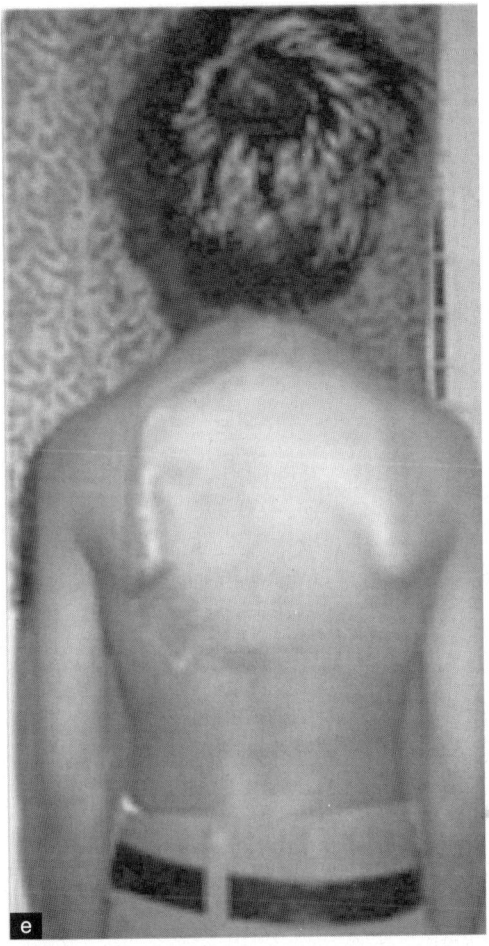

An 11-year-old boy with spinal tuberculosis of D4–D6 with kyphosis and without neurological deficit. Lateral radiograph (Fig. a) shows destruction of D4–D6 vertebrae. Sagittal reconstructed image on CT scan (Fig. b) shows destruction of D4–D6 vertebrae with D5 completely destroyed leading to dorsal kyphosis. Anterolateral decompression along with posterior instrumentation and deformity correction was performed by extrapleural anterolateral approach via C shaped incision. Immediate postoperative radiograph (Fig. c) shows correction of kyphosis. The follow-up radiograph (Fig. d) at two years shows bony fusion and maintained correction. Clinical photograph (Fig. e) at two years follow-up shows correction of kyphosis and scar of classical 'C' shaped incision.

Case 25: TB of lumbar spine with kyphotic deformity

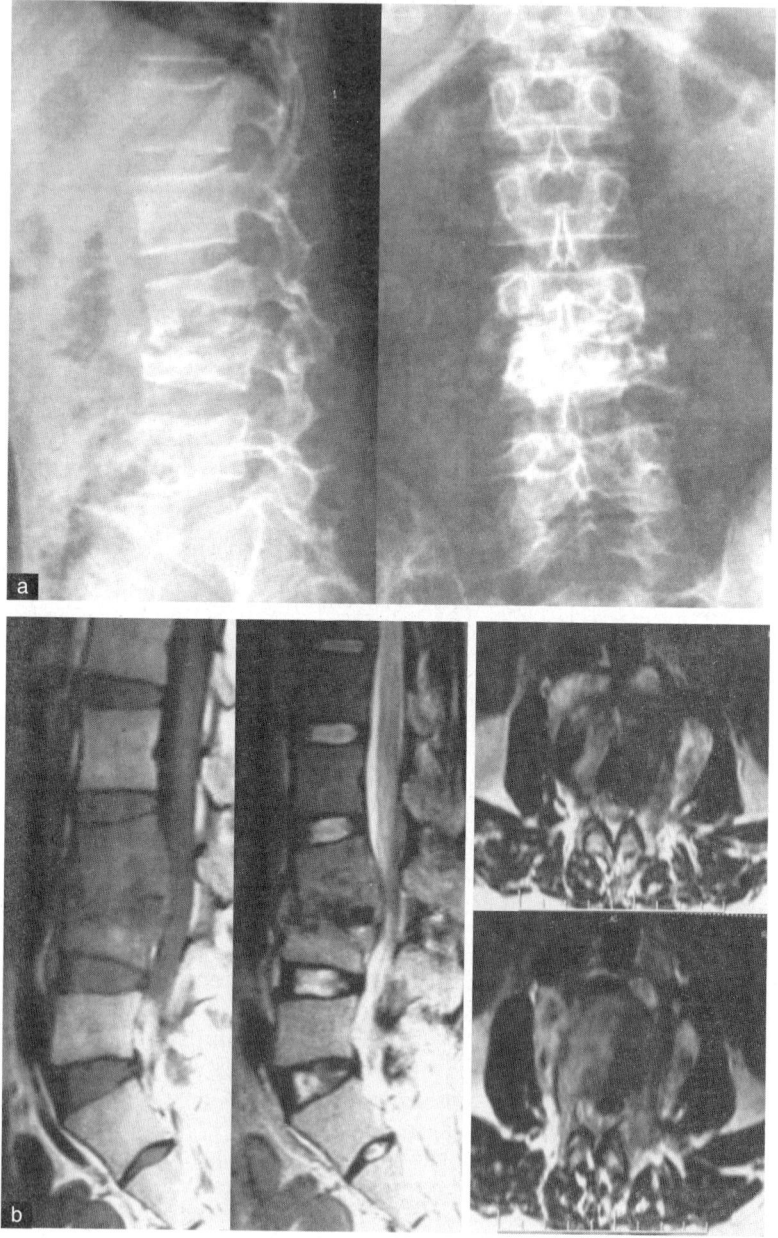

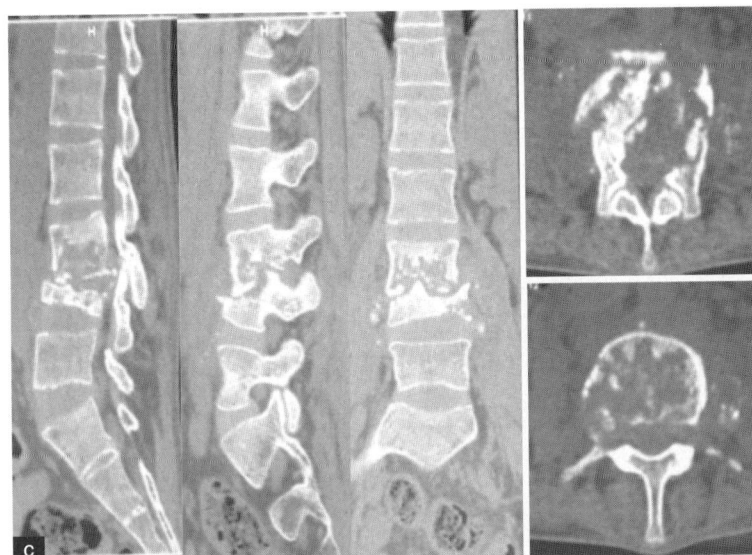

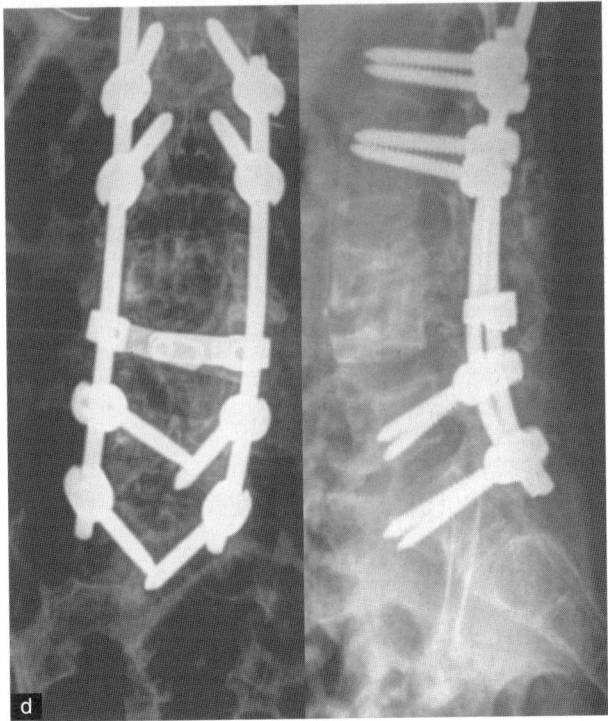

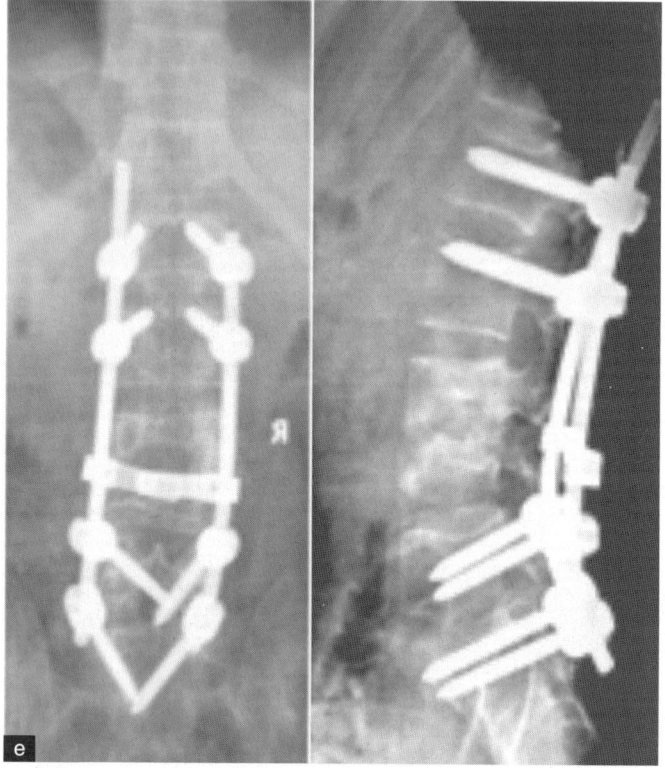

A 24-year-old male presented with complaints of low back pain for past 18 months and decreased sensation in bilateral lower limbs for past 6 months. He had associated constitutional symptoms (fever and decreased appetite with weight loss). On examination, there was lumbar kyphus at L3 and L4 levels with tenderness with no palpable swelling. On neural examination, motor system was intact, with mute plantars. Tone was normal but there was sensory deficit below L1. Bladder and bowel were not involved. Patient was on ATT for past 2 months. Plain X-ray (Fig. a) showed localized osteopenia, obliteration of the disk space between L3 and L4 and reduction in height of both vertebral bodies producing kyphotic deformity. MRI mid-sagittal T1WI, T2WI and axial T1WI and T2WI images (Fig. b) showed features suggestive of infective pathology with reduced canal diameter causing thecal compression. CT (Fig. c) showing features of tuberculosis with fragmentary type of destruction. Patient was taken for posterior decompression by laminectomy, posterior stabilization and deformity correction using pedicle screws stabilization system (Fig. d). At 1 year follow-up (Fig. e), there was no loss of correction and showed radiological features of healing.

Case 26: TB spine in a child with kyphotic deformity

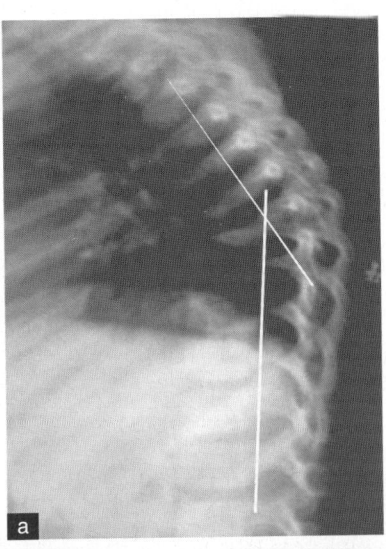

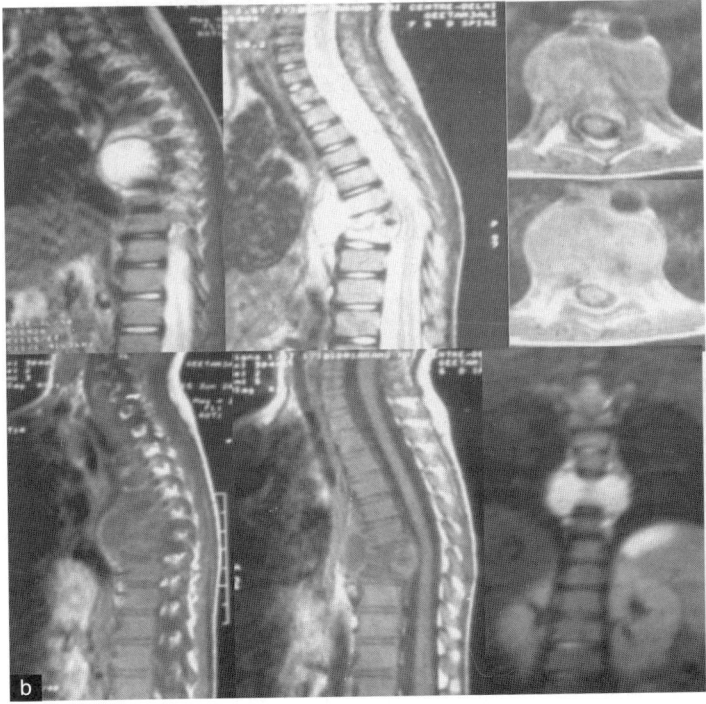

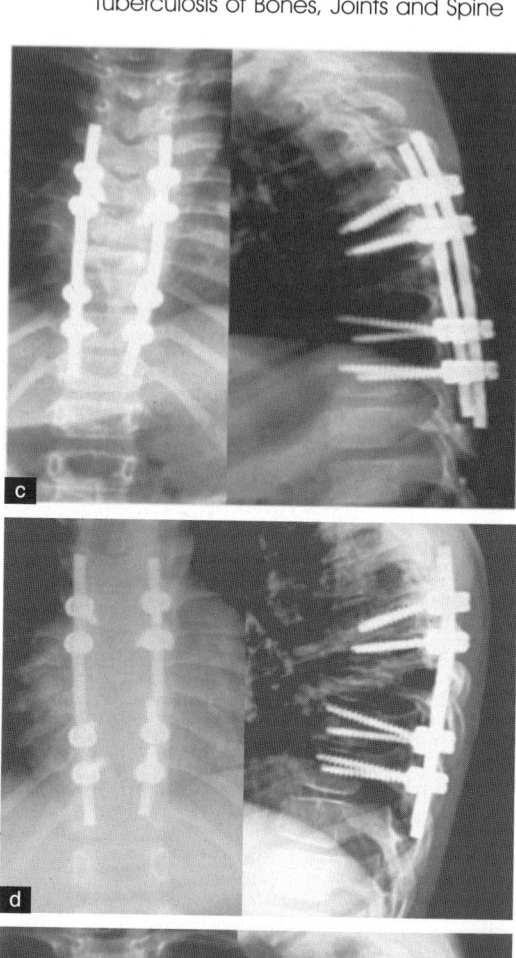

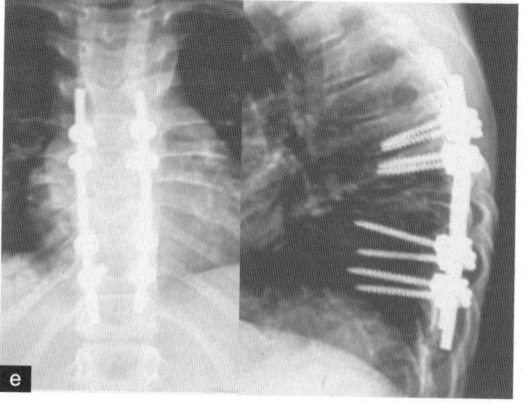

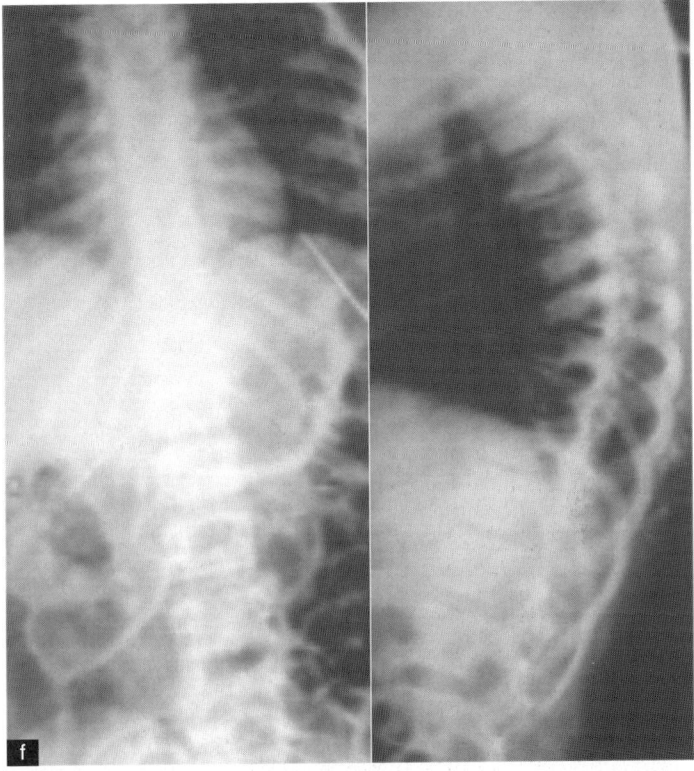

A 5-year-old female presented with complaints of pain in mid-back for past 6 months and deformity in back for past 2 months. Patient was started on ATT at another setup and was on bed rest, but the deformity was increasing progressively. On clinical examination, patient had an angular kyphus at D7 and D8 levels which was tender on palpation. Patient had no neurological deficit. Plain radiograph (Fig. a) AP and lateral view showed decreased disk space between D6 and D8 with loss of D7 with kyphotic deformity. On MRI (Fig. b), T1WI and T2WI show hypointense and hyper-intense paravertebral collection extending from D5 to D9. Axial and coronal sections also were suggestive of infective etiology. In view of the progression of kyphus, patient was operated for kyphus correction with stabilization by pedicle screws (Fig. c). Patient was continued on ATT with no neural deficit post-operatively. Lesion healed after 18 months of ATT. Patient had complaints of implant impingement (Fig. d) which were removed after 5 years of primary surgery (Figs. e, f). One could appreciate increase in the anterior body height with growth as growth potential of vertebral body was not deranged.

Case 27: TB spine dorsolumbar junction with kyphotic deformity

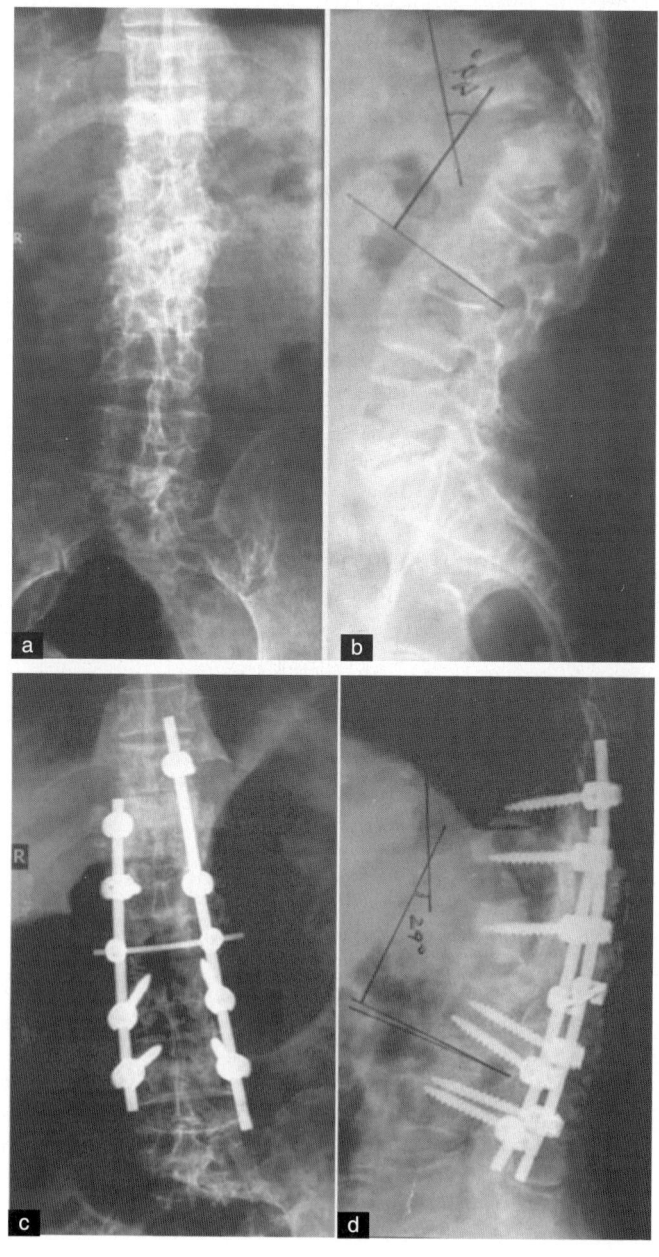

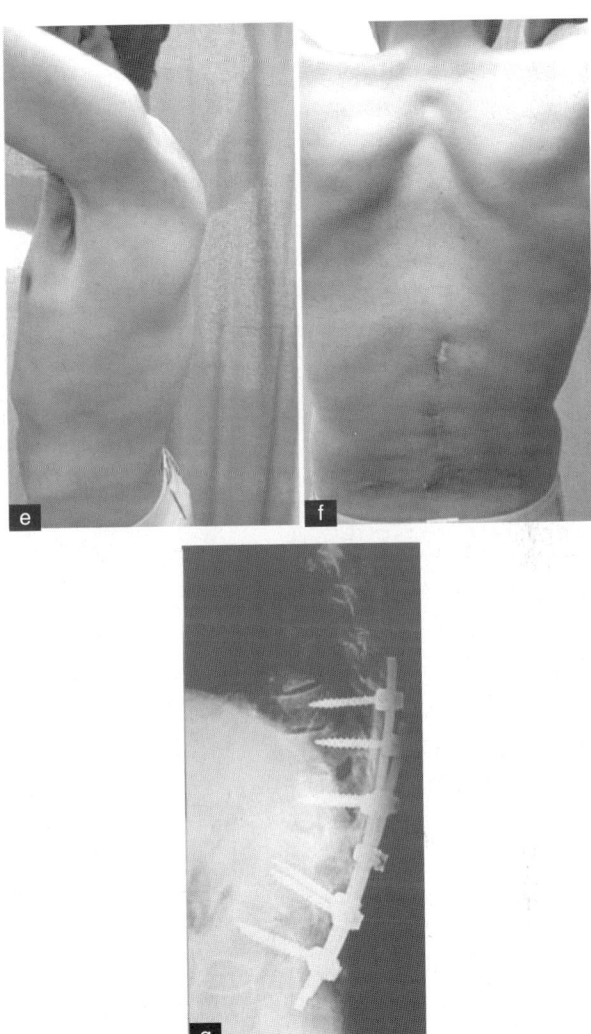

A 46-year-old male of spinal tuberculosis D11–L4 region with grade III paraplegia. AP and lateral radiographs (Figs a, b) show destruction of multiple vertebrae at dorsolumbar junction with kyphosis of 49°. The patient was operated by midline posterior approach, posterior column shortening and internal fixation with posterior pedicle screw instrumentation. Post-operative AP and lateral radiographs (Figs c, d) show corrected angle of 29°. Clinical photographs (Figs e, f) at one year follow-up showing correction of kyphosis. Radiograph at 3 years follow-up (Fig. g) shows fusion of affected vertebrae.

Case 28: TB spine with presumptive drug resistance

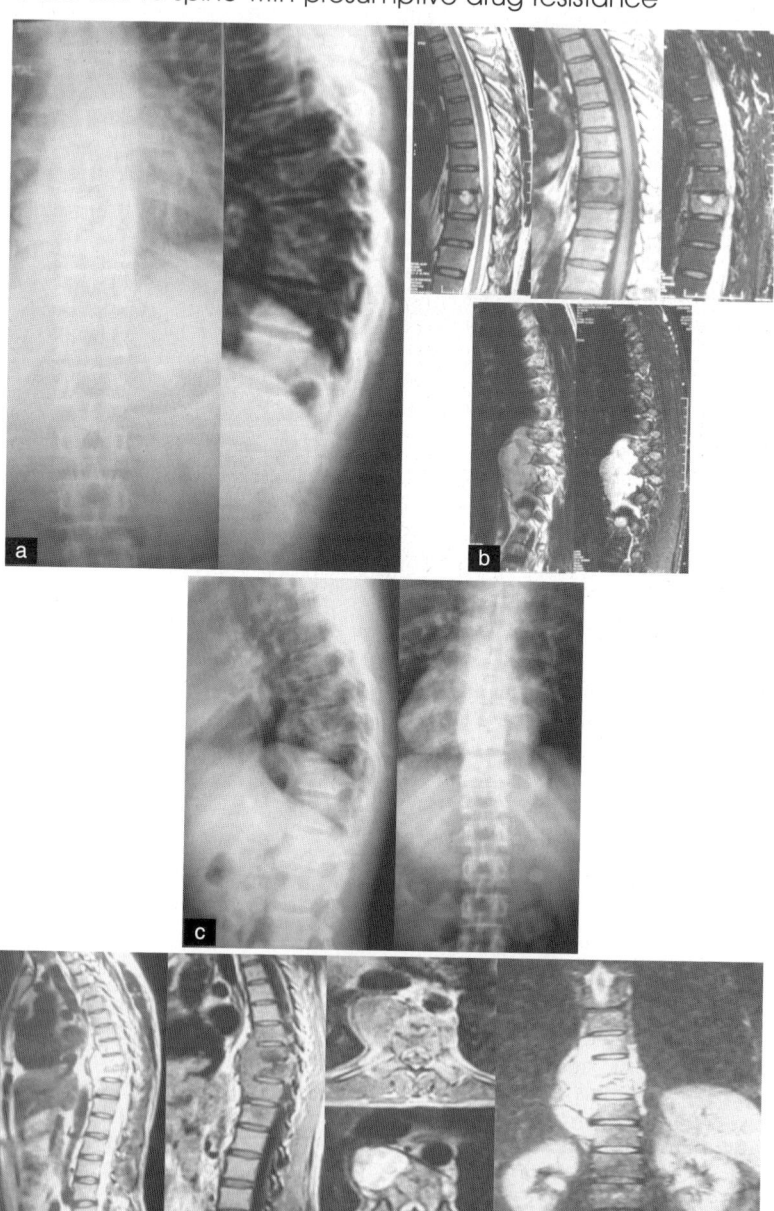

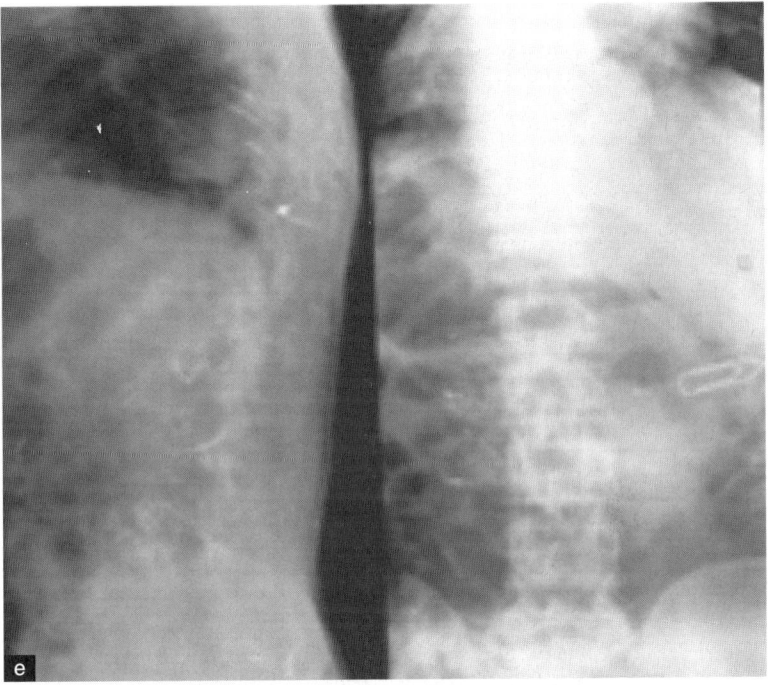

A 32-year-old male patient had history of pulmonary tuberculosis for which he took ATT for 6 months. Just after completion of his treatment, he developed low back pain. Plain X-rays (Fig. a) showed reduced disk space between D9 and D10 with regional osteopenia. His MRI (Fig. b) T2WI and T1WI showed marrow edema in the body of D10 involving the disk space between D9 and D10. There was associated collection in paravertebral space (hypointense on T1WI and hyperintense on T2WI). With the classical features of TB spine, a presumptive diagnosis was made and the patient was continued on ATT. After one year of back pain, patient presented at GTBH. The pain was persistent, more during night and associated with low grade fever. His ESR was 52 mm/hr with positive CRP. Patient had no known co-morbidities. There was no neural deficit or deformity. A repeat X-ray (Fig. c) and MRI (Fig. d) showed no signs of healing and increase in the size of collection (on MRI). Considering it to be therapeutically refractory, costotransversectomy was performed draining 30 ml of thick straw-colored pus (Fig. e, postoperative X-rays). It was sent for DST which proved drug resistance for rifampicin and INH and patient has been started on second line ATT as per sensitivity studies.

Case 29: TB spine with clinical drug resistance

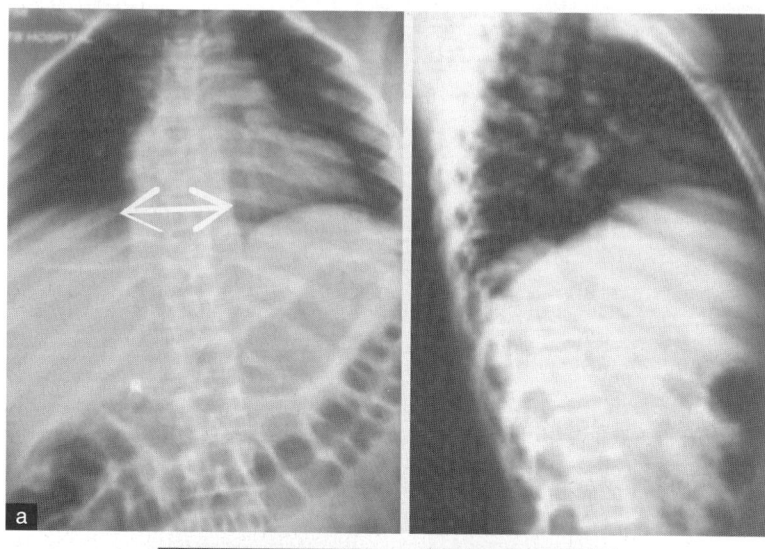

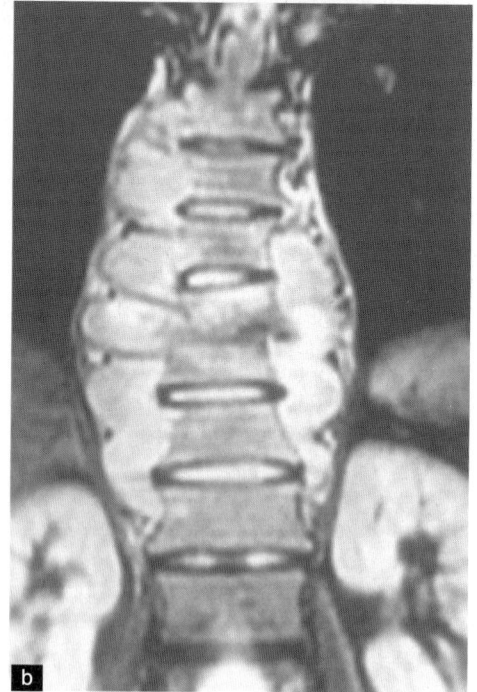

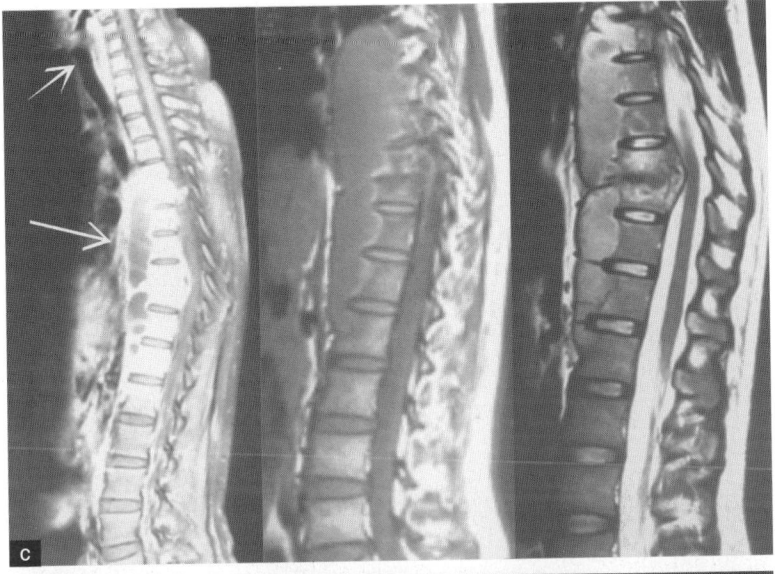

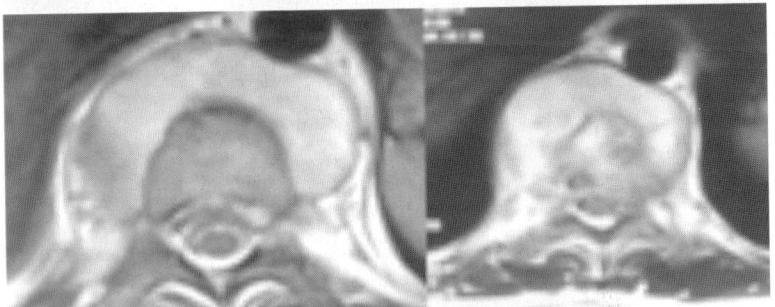

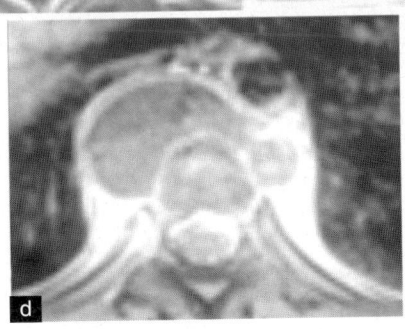

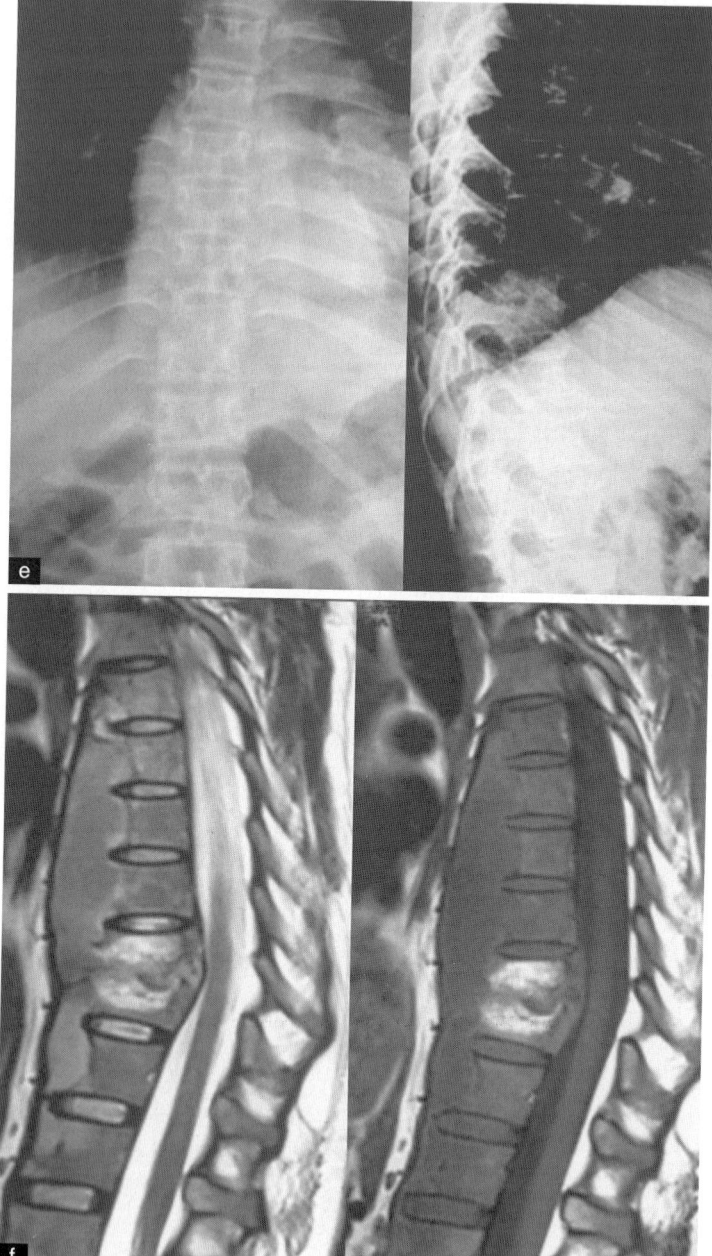

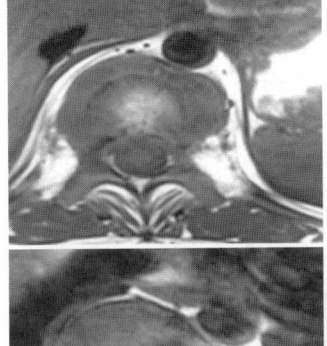

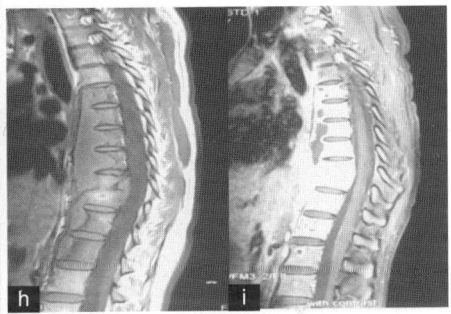

An 18-year-old female patient presented with complaints of low backache for past 1½ years. There was associated low grade fever, decreased appetite and loss of weight. History of night cries was present. On examination, there was tenderness present at D9 and D10 levels with a palpable knuckle. There was no neural deficit. On plain X-ray (Fig. a) showed increased paravertebral shadow, reduced disk space between D9 and D10 and regional osteopenia. MRI showed (Figs b–d) contagious vertebral body disease with preserved intervertebral disk spaces, with large pre- and paravertebral loculated collection which was hypointense on T1WI and hyperintense on T2WI. The patient was started on ATT and advised bed rest with a presumptive diagnosis of TB spine. After 8 months of ATT, the paravertebral shadows persisted (Fig. e) and no sings of radiographic and MRI features of bone healing were noted. Considering the patient to be therapeutically refractory, costotransversectomy at D10 level was done and the tissue procured was sent for DST. But DST failed to prove drug resistance following which, patient was started on second-line ATT as clinical drug resistance. After 1½ years of presentation, a repeat contrast enhanced MRI (Figs f–i) showed persistence of disease. Hence, antero-lateral decompression was done and 10–15 ml of seropurulent fluid was evacuated and sent for repeat DST. But, no organism was grown on culture. Patient was kept on second-line ATT for 30 months as she showed improvement in general condition, back pain and ESR. Patient is still under follow-up.

Case 30: TB spine dorsolumbar spine with drug resistance

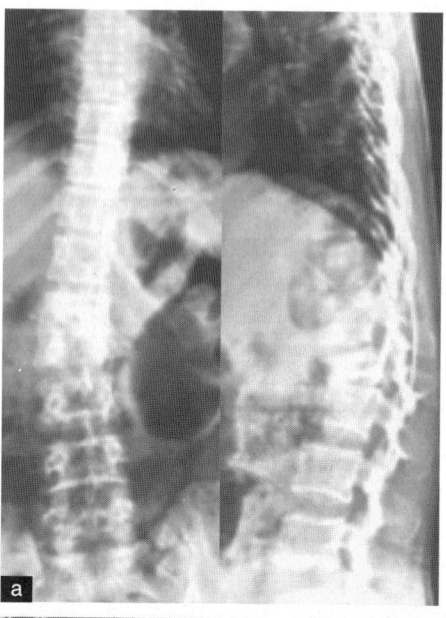

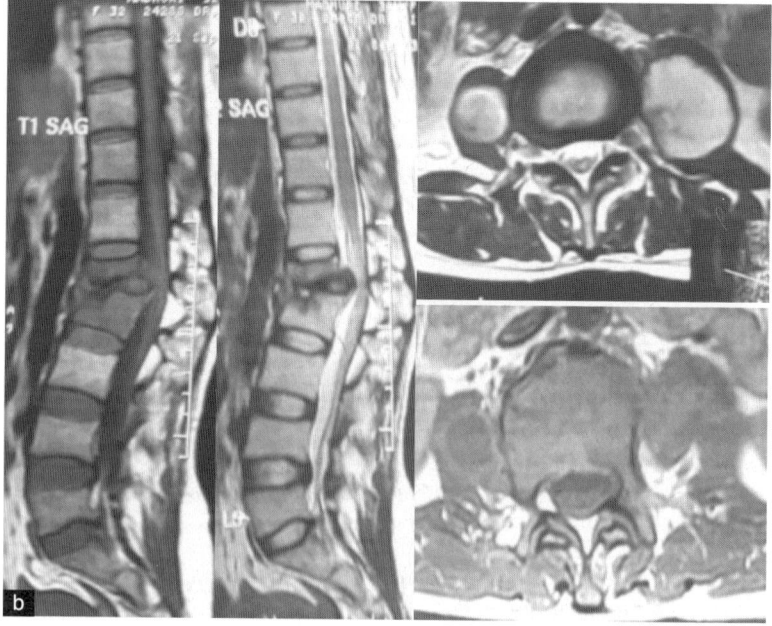

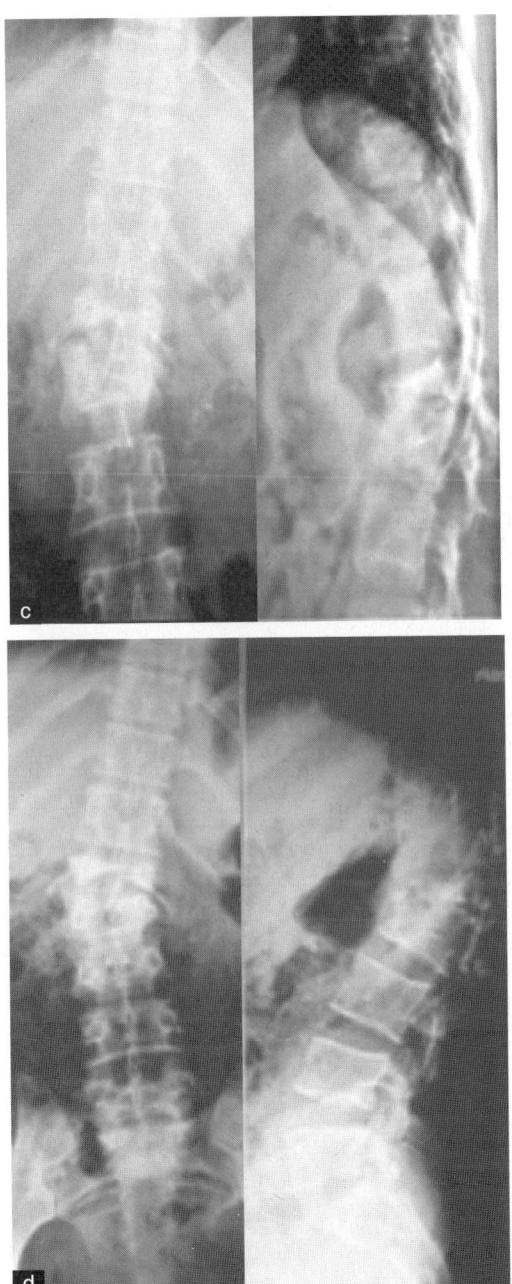

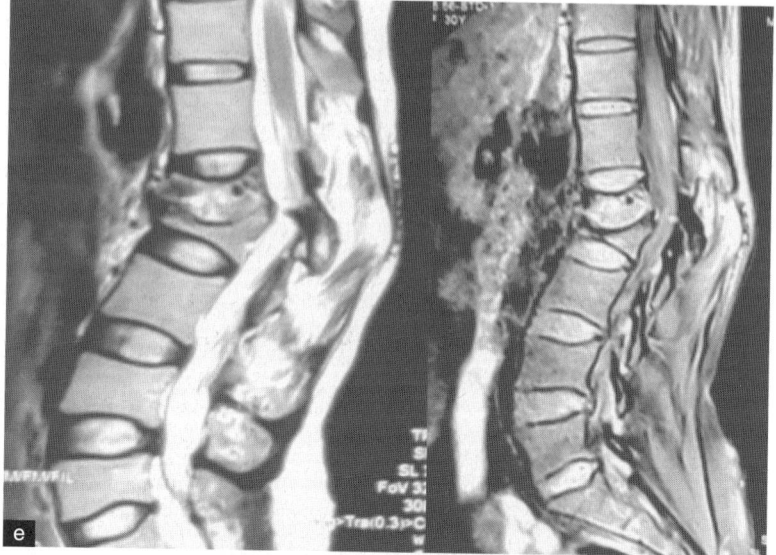

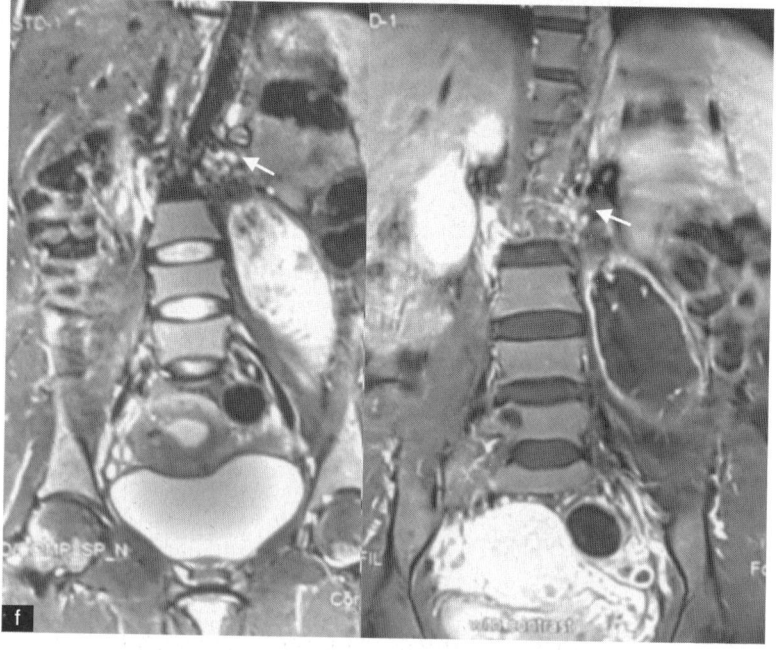

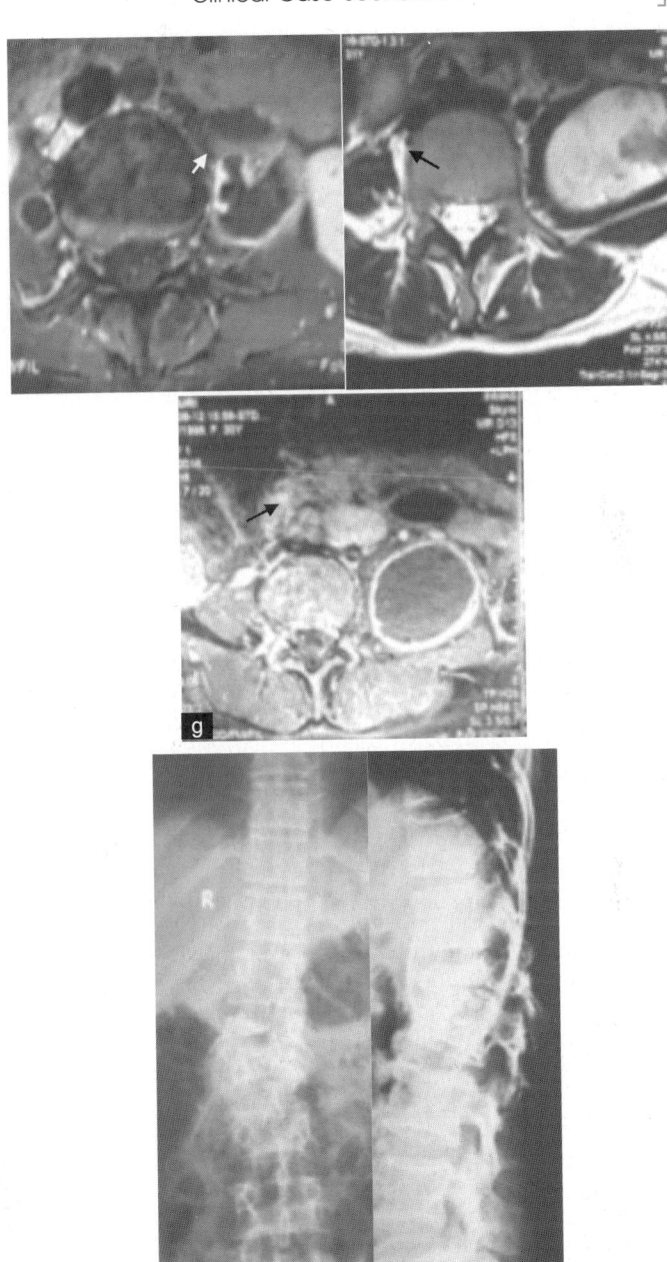

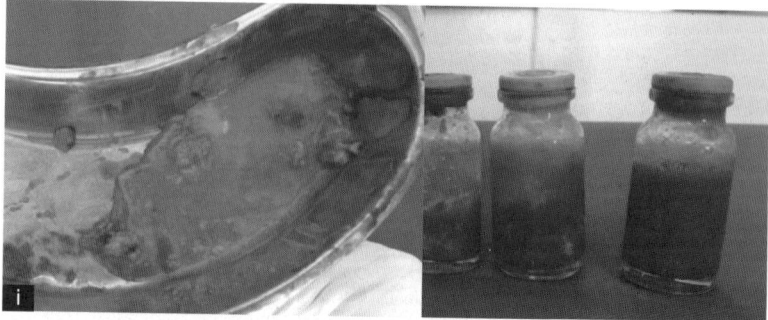

A 32-year-old female presented with complaints of low backache for past one and half years, low grade fever with loss of appetite. There was no history of trauma, tuberculosis or any co-morbidities. Patient was on ATT for past 1 year, started by an orthopedic surgeon in other institute, on the basis of clinicoradiological picture. On examination, she had tenderness at L1–L3, with loss of lumbar lordosis and no neural deficit. Her previous X-rays (Fig. a) showed regional osteopenia, with loss of disk space between L1 and L2 and loss of height of both vertebral bodies, producing kyphosis. Her new X-rays after one year of ATT intake (Fig. c) showed persistent findings with increase in kyphosis. The MRI (Fig. b) mid-sagittal and axial sections;T1WI and T2WI showed destruction of L1 and L2 with anterior collapse, with altered marrow signals which are hypointense on T1WI and hyperintense on T2WI with end plate irregularity, causing cord compression and canal stenosis. With the diagnosis of TB spine, patient was advised strict bed rest and continued on ATT. After 2 years of total ATT intake, repeat X-rays (Fig. d) showed progression of kyphus, persistence of osteopenia, suggesting inadequate healing. Patient's deformity increased with radicular pain in right lower limb. Tenderness had reduced only partially with a palpable knuckle, but no neural deficit. Her ESR was 49 mm/hr while CRP was positive. Fresh MRI mid-sagittal T1WI and T2WI scan (Fig. e) showed progression of disease with increased destruction of L1 and L2, and increased collection. On administration of contrast, the paravertebral abscess showed rim enhancement (arrow; Fig. f, g). The clinicoradiological picture was suggestive of therapeutically refractory TB spine, hence anterior retroperitoneal decompression was done, 50 ml of thick pus was evacuated and bone graft from posterior iliac crest was placed between L1 and L2 (Fig. h). The pus (Fig. i) was sent for histopathological and drug sensitivity testing (DST). DST confirmed drug resistance to rifampicin and patient has been started on second-line drugs. She had no postoperative neural deficit. Her radicular pain has reduced substantially at 3 months follow-up.

Case 31: TB spine with delayed presentation (severe kyphotic deformity and severe paraplegia)

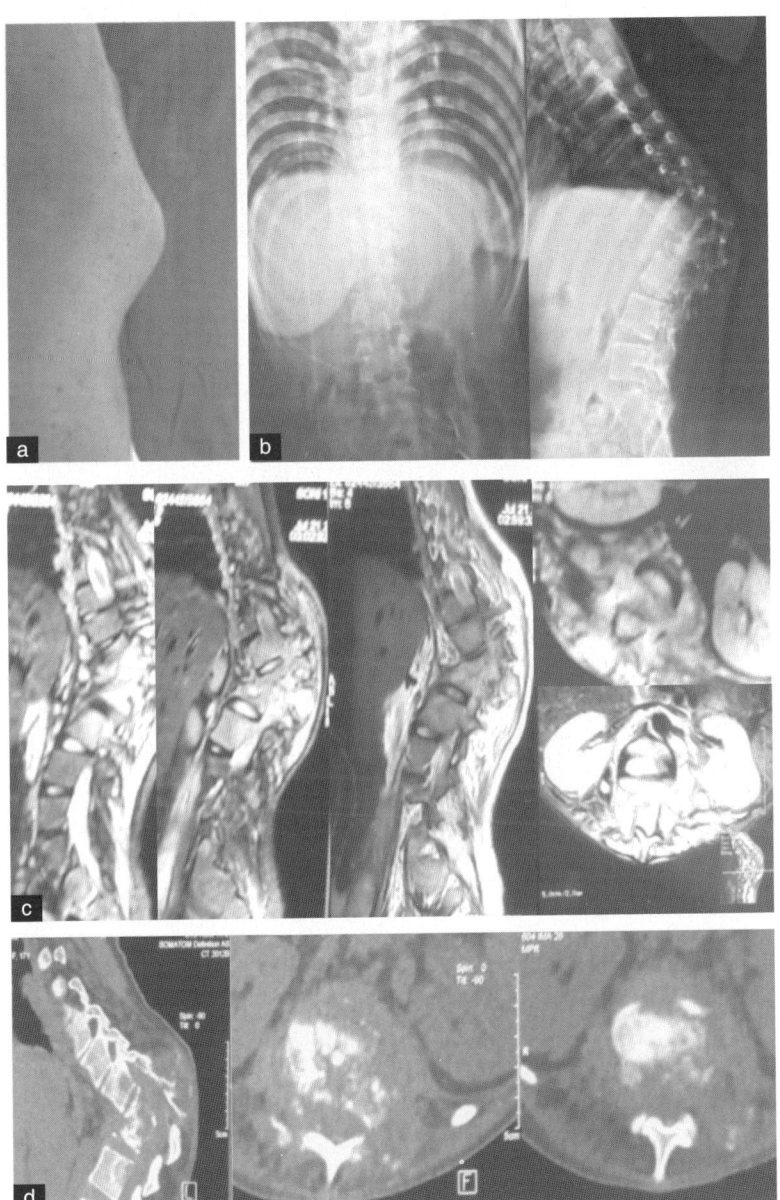

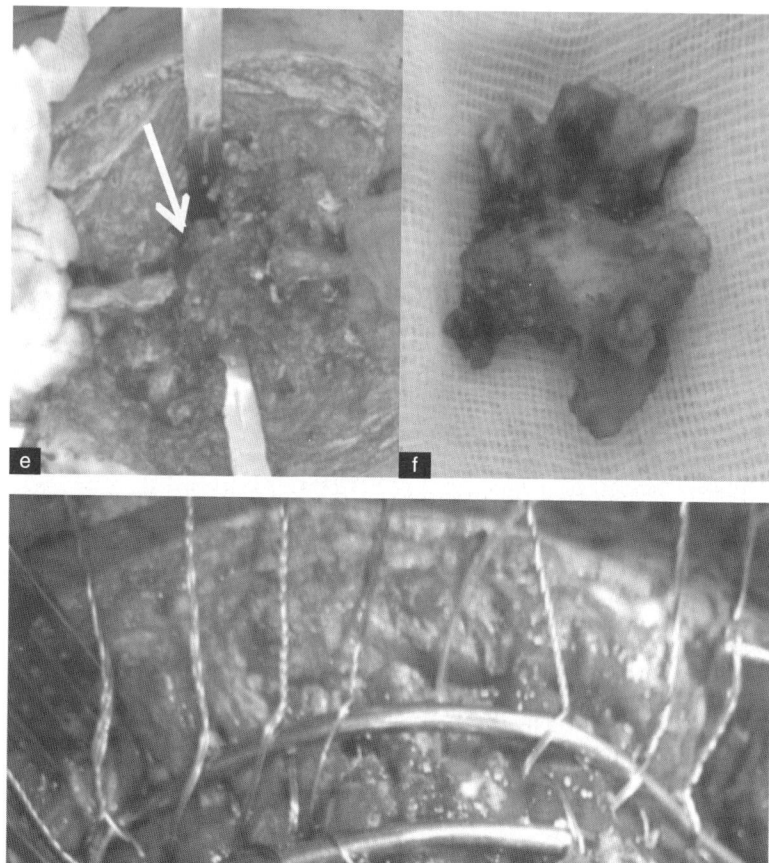

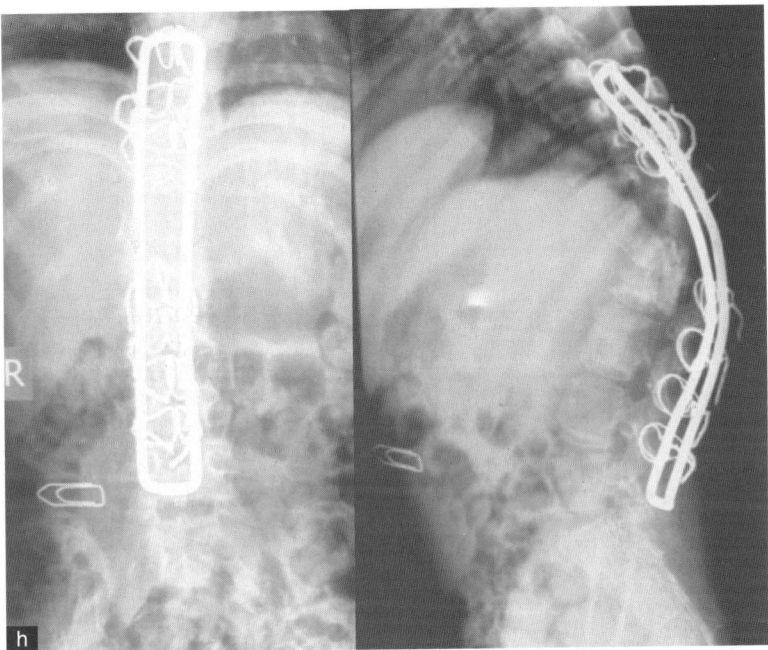

A 17-year-old female presented with complaints of pain over mid-back for past 2 years, progressively increasing kyphotic deformity for past 18 months, weakness with decreased sensation in bilateral lower limbs for past 3 months with urinary incontinence. She had no previous history of tuberculosis. She took ATT for spinal tuberculosis for 9 months which was stopped 6 months back. On examination, there was a gibbus in mid-back (Fig. a) with grade IV flaccid paraplegia (no power in lower limbs, 90% sensory loss below L1 with bladder bowel involvement, no bedsores). X-rays (Fig. b) showed regional osteopenia, with destruction of multiple vertebrae D11, D12, L1 and L2 with no disk space visible between them and resultant kyphotic deformity. MRI (Fig. c) also showed panvertebral involvement with destruction of D12, L1 and their collapse and associated cord compression. CT (Fig. d) confirmed the findings with fragmentary type of destruction. Patient was advised for decompression, instrumented stabilization and if possible, deformity correction which needed pedicle screws, but the arrangement of the same was not possible due to financial constraints. She was taken up for posterolateral decompression (Fig. e), after removing the 12th rib, posterior element of the D12 was necrotic and could be removed as one piece (Fig. f). Posterior fusion and fixation using Hartshill rectangle and sublaminar wires were performed (Fig. g). A deformity correction of up to only 30° was possible (Fig. h)). Postoperatively patient showed almost 80% sensory recovery in both lower limbs with fair power in bilateral hip and knee but weak power in muscles of foot and ankle. Patient is free of urinary catheter with occasional stress incontinence. She is now 4 months postoperative and still on ATT and making good progress.

Case 32: TB spine in a child with severe kyphotic deformity at dorsolumbar spine

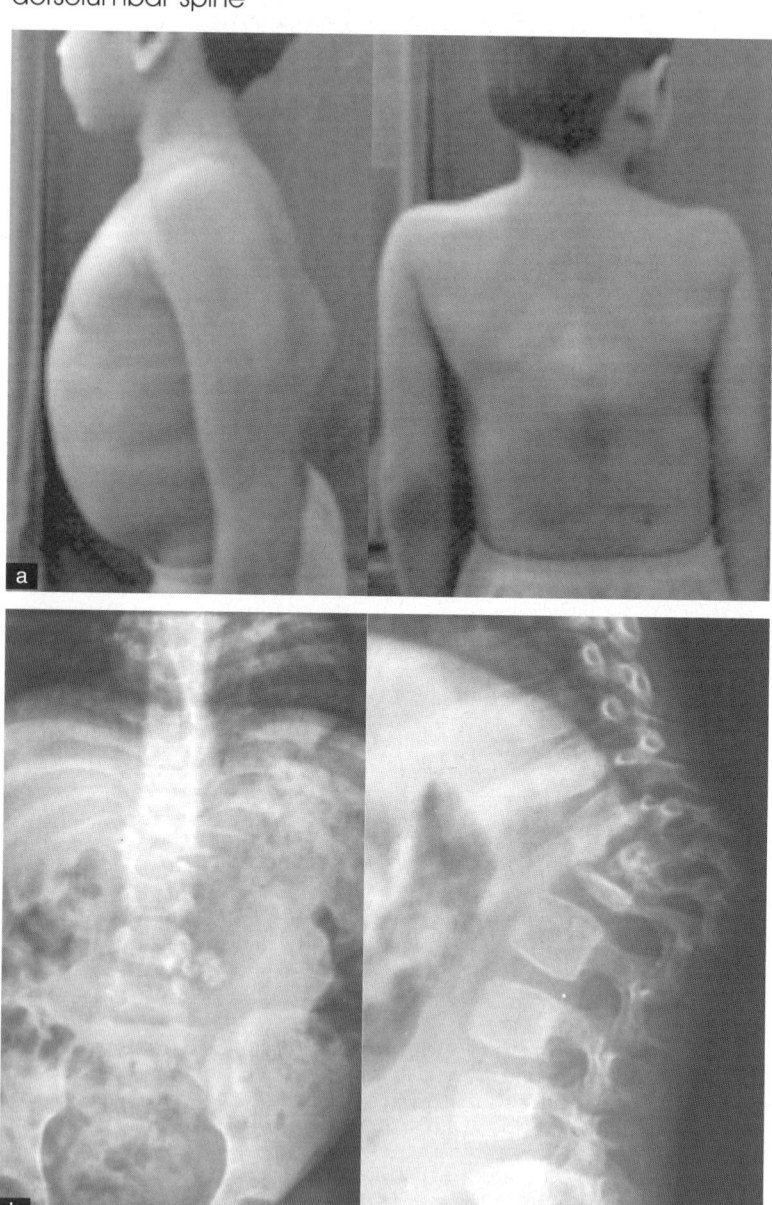

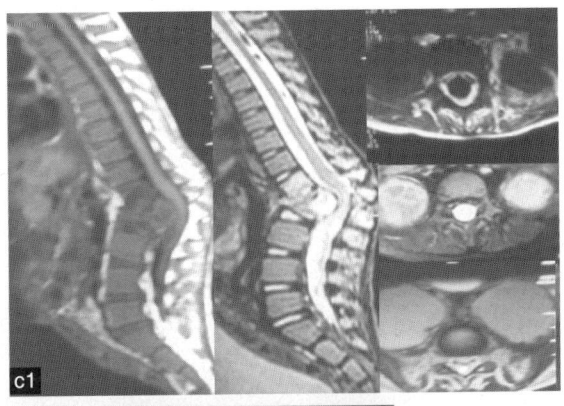

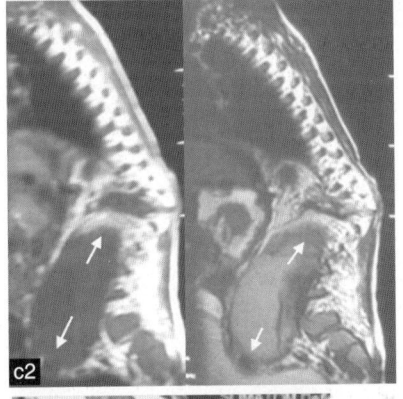

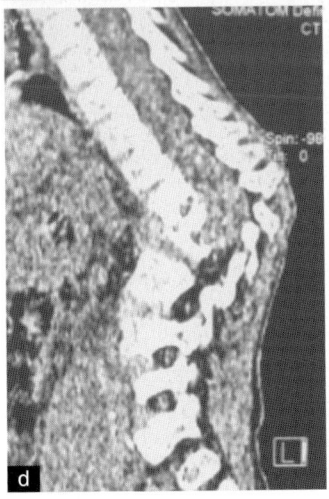

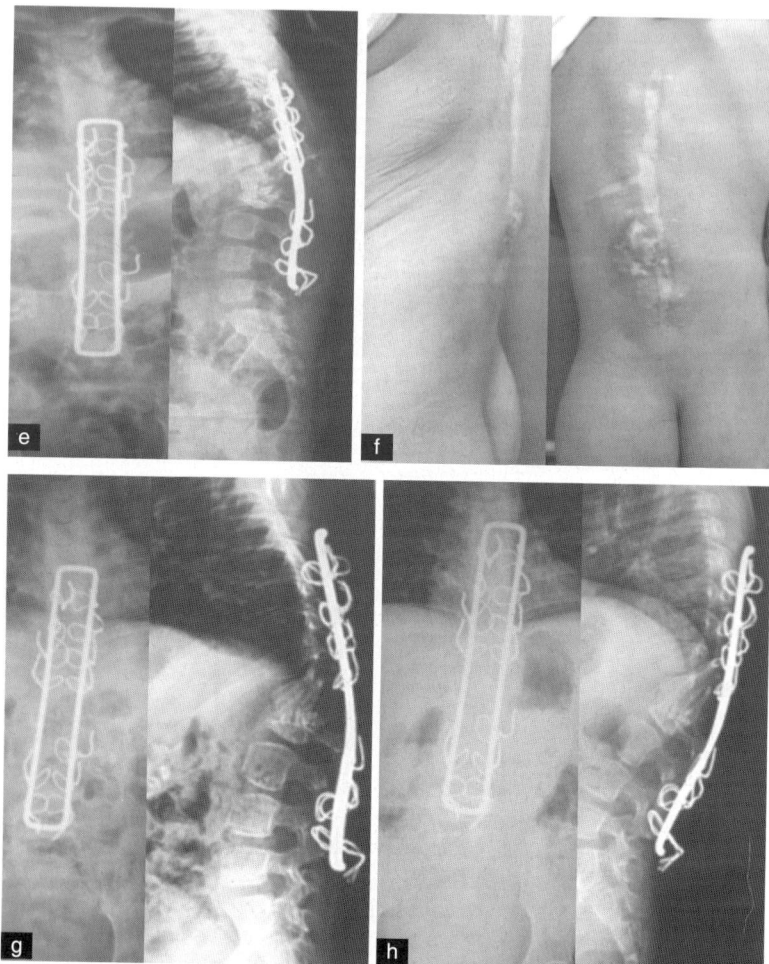

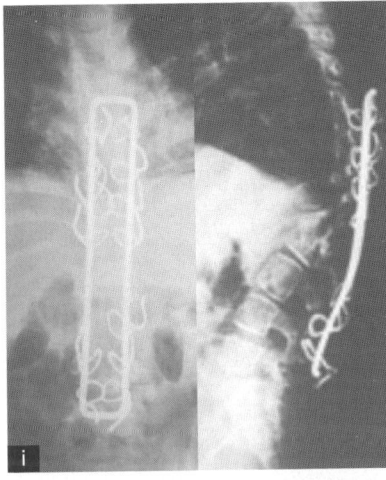
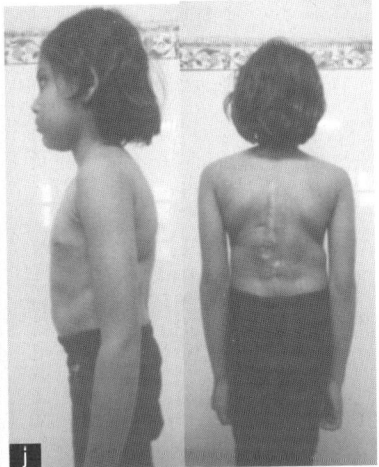

A 4-year-old girl was brought by her parents with complaints of pain in mid-back for past 7–8 months and deformity in mid back for 1 year. There was no history of weight loss/appetite/fever. Patient was on ATT for past 8 months from another hospital. On general and systemic examination, no significant findings were seen. Patient came walking with both hands on knee (like cantilever) and had non-tender kyphotic deformity (Fig. a) present at dorsolumbar junction. No paraspinal spasm/scar/sinuses/bedsore was seen. There was no neural deficit. Her X-rays (Fig. b) showed destruction of vertebral bodies of D12, L1 and L2 with reduced disk spaces and residual kyphus due to anterior disease and lateral translation of proximal spine over distal. MRI [(Fig. d) T1WI, T2WI sagittal and axial scan (Fig. c1)] show vertebral destruction from D11 to L2 with altered marrow signals (hypointense on T1WI and hyperintense on T2WI) with associated pre- and paravertebral collection with similar signals causing cord compression. Bilateral psoas abscesses were also seen (Fig. c2). CT scan (Fig. d) also confirmed the findings of X-rays and MRI. Patient was continued on ATT, strict bed rest, nutrition supplementation with back care and general hygiene. Patient underwent kyphus correction by midline posterior approach and stabilized with Hartshill rectangle and sublaminar wires and posterior fusion with bone grafting (Fig. e) from posterior iliac crest. 2 weeks later, anterior fusion was performed using extrapleural anterolateral approach. A plaster (POP) jacket was given after suture removal for 3 months. Patient developed gluteal abscess after 2 months of surgery which was later drained and pus showed sensitive *Mycobacterium* to Rcin and INH. All wounds healed uneventfully with (Fig. f) ATT for 18 months. Anterior fusion was obtained as seen on postoperative and follow-up. X-rays (Fig. g–i). Patient continue to grow in height (Fig. j) and has no complaints. She is being planned for implant removal under ATT cover.

Case 33: TB spine with lumbosacral kyphosis

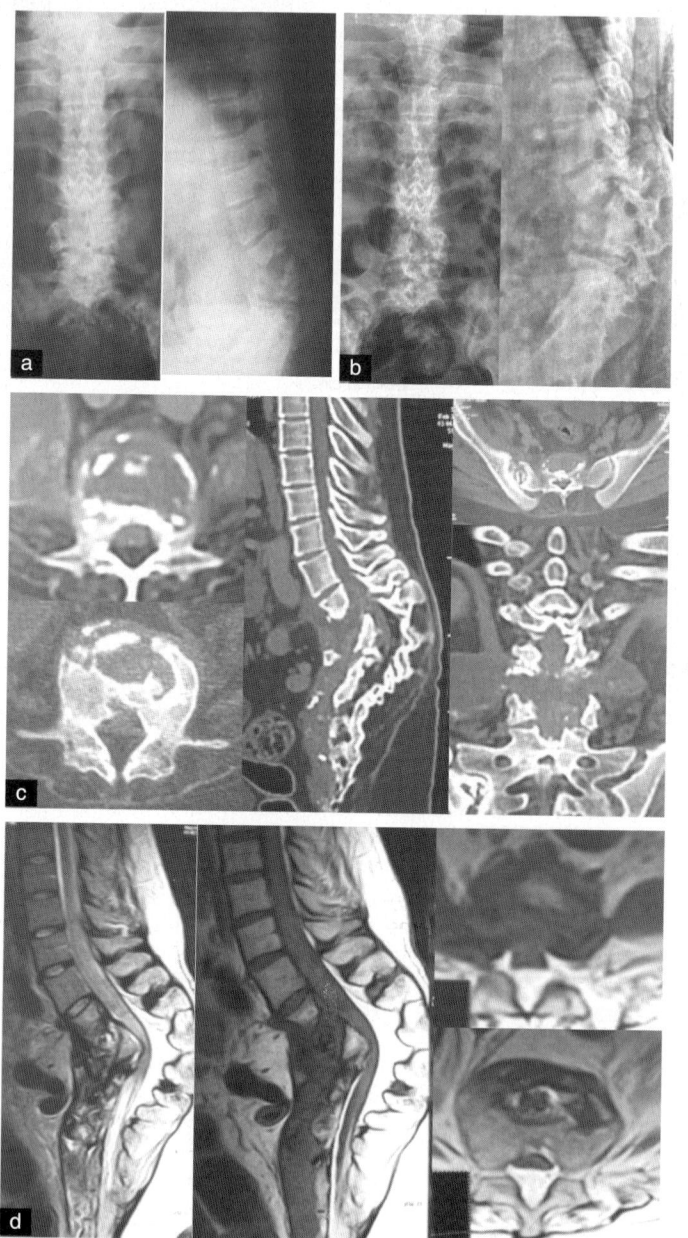

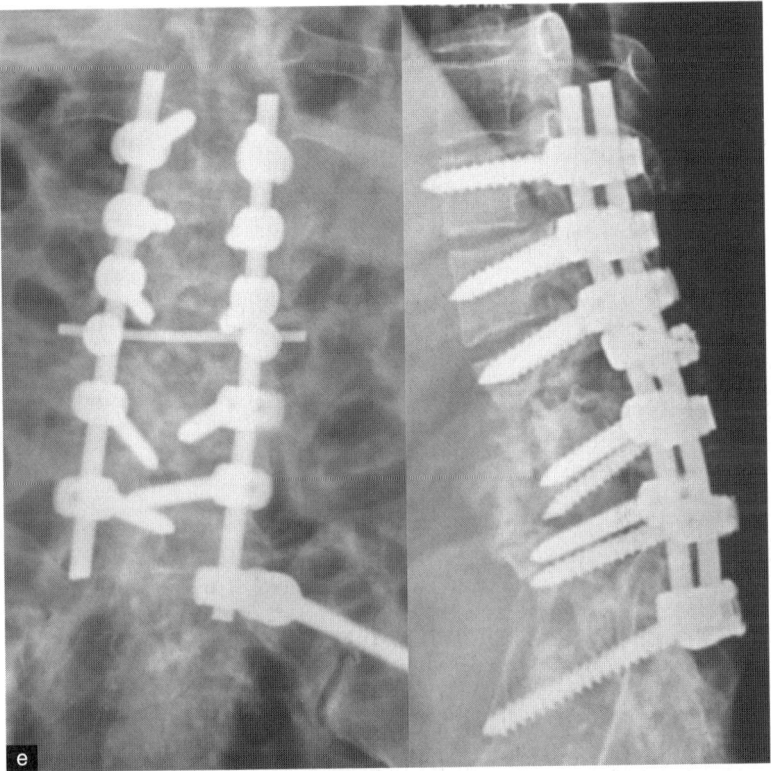

e

A 30-year-old female presented with severe backache and lumbar kyphosis with no neurological deficit. Patient was on category 1 ATT for 6 months before reporting to GTB hospital. Initial plain X-rays (Fig. a) AP and lateral preoperative radiographs show complete involvement and destruction of L3–L5 vertebrae with partial involvement of L2 vertebra with significant lumbar kyphosis. X-rays on presentation (Fig. b) showed progression of kyphosis with persistent disease. Preoperative CT scan (Fig. c) shows fragmentation of vertebral bodies at multiple levels in axial images, kyphosis at lumbar level in sagittal reconstructed image and panvertebral involvement in coronal image. MRI (Fig. d; sagittal and axial; T2WI and T1WI) which confirms destruction extending up to sacral region. Due to extensive involvement with lumbar kyphus and non-responding pain; patient was operated by posterior instrumentation and deformity correction with pedicle screw fixation at lumbosacral level using midline posterior approach along with iliac screw on one side. Plain X-rays (Fig. e), AP and lateral radiographs show correction of kyphosis with sound fixation of lesion. Patient remained neurologically intact after surgery and attained healed status.

Case 34: Various types of presentation of TB hip

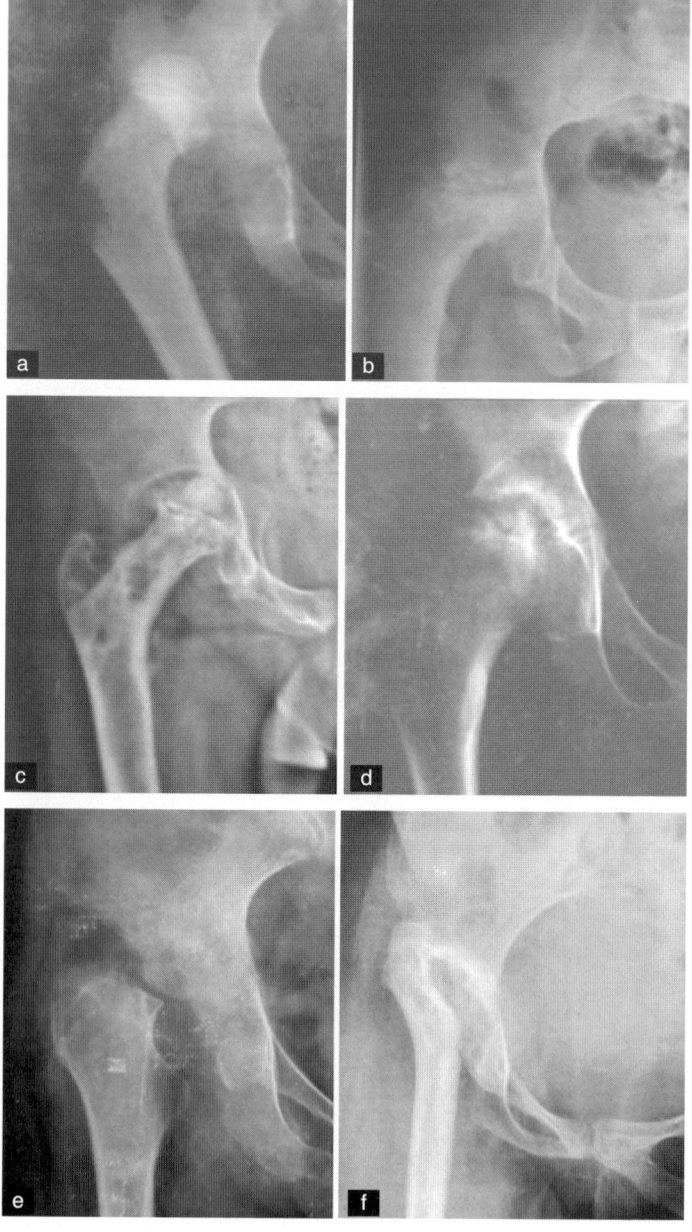

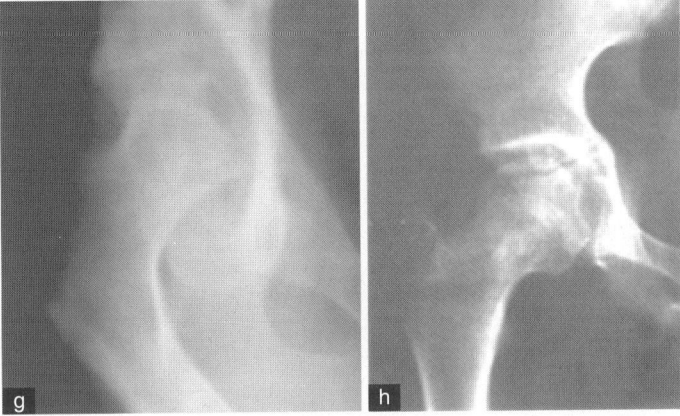

Figures showing X-rays of various radiographic presentations of tuberculosis of the hip:

Fig. a. Dislocation type.

Fig. b. Wandering acetabulam with destroyed femoral head.

Fig. c. Mortar and pestle type lesion while on treatment.

Fig. d. Perthes like lesion.

Fig. e. Destroyed head and neck due to tuberculosis where joint debridement and excisional arthroplasty was performed.

Fig. f. X-rays of a case where the Bacheolar's osteotomy is performed following one world girdlestone excisional arthroplasty.

Fig. g. Mortar and pestle type which is present once the lesion has healed.

Fig. h. Normal type, the patient has contained head with irregular joint surfaces. The patient attained fairly preserved arc of motion at the hip joint.

Case 35: TB hip with sequelae

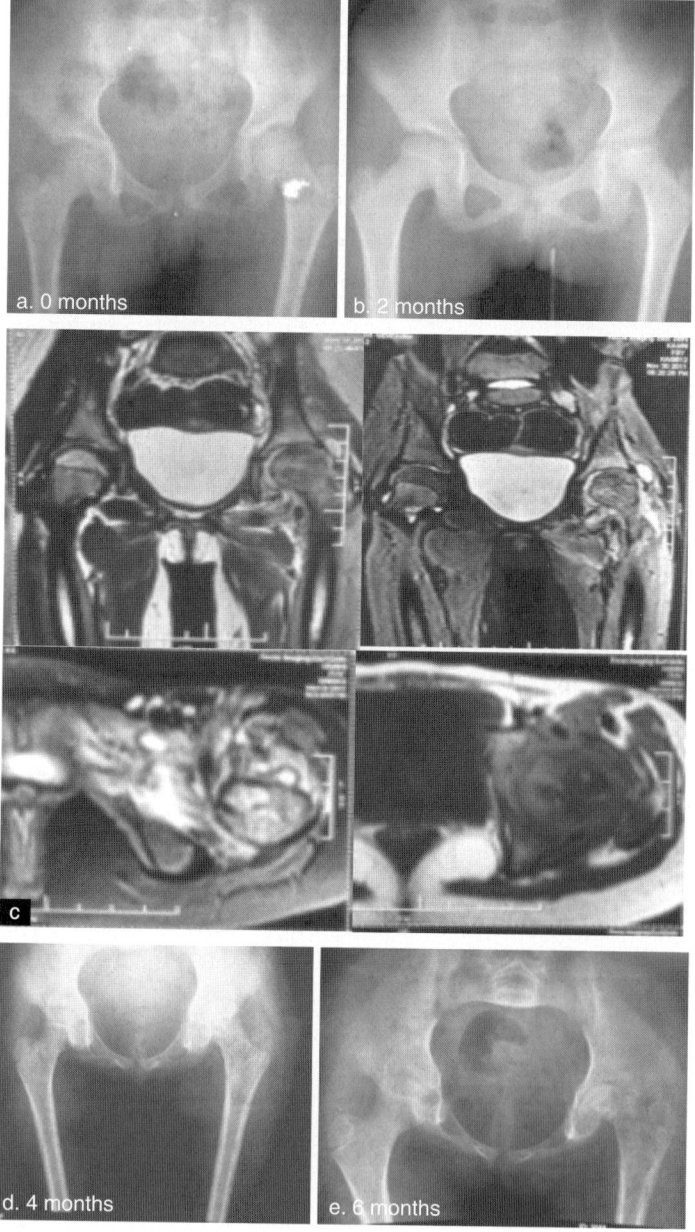

a. 0 months
b. 2 months
c
d. 4 months
e. 6 months

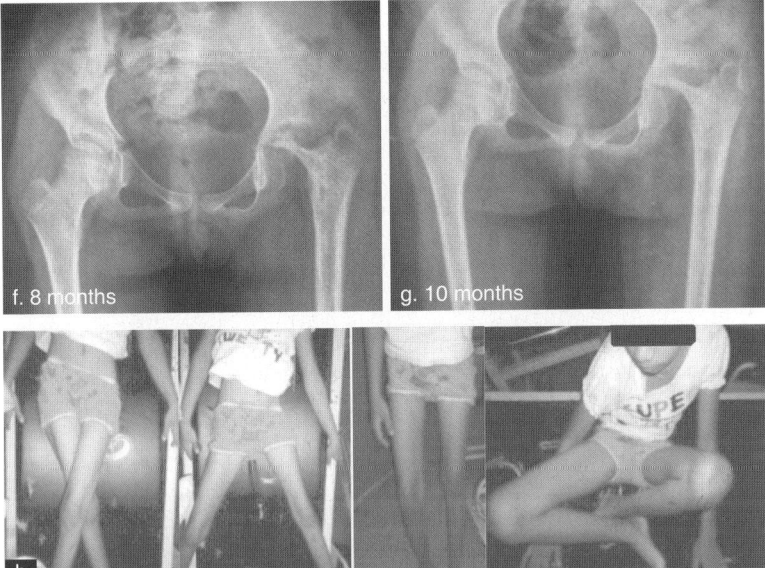

f. 8 months   g. 10 months

h

A 9-years-old female child presented with complaints of pain in left hip for past 2 months with an associated limp. It was insidious in onset and gradually progressive. The complaints had progressed to the extent that she was bedridden. She was taken to a local hospital where some surgical intervention of hip (? Incision and drainage) was done. In spite of it, there was no improvement in pain. There was no associated history of fever or any constitutional symptoms. On examination, she was malnourished thin built. Her left lower limb was in the attitude of abduction, external rotation with both ASIS at the same level. There was exaggerated lumbar lordosis. A healed surgical scar was present at the anterior aspect of thigh. There was tenderness present in the Scarpa's triangle with painful gross restriction (almost nil) of movements. There was no limb length discrepancy. Her blood investigations were within normal limits with ESR of 24 mm/hr. Initial X-ray (Fig. a) showed irregular femoral joint surface with? Lesion in femoral neck with associated osteopenia. X-ray on presentation (Fig. b) showed reduced joint space of left hip. MRI (Fig. c) showed hip joint involvement with distended joint capsule. She was started on ATT and given skeletal traction using upper tibial pin. In spite of the conservative management, pain continued to worsen, therefore, patient was operated for hip joint debridement. Tissue was sent for culture and histopathological examination which confirmed the diagnosis of TB. Sequential X-rays (Figs d–g) showed increase in the bone density with the progression of hip morphologically to mortar and pestle type of disease sequelae. At completion of treatment, patient had fair preservation of hip movements (Fig. h). However, patient will need reconstruction of the hip at a later age.

Case 36: TB of hip

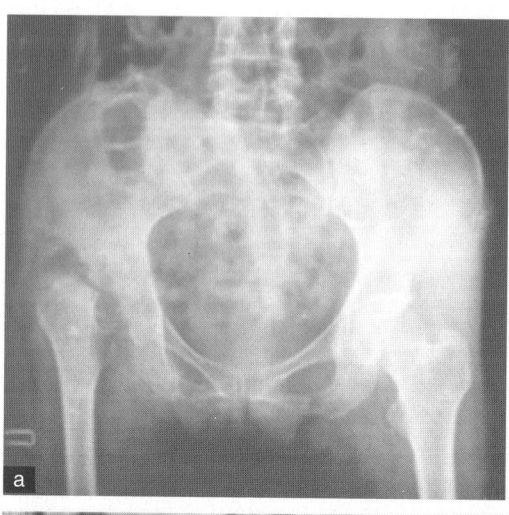

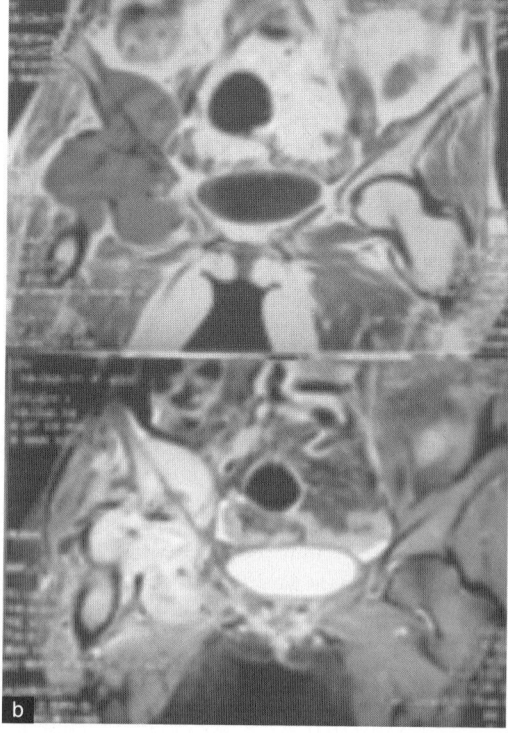

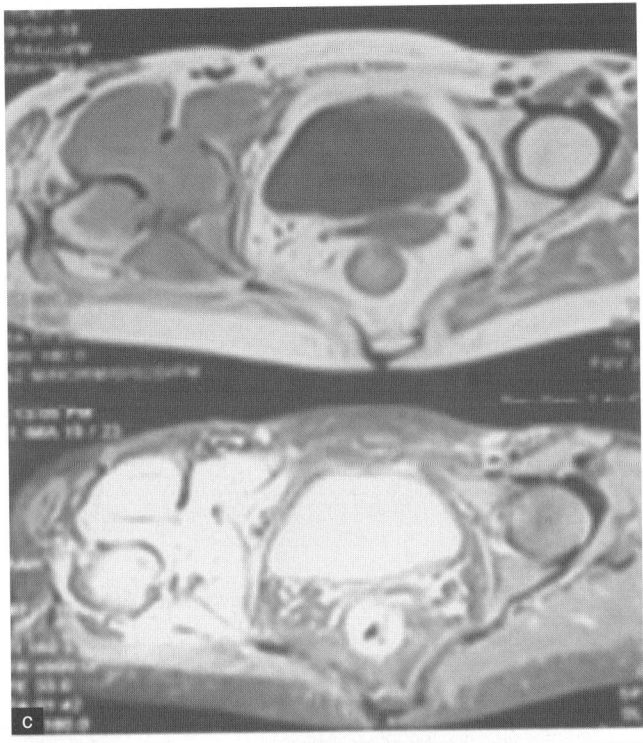

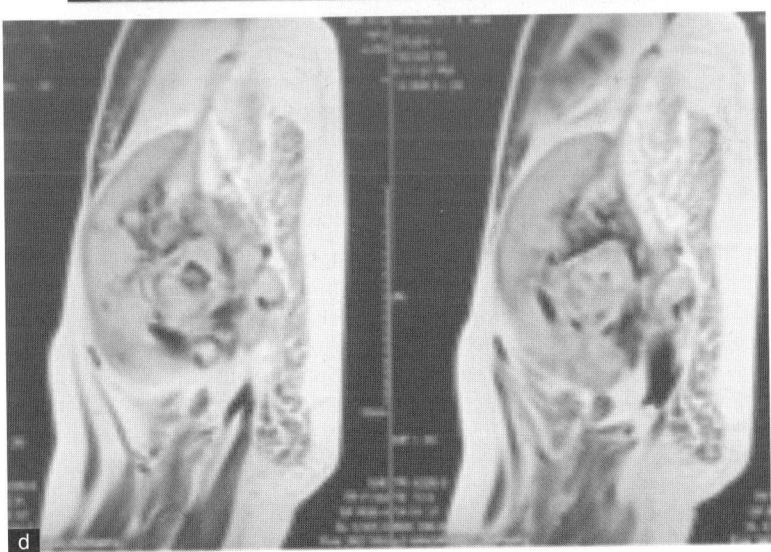

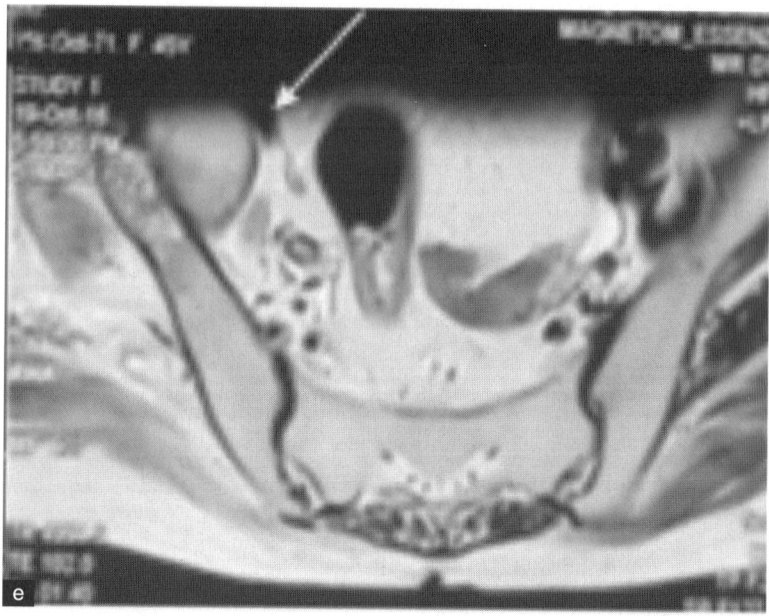

A 43-year-old female patient presented with complaints of pain over right hip and limp for past 3 months. The pain was more severe at nights and was also present on rest. There was no history of trauma or tuberculosis. Patient had no known co-morbidities. History of loss of appetite and weight with low grade fever was present. On examination, patient had a bipedal, antalgic gait with Trendelenburg component. She had fullness and tenderness over right Scarpa's triangle. Vascular sign of Narath was present. There was no associated deformity but the movements at hip were associated with pain and spasm. Flexion was restricted up to 90°, while other movements were nearly comparable with the normal side. Telescopy test was positive. X-ray of bilateral hip joints (Fig. a) with pelvis showed break in the Shenton's line with proximally migrated greater trochanter. The femoral head and neck were destroyed, acetabular margins was fuzzy and regional osteopenia was present. MRI (Figs b–d) showed destruction of femoral head and neck with hypointense on T1WI and hyperintense on T2WI collection in the hip joint which was communicating with the iliacus (arrow, Fig. e). Hip aspiration yielded frank straw-colored pus which was sent for microbiological and pathological investigations. Patient was started on ATT and skeletal traction. In view of the disease load and destroyed joint, patient was taken for excisional arthroplasty. The patient is still on treatment.

Case 37: Sequelae of TB hip—THR

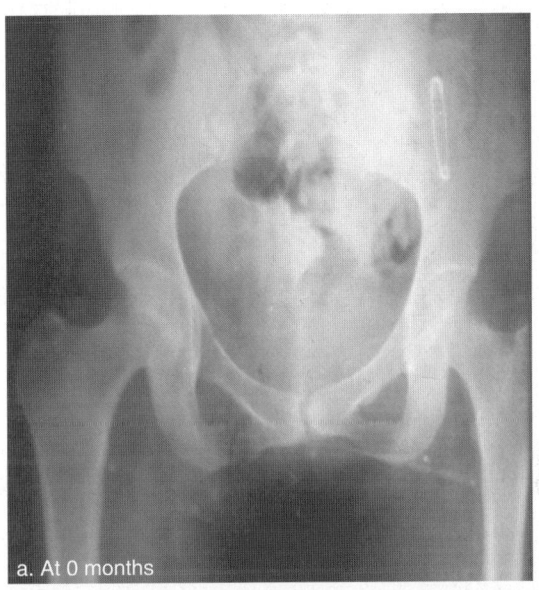

a. At 0 months

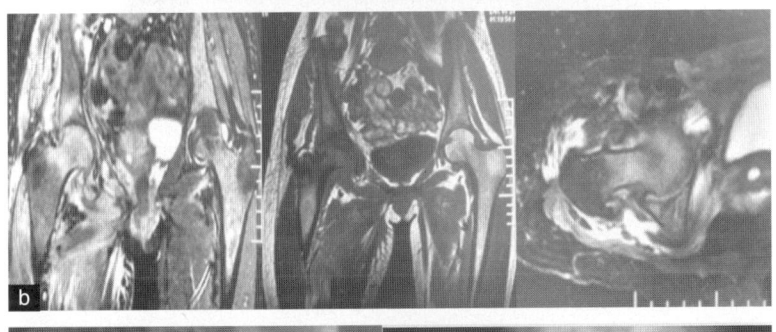

b

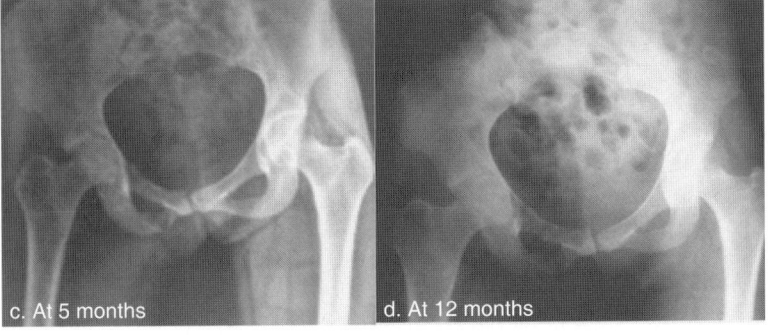

c. At 5 months

d. At 12 months

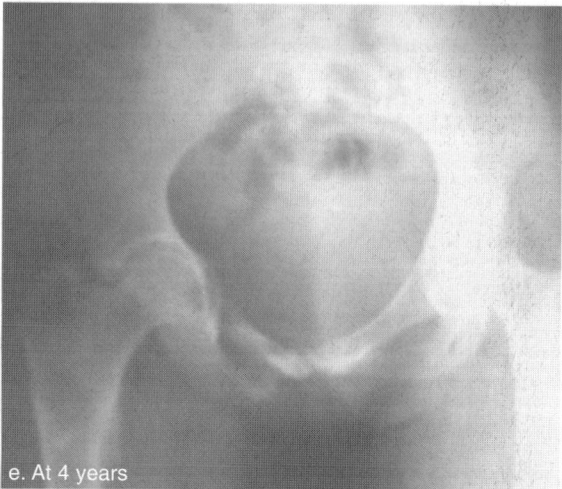

e. At 4 years

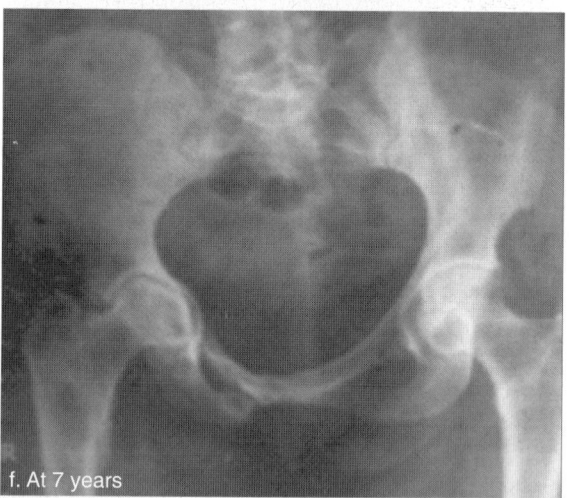

f. At 7 years

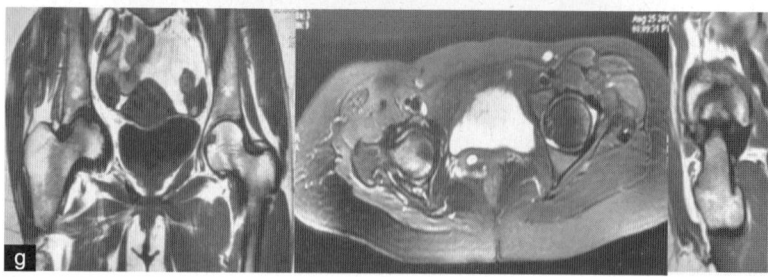

g

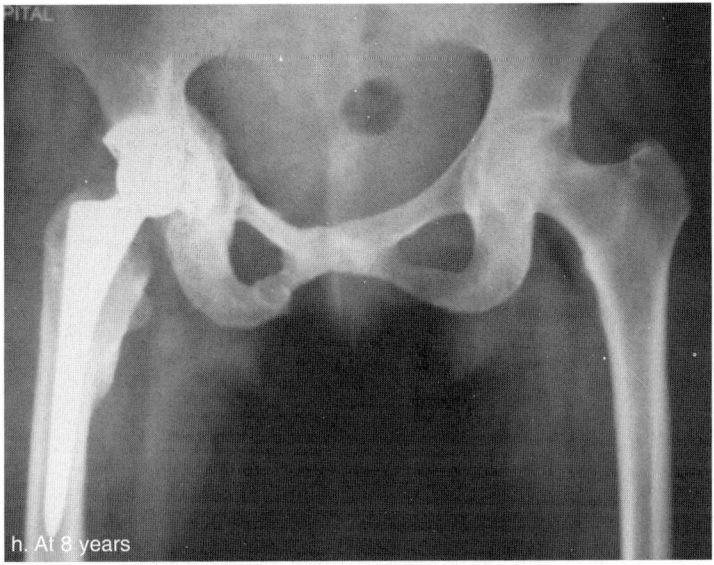

h. At 8 years

A 34-year-old female presented with complaints of pain over right hip and limp for past 4 months. The pain was insidious in onset and gradually progressive. There was no history of trauma or tuberculosis or any co-morbidities. Low grade fever was associated with these complaints. The gait was antalgic, with tenderness present over Scarpa's triangle. There was fixed flexion deformity at hip of 30° with further flexion up to 90°. All movements were painfully restricted and associated with spasm. Telescopy was absent, with proximal migration of greater trochanter and true shortening of 1 cm. X-rays (Fig. a) showed regional osteopenia and reduced right hip joint space. MRI (Fig. b) shows involvement of both femoral and acetabular surfaces with associated collection which was hypointense on T1WI and hyperintense on T2WI. With a presumptive diagnosis of TB hip, patient was started on ATT and skeletal traction using upper tibial steinmann pin. Sequential X-rays (Figs c, d) showed healing response in the form of reconstitution of bone density, sharpening of articular margins. Patient was given ATT for 18 months. But patient had painful restriction of movements. She was able to carry out her activity of daily livings but with difficulty. X-rays (Figs e, f) showed protrusion type changes in hip joint as a sequelae to TB. Patient continued with her activities, but by 7th year she had regular pain and needed analgesics. Patient was advised THR for the same. An MRI (Fig. g) was performed to rule out any residual disease or reactivation. Patient was started on ATT prophylactically, and an uncemented THR was performed (Fig. h). Patient has improved symptomatically and now mobilized and was given ATT for 6 months.

Case 38: TB hip (sequelae)

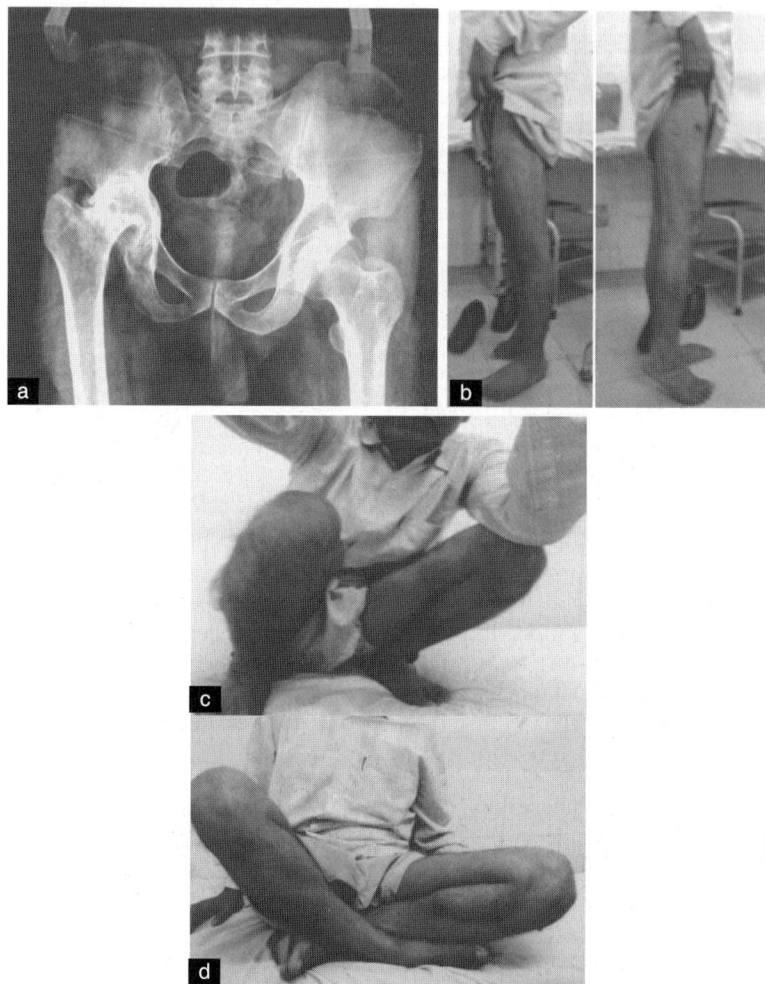

Figure (a) X-ray of a case of sequelae of tuberculosis of the hip, with proximally migrated femur and a destroyed acetabulum. Clinically (Fig. b) patient has shortening and mild restriction of mobility. He can squat (Fig. c) and sit cross-legged (Fig. d). This shows that in spite of the bad radiographic picture patient has fairly preserved range of motion at hip and the patient from agricultural background was happy with the function achieved and was not keen for chair bound lifestyle following replacement/arthroplasty. However, at any stage, patient may be offered total hip arthroplasty.

Case 39: TB hip in a child with suspected drug resistance

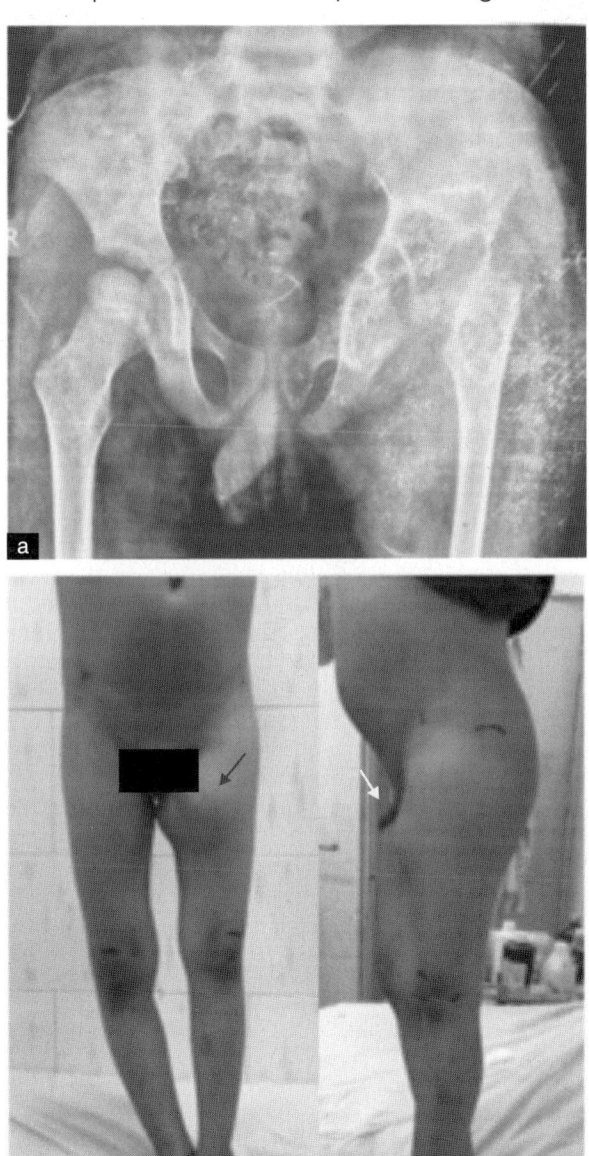

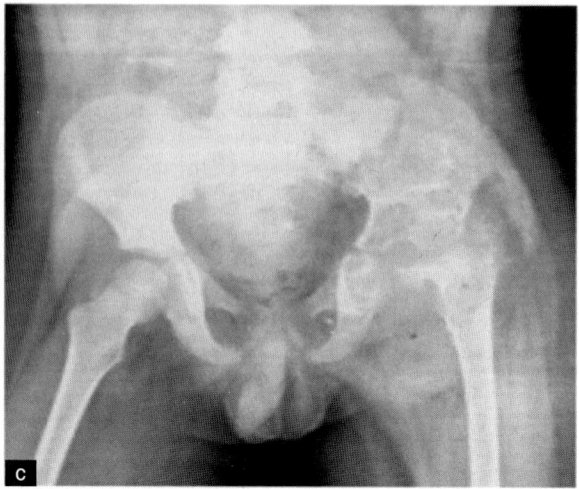

A 5-year-old boy presented with complaints of pain in left hip and limp for 1 year. History of night cries was present along with low grade fever. Child was taking medicines from local practitioner on and off. On examination, there was fullness and tenderness at base of Scarpa's triangle with global restriction of movements at hip associated with sever pain and spasm. The limb was in attitude of flexion, abduction and external rotation. X-rays (Fig. a) showed lytic lesions in proximal femur and acetabulum with inconspicuous femoral head. The greater trochanter was proximally migrated with wandering acetabulum like picture. With a presumptive diagnosis of TB hip, child was started on ATT and traction. After 7 months of ATT, child developed swelling on the anterior aspect of thigh (Fig. b), while the shortening and global restriction of movements persisted, with no significant radiological signs (Fig. c) of healing. A diagnosis of therapeutic refractory TB hip was made. Patient was advised for joint debridement and send samples for histological, cytological and culture-sensitivity studies for *Mycobacterium*.

Case 40: TB knee with triple deformity

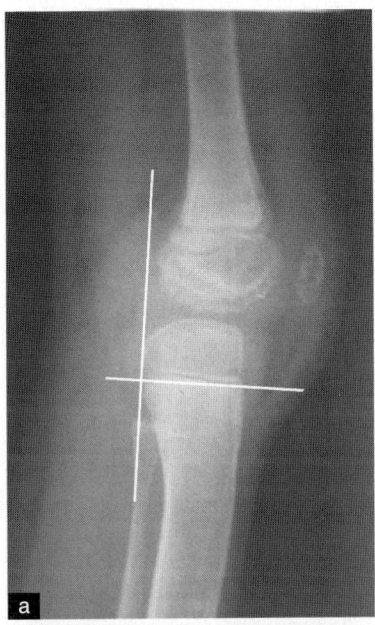

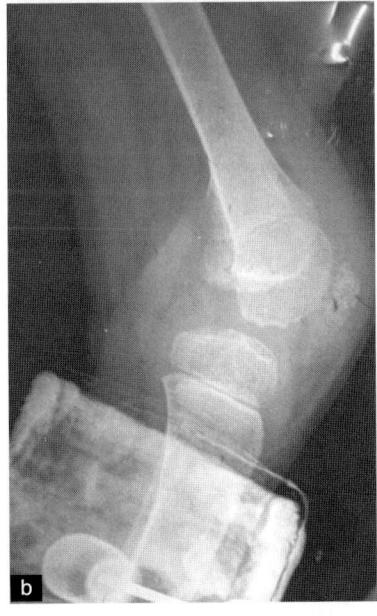

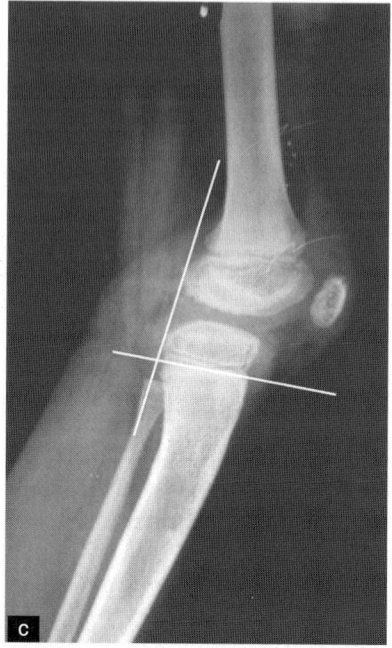

A 7-year-old male child presented with complaints of pain and deformity in right knee for past 6 months. There was no history of trauma, tuberculosis in the family or any bleeding diathesis. Child had flexion deformity at knee of 20° with further flexion (painful) up to 70°. The local temperature was raised and synovium was thickened. Knee effusion was present. There was associated posterior subluxation (Fig. a), external rotation of tibia over femur and minimal valgus. Inguinal lymph nodes were significantly enlarged. A diagnosis of tuberculosis of knee with secondary triple deformity was made. Child was started on ATT and kept on modified Russell's traction (Fig. b). Gradually, the posterior subluxation and flexion deformity reduced. Then patient was given a groin to toe cast, which was removed 2 months later. Patient's deformity reduced (Fig. c) and has a near normal range of motion 5° to 150°.

Case 41: TB of metatarsal

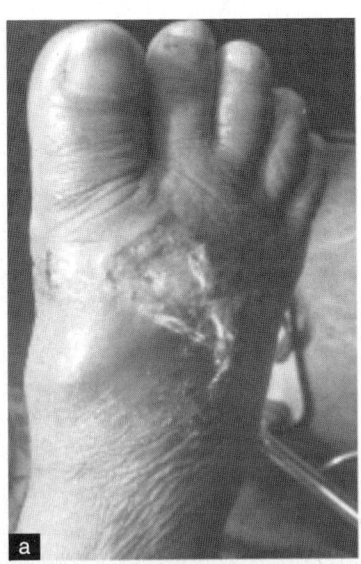

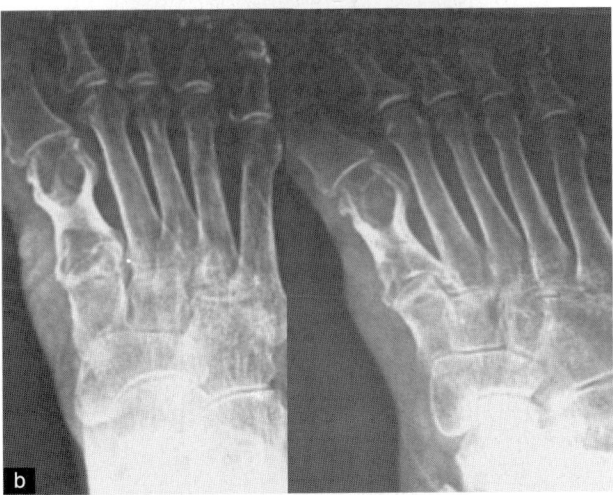

A 40-year-old male presented with history of pain and swelling over foot for past 6 months with pus discharging ulcer (Fig. a) over dorsum of foot for past 6 weeks. X-rays (Fig. b) showed regional osteopenia with lytic lesion in first metatarsal. There was no associated periosteal reaction. Patient was started on ATT after taking edge biopsy which proved it to be tubercular in origin.

Case 42: TB of metatarsal

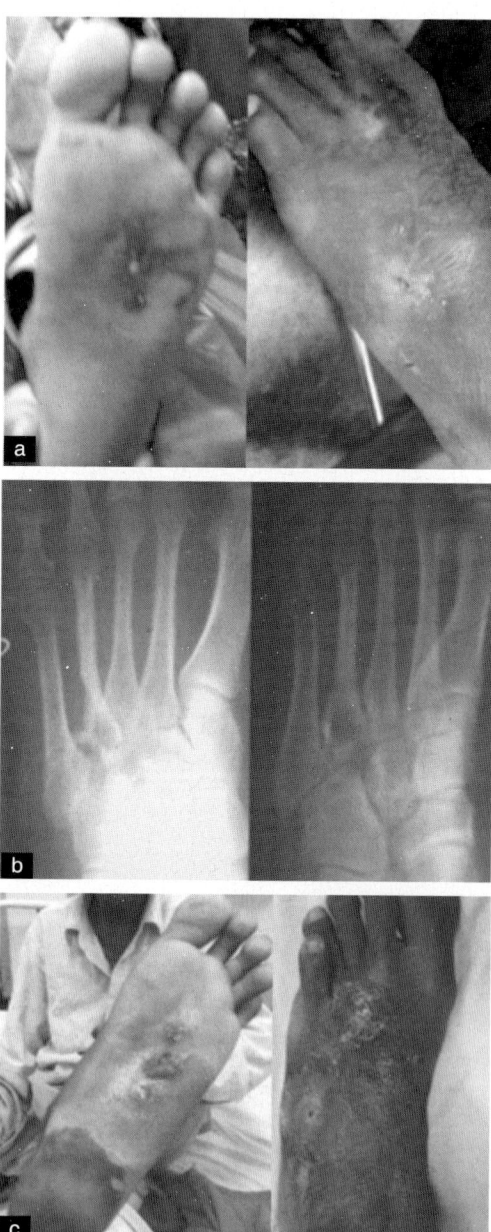

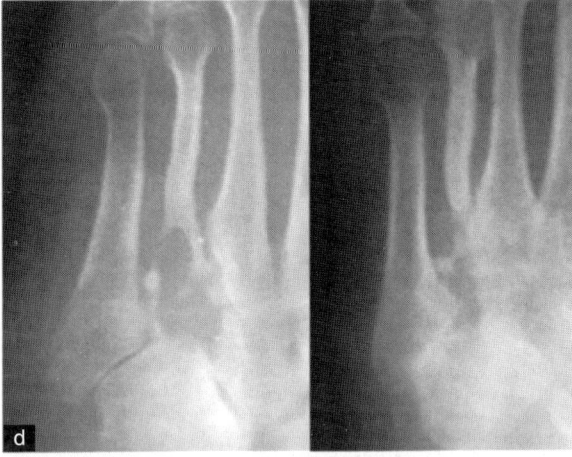

A 28-year-old male patient presented with complaints of pain and swelling in left foot for past 2 years along with multiple discharging sinuses from both surfaces of left foot for 18 months. Patient has no history of constitutional symptoms. On examination (Fig. a), there was a 4 × 2 cm sinus tract opening over dorsum of left mid-foot, 4 cm from lateral margin with no active pus discharge. There was another 5 × 4 cm sinus tract opening over plantar surface of left mid-foot 8 cm from lateral margin with no active pus discharge. Signs of multiple healed sinuses were present over both surfaces. Plain X-rays (Fig. b) showed lytic lesion in the base of fourth metatarsal with no associated periosteal reaction. He was started on ATT with a presumptive clinicoradiological diagnosis of TB. But even after 9 months of ATT, sinuses persisted (Fig. c) and radiologically, the bony destruction increased in size without any signs of healing (Fig. d). It is a case of presumptive drug resistance and the lesion needs to be surgically evacuated and tissue to be sent for cytological evaluation, histopathology, molecular diagnosis and culture sensitivity studies for aerobic, anaerobic, TB, fungus.

Case 43: TB shoulder

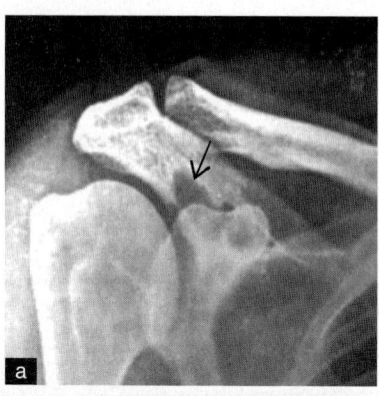

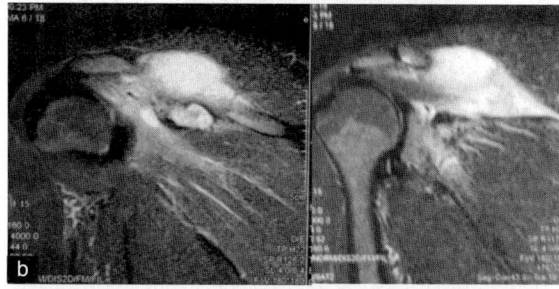

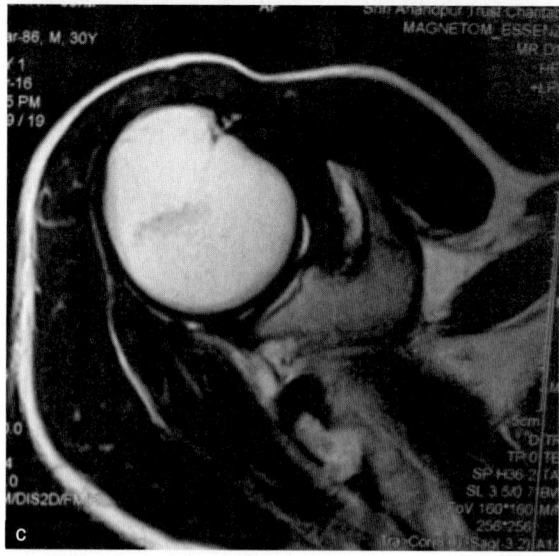

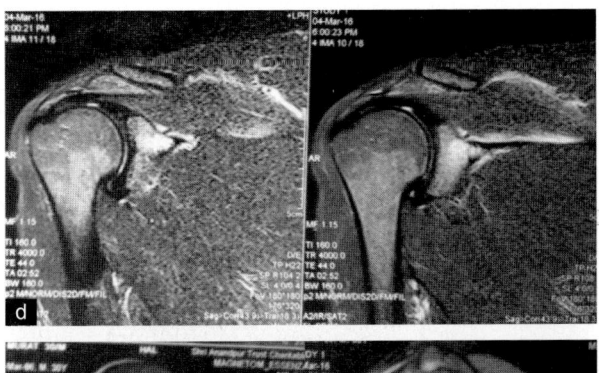

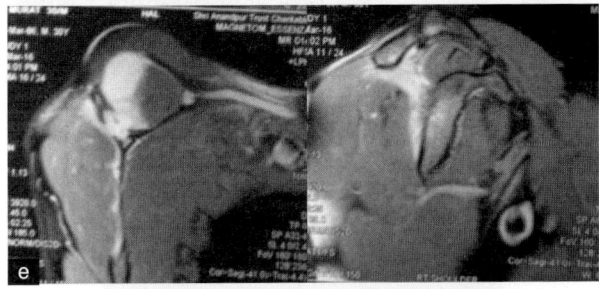

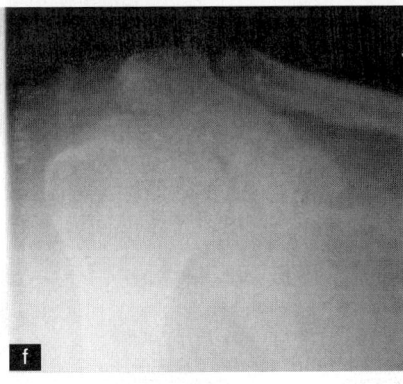

The plain radiographs of a 30-year-old male teacher who presented with complaints of pain near right shoulder and difficulty in lifting weight. X-ray (Fig. a) showed normal glenohumeral joint but there was an associated lytic lesion (geographic) in the spine of scapula. It had a narrow zone of transition. MRI images (Figs b–e) showed a lesion in the scapular spine which was hypointense on T1WI (Fig. d) and hyperintense on T2WI (Fig. b). The lesion was clinically not well defined, hence, a CT-guided biopsy was performed. It showed necrotic granulomas suggesting a tubercular lesion. The patient was started on ATT. 6 months post-treatment resolution of lytic area (Fig. f) was noted. Patient is continuing on his ATT.

Case 44: TB of shoulder with proven drug resistance

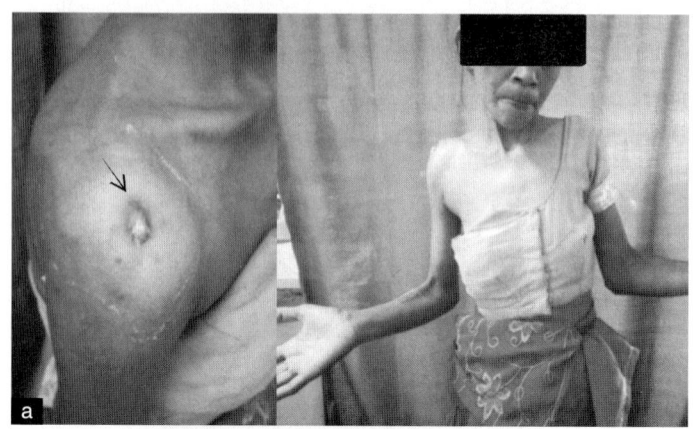

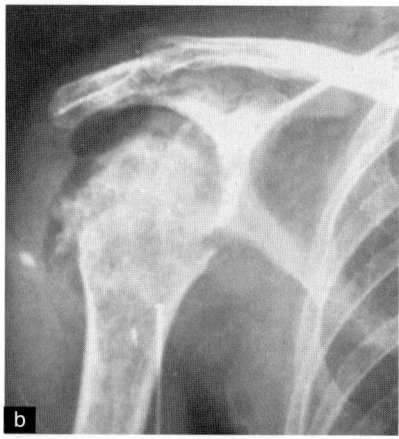

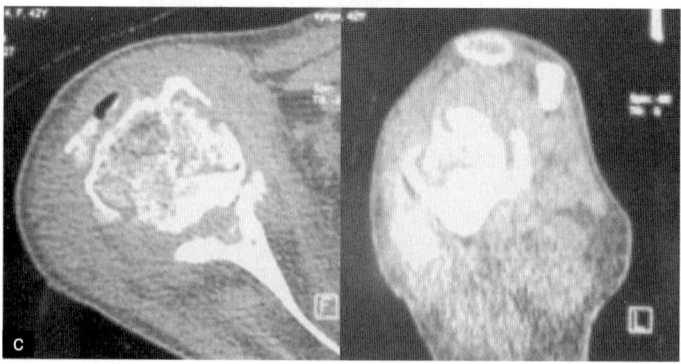

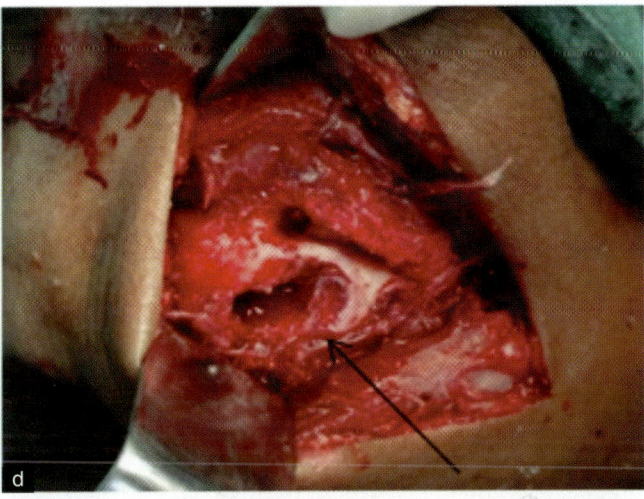

Clinical images (Fig. a) of a 42-year-old female who presented with complaints of pain in right shoulder for 2 years with pus discharging sinus for past 7 months. She had associated fever and other constitutional symptoms for past 11 months. The shoulder was tender with gross, global and painful reduction of movements at shoulder joint. A pus discharging sinus with classical bluish margins (arrow) was present on the anterolateral aspect of the shoulder. Plain radiographs (Fig. b) showed destroyed humeral head and glenoid with reduced joint space. Regional osteopenia was also noticeable. Similar findings were seen on CT scan images (Fig. c) which showed fragmented humeral head, destroyed glenoid margins and calcific densities outside the humeral head. Patient was on ATT for past 14 months. Her ESR on presentation was 62 mm/hr with CRP positive (Note: quantitative CRP values are preferred). With a diagnosis of therapeutic refractory disease, patient was taken for debridement and procurement of tissue for culture and sensitivity studies. Intraoperatively (Fig. d), a lesion was seen in the humeral head with seropurulent fluid in the joint cavity. The tissue and fluid obtained were sent for CB-NAAT and DST using Line Probe Assay. Patient was proven to be MDR-TB case (resistance to Rcin and INH) and was started on second-line ATT.

Case 45: TB shoulder with proven drug resistance

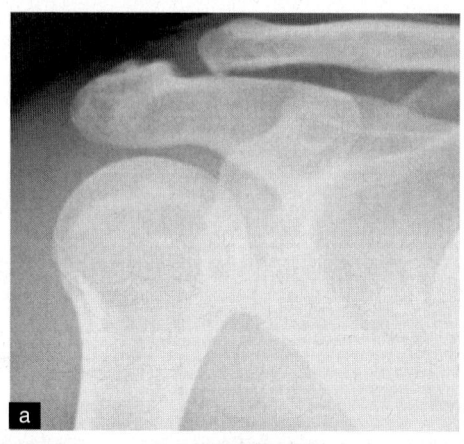

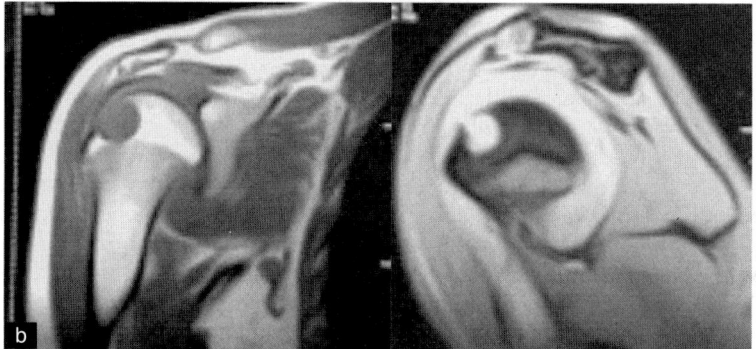

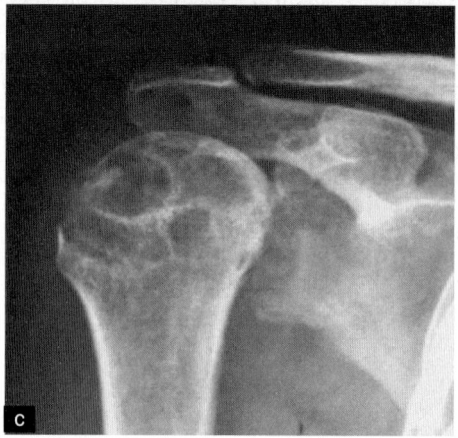

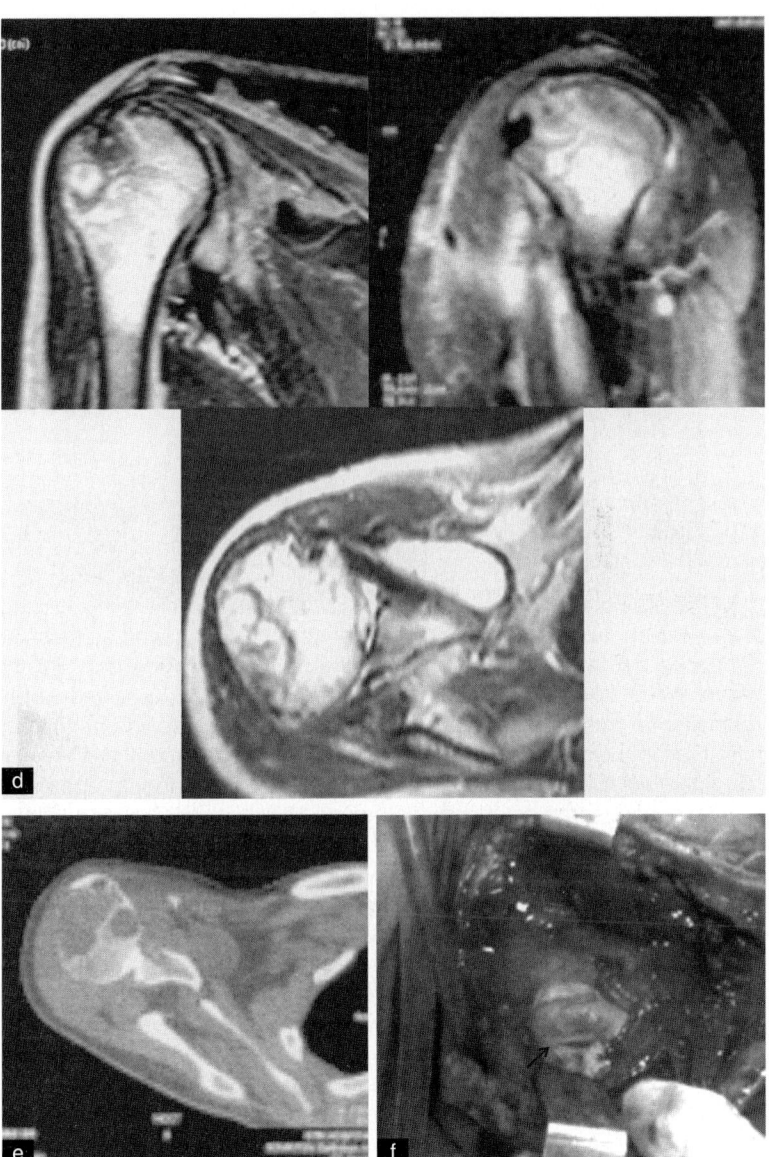

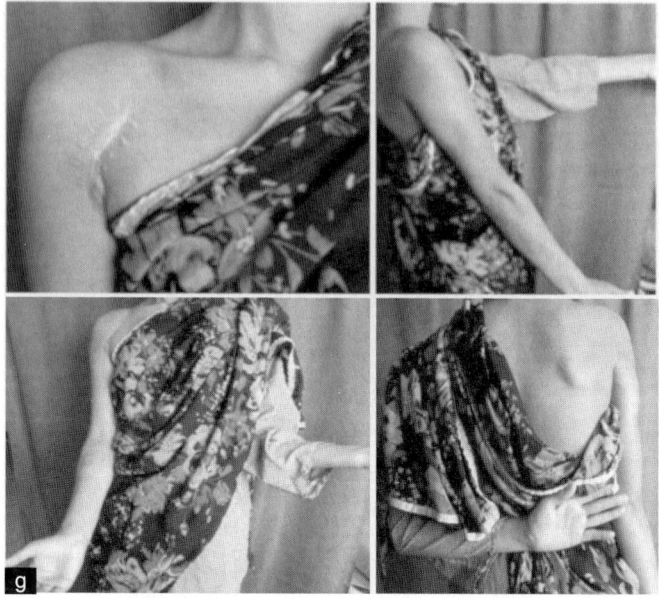

A 24-year-old female presented with complaints of pain and stiffness in right shoulder for past 6 months. She had history of pulmonary TB for which she received ATT for 6 months, 18 months back. She had global restriction of movements with tenderness in anterior aspect of shoulder joint. Patient was taking Cat II ATT (HRZES) for past 3 months in view of shoulder joint tuberculosis. Her X-rays at presentation (Fig. a) appeared normal except some osteopenia, although MRI (Fig. b) showed a lesion in greater tuberosity of proximal humerus which was hypointense on T1WI and hyperintense on T2WI. Patient was continued on ATT and shoulder was mobilized once pain was reduced. After 18 months of ATT, patient's pain had reduced partially with stiffness in the joint was persisting. X-ray (Fig. c) showed multiple lytic lesion in the proximal humerus with regional osteopenia. MRI (Fig. d) also showed multiple lesions in the proximal humerus collection in subscapularis which was hypointense on T1WI and hyperintense on T2WI. CT (Fig. e) also showed multiple lytic lesions in the humeral head and greater tuberosity. With a diagnosis of presumptive drug resistance, patient underwent joint debridement and tissue samples were sent for DST, histopathology and cytopathology. Frank pus was drained (arrow, Fig. f) from the cavities of the lesions in the humeral head. Drug resistance (resistance to Rcin and INH) was proved on Line Probe Assay and CB-NAAT/GeneXpert and patient was started on second-line ATT. The stiffness in joint persisted but patient had pain relief and is still under follow up (Fig. g).

Case 46: TB of elbow

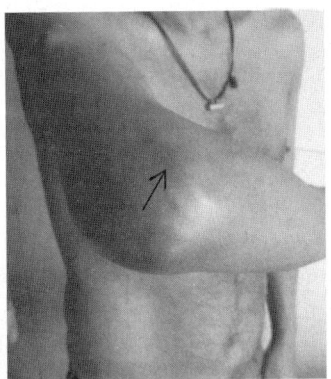

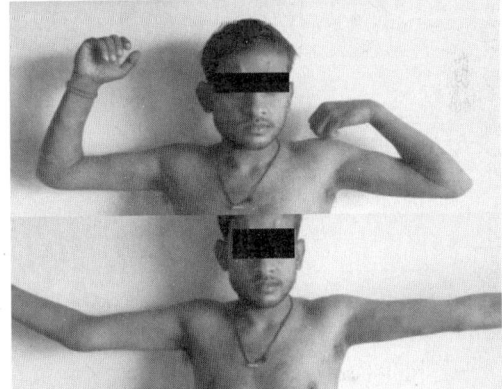

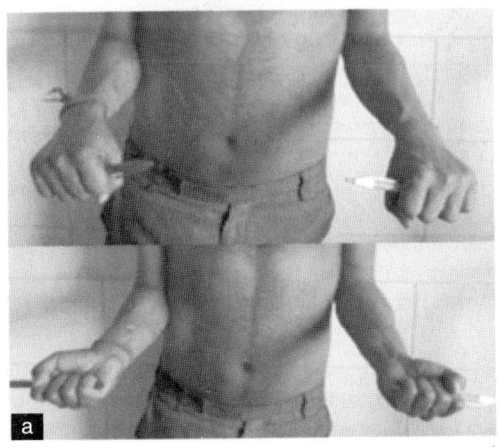

a

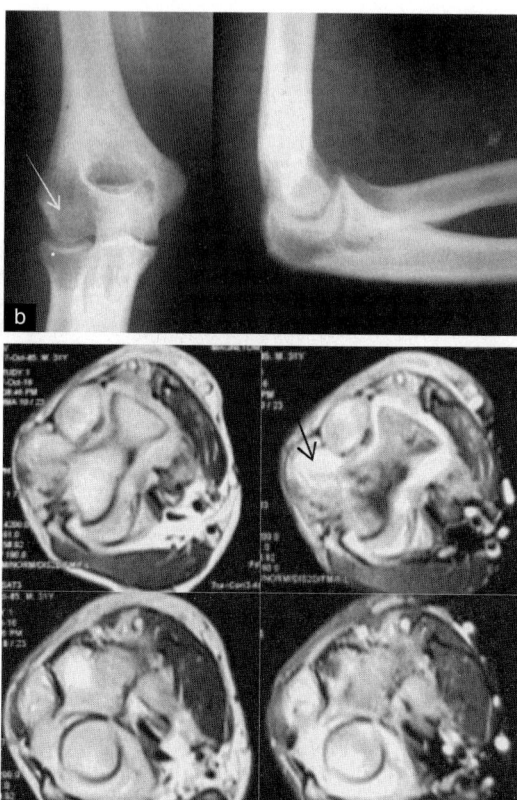

A 24-year-old male who presented with complaints of pain and swelling over right elbow for past 3 months. The swelling was chiefly around posterolateral aspect of the elbow (arrow; Fig. a). He had painfully reduced movements at the elbow with a fixed flexion deformity of 30°. Prono-supination were fairly preserved. Supratrochlear lymph nodes were enlarged and palpable. Plain X-rays (Fig. b) showed regional osteopenia especially in the lateral humeral condyle. Joint space was preserved. MRI (Fig. c), T1WI and T2WI axial sections, showed lesion in the lateral humeral condyle with collection around the proximal radius(arrow). Patient with a presumptive diagnosis was started on ATT. The aspirate from the most fluctuant part (arrow) yielded pus which was sent for AFB smear, culture, molecular diagnosis and cytology.

Comments: The epitrochlear lymph nodes can also be a source of tissue for ascertaining the diagnosis. Since the lesion is juxta-articular which has opened into the joint, the patient is likely to have good clinical outcome.

Case 47: TB of elbow

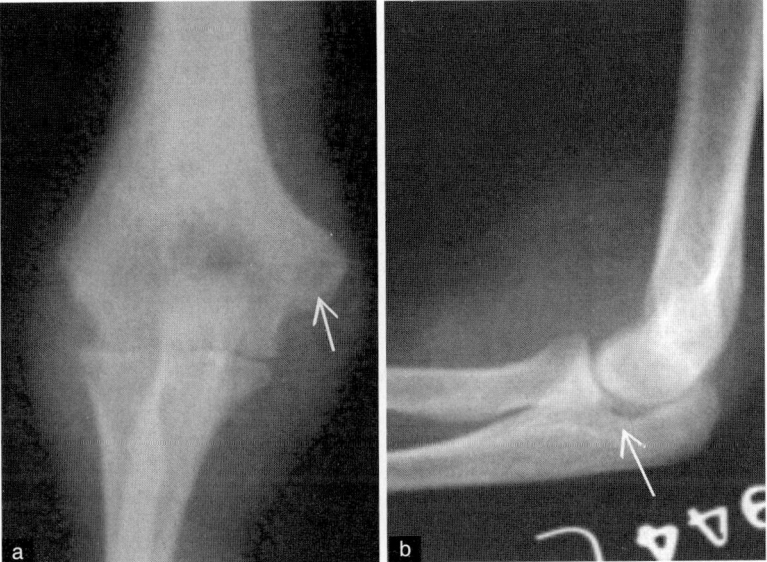

A 20-year-old female presented with pain and swelling in left elbow for past 8 months. On examination, there was fullness in the posteromedial aspect of elbow, with raised local temperature. The muscles of arm and forearm were wasted and there was stiffness in elbow (ROM 30–90°). The lymph nodes were not palpable. X-ray (Fig. a) showed well-defined lytic zone in the medial epicondyle of humerus, with no associated periosteal reaction. Lateral view (Fig. b) showed a similar lesion in subchondral region of ulna. The joint was aspirated, a cytopathological evaluation showed AFB. The patient was started on ATT and an above elbow slab for temporary splintage.

Case 48: TB of elbow—outcome

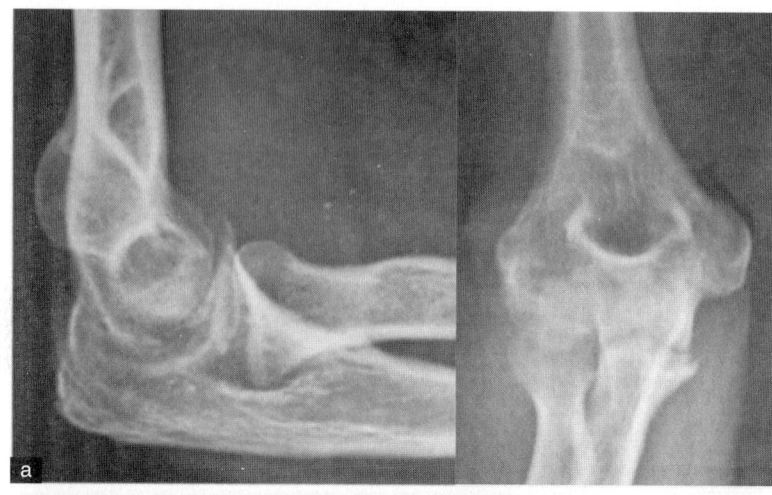

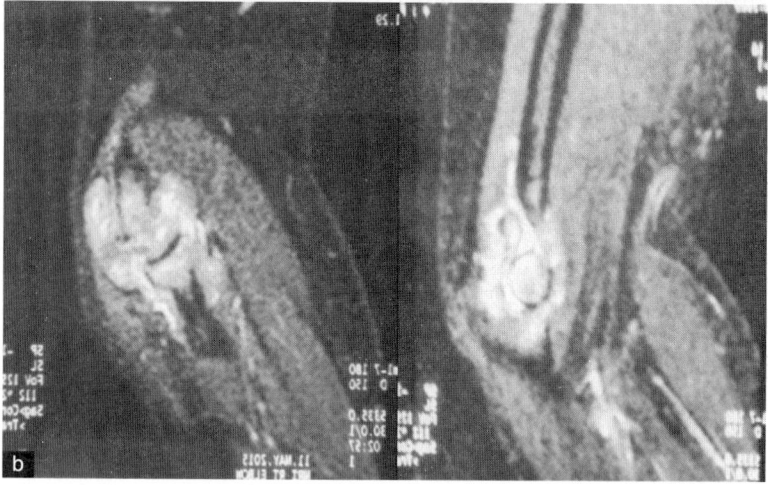

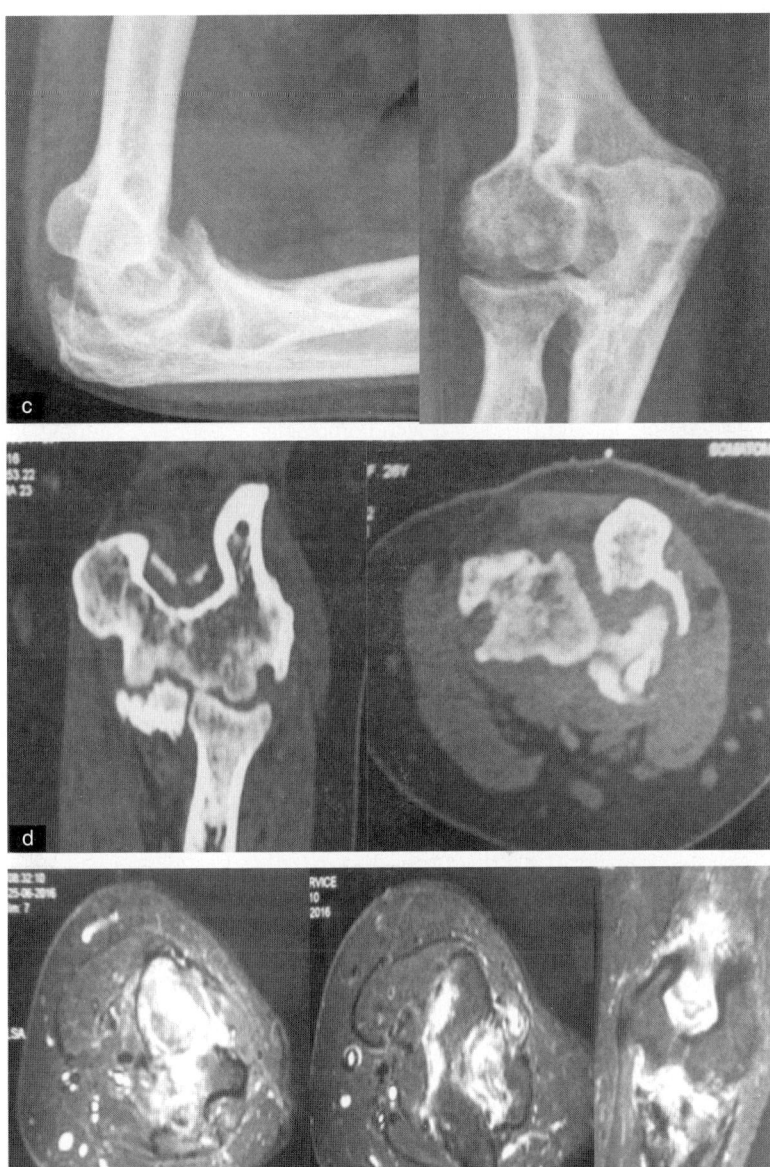

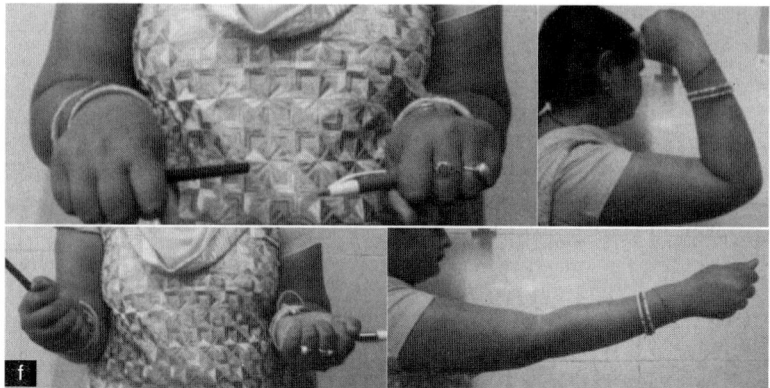

A 24-year-old female presented with complaints of pain and stiffness in her right elbow for past 4 months. The pain was insidious in onset and gradually progressive. It was more in morning but she had no history of night cries or any other joint pains. On examination, she had fullness on the postero-lateral aspect of the right elbow with tenderness over the lateral humeral condyle. The elbow range of motion was restricted from 30° to 80° with associated pain and spasm. X-rays (Fig. a) showed regional osteopenia, with decreased ulnohumeral joint space and fuzziness of the joint margins. MRI (Fig. b) showed marrow edema in distal humerus (hypointense on T1WI and hyperintense on T2WI) with collection in the ulnohumeral joint capsule. With the diagnosis of TB elbow, patient was started on ATT with an above slab for initial 3 weeks. Once patient was pain free, patient's elbow was mobilized by active elbow ROM and prono-supination exercises. The pain reduced and range of motion improved. After 18 months of ATT, there were partial signs of healing, with destroyed articular surface (Fig. c). CT (Fig. d) and MRI (Fig. e) confirmed about the articular damage and persistence of areas of activity. But patients functional picture (Fig. f) showed good results. Her ESR was 46 mm/hr with CRP 12 mg/dl (raised). The patient is continuously showing an improvement and may require ATT for longer duration.

[

Case 49: TB of wrist

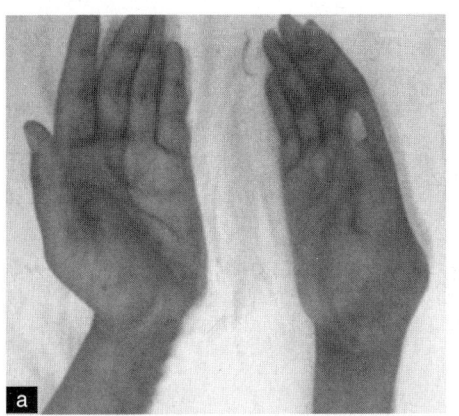

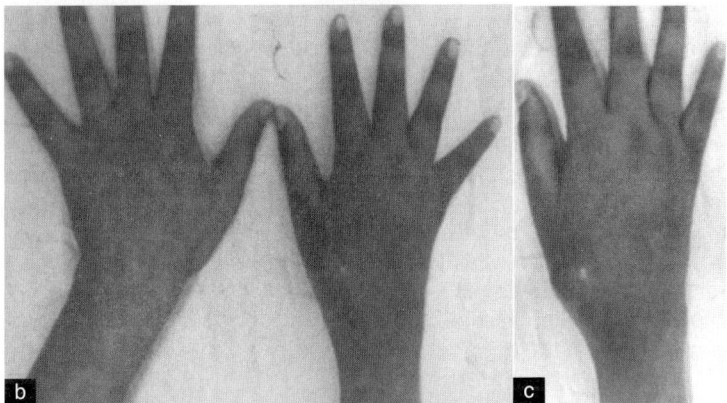

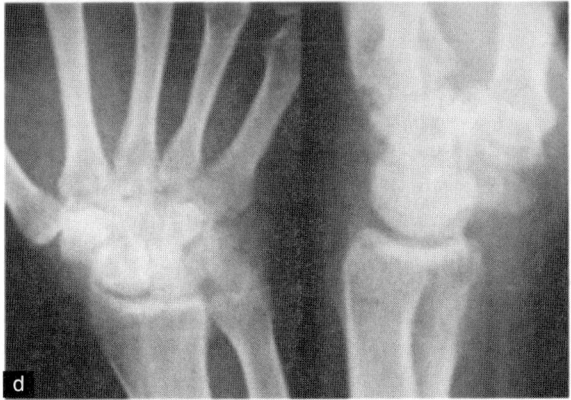

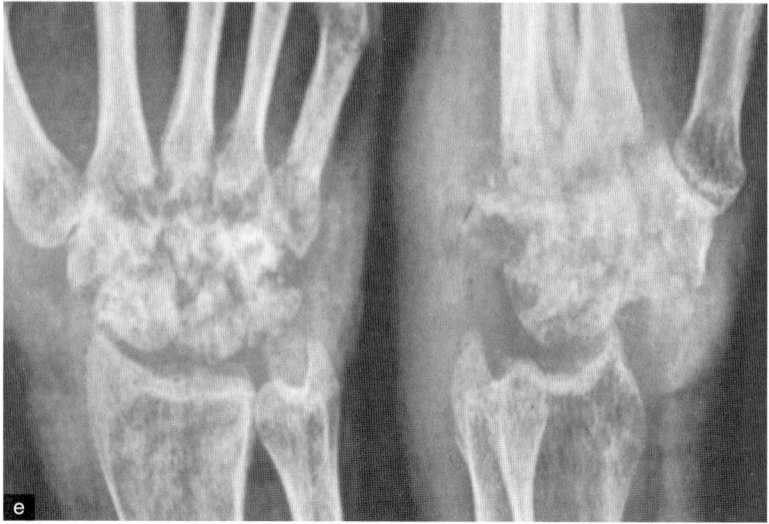

A 22-year-old male presented with complaints of pain, swelling and restriction of movements in right wrist for past 5 months. There was erythematous swelling present on the dorsolateral aspect of the wrist (Figs a–c). No other joint was involved. Initial radiographs (Fig. d) showed decreased intercarpal joint space. X-ray (Fig. e), AP and lateral view, of patients 3 months post-presentation showed improved bone density of all carpals and distal forearm bones. The margins were fuzzy and joint spaces (radiocarpal and intercarpal joint) were lost. There was associated volar subluxation of radiocarpal joint. Patient was continued on ATT and below elbow slab in neutral position.

Case 50: TB of hand bones

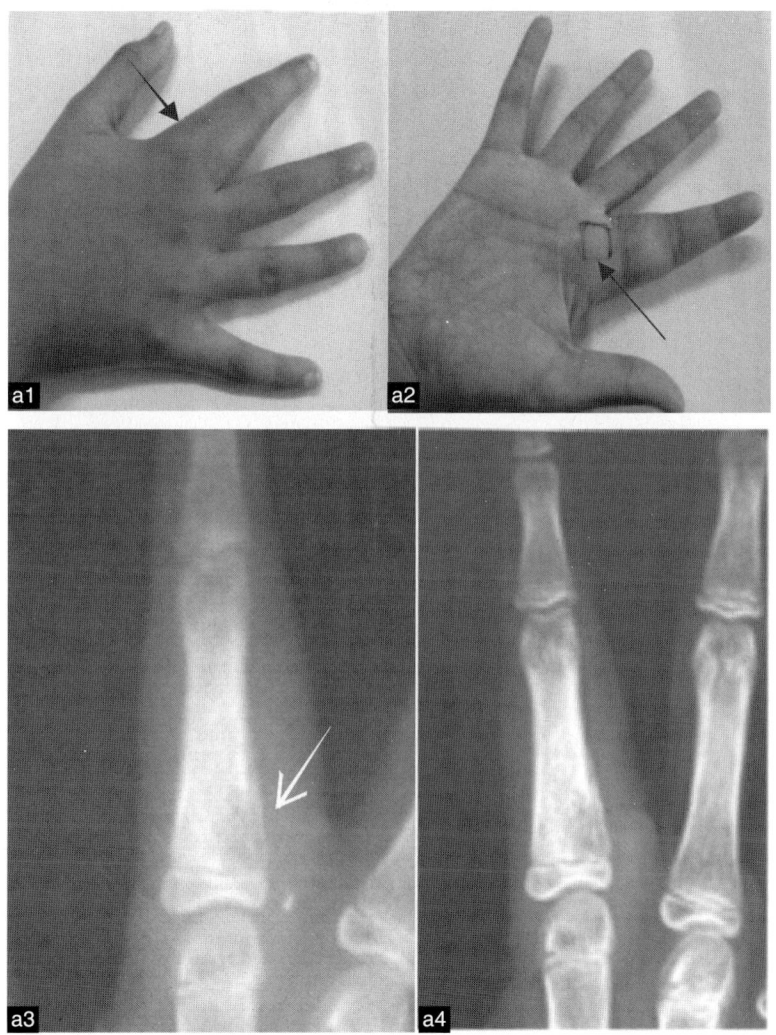

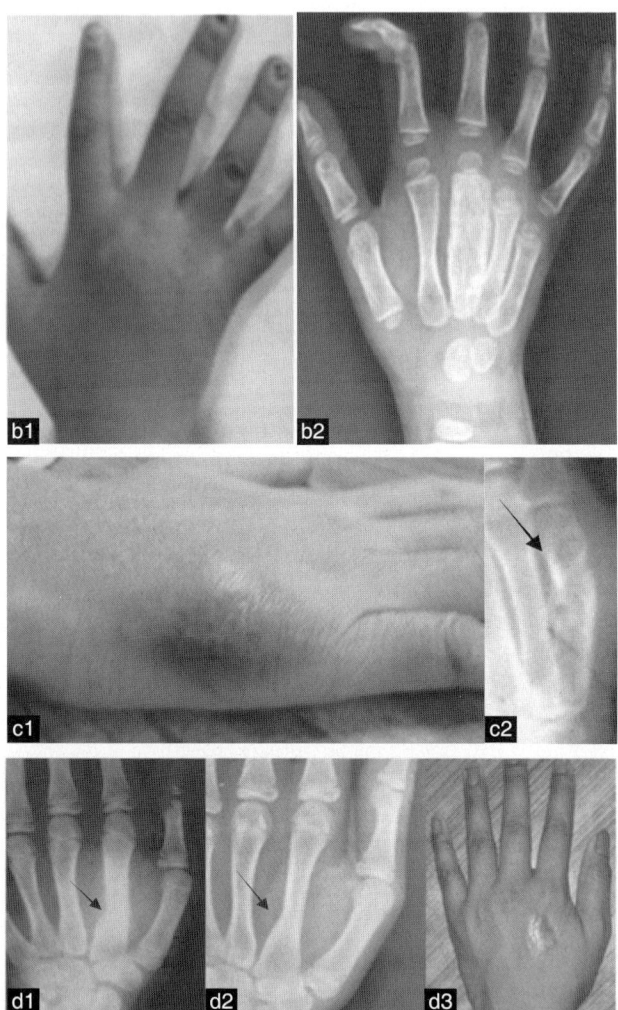

Various presentations of tuberculosis involving bones of hand. Figure (a) shows clinical picture and radiographs of a 10-year-old child who presented with swelling in index finger for 2 months. The radiographs showed expansion of the proximal phalanx with a lytic lesion on its ulnar base. Figure (b) shows clinical and radiographic picture of 9-year-old boy with TB dactylitis of third metacarpal. Figure (c) shows tuberculosis affecting fifth metacarpal neck while proximal shaft of second metacarpal is seen in Figure (d).

Index